APPLICATIONS AND CASE STUDIES IN CLINICAL NUTRITION

Isabelle Giroux, Ph.D., R.D., B.Ed., P.H.Ec.

Associate Professor and Dietetics Program Director
Brescia University College,
affiliated with the University of Western Ontario

Wolters Kluwer | Lippincott Williams & Wilkins
Health

Philadelphia • Baltimore • New York • London
Buenos Aires • Hong Kong • Sydney • Tokyo

Acquisitions Editor: David Troy
Managing Editor: Matt Hauber
Marketing Manager: Marisa O'Brien
Production Editor: Gina Aiello
Designer: Holly McLaughlin
Compositor: Nesbitt Graphics
Printer: Data Reproduction Corp.

Library of Congress Cataloging-in-Publication Data

Giroux, Isabelle.
  Applications and case studies in clinical nutrition / Isabelle Giroux.
      p. ; cm.
  Includes bibliographical references and index.
  ISBN-13: 978-0-7817-4674-8
  ISBN-10: 0-7817-4674-4
  1. Diet therapy–Case studies. 2. Diet therapy–Problems, exercises, etc. I. Title.
  [DNLM: 1. Nutrition Physiology–Programmed Instruction. QU 18.2
G528a 2007]
  RM216.G59 2007
  615.8'54–dc22
                                          2006101663

The publishers have made every effort to trace the copyright holders for borrowed material. If they have inadvertently overlooked any, they will be pleased to make the necessary arrangements at the first opportunity.

To purchase additional copies of this book, call our customer service department at (800) 638-3030 or fax orders to (301) 223-2320. International customers should call (301) 223-2300.

Visit Lippincott Williams & Wilkins on the Internet: http://www.LWW.com.
Lippincott Williams & Wilkins customer service representatives are available
from 8:30 am to 6:00 pm, EST.

06 07 08 09 10
1 2 3 4 5 6 7 8 9 10

DEDICATION

*To my adorable daughters, Amanda Chantale and Emma-Catherine,
and my loving husband for your endless patience and support.*

To my caring parents and friends, professional colleagues, and guiding mentors.

To my students, who are avid to learn, energetic, and full of potential.

PREFACE

PURPOSE AND OBJECTIVE

Applications and Case Studies in Clinical Nutrition is designed to provide a practical educational resource in clinical nutrition to complement the classical textbooks and references widely used in the field of dietetics both in the United States and Canada. This ancillary educational resource has been written primarily for university-level nutrition students and has been constructed to serve as a hands-on book to accompany the student's core clinical and life cycle nutrition textbooks and courses. Therefore, it is a comprehensive resource suitable for use with a variety of texts and courses, creating a great deal of flexibility for course instructors, dietetic educators, and dietetic programs.

In addition to being especially useful to undergraduate nutrition students, this book is also very helpful to many others, including nutrition graduates preparing for work or dietetic internship, dietetic interns, nutrition assistants, dietetic technicians, dietitians coming back to practice, candidates pursuing graduate studies in human nutrition, health professionals including physicians and nurses, dietitians wanting to update themselves, and many others who believe in lifelong learning and have a passion for nutrition.

The objective of this book is to actively engage the learner in progressively acquiring the essential basis in preparation for work in clinical nutrition.

PEDAGOGY

Applications and Case Studies in Clinical Nutrition utilizes a unique, progressive pedagogic approach to assist students to learn in a practical way, as well as to support and stimulate them in their learning. This teaching approach helps candidates to review the information they have learned from previous introductory university core science and basic nutrition courses, understand new information and concepts relevant to clinical nutrition, integrate their previous knowledge with the new learning, and ultimately apply key concepts of clinical nutrition in challenging practical situations such as real-life case studies.

Each section of the book has been designed based on this progressive learning approach, and includes the following teaching template: Review the Information, Understand the Concepts, Integrate Your Learning, and Challenge Your Learning. Because of this progressive learning strategy, this book can be used to accompany and complement courses or used on its own as a self-directed learning tool. No matter how the book is used, it is sure to keep the learner alert, thinking, practicing, and integrating.

PARTS AND RESOURCES

This educational resource is divided into seven parts covering the main essential basic areas necessary to support the formation of the future dietitian working in clinical nutrition: (1) Dietary Constituents and Energy, (2) Alimentary Tract and Nutrition, (3) Nutrition Throughout the Human Life Cycle, (4) Nutrition in Diverse Cultures and Communities, (5) Nutrition Care Process, (6) Regular and Modified Diets, and (7) Prevention and Management of Disease. The seven parts build on one another; therefore, Part 7 allows an integration of concepts acquired in Parts 1 through 6. Each part of this book contains many sections allowing the reader to explore varied areas of care and aspects of the work of dietitians through a progression of practical applications and case studies.

Appendices contain useful reference tables: Unit Conversion Factors and Summary Tables of Main

Dietary Reference Intake (DRI) Recommendations. They also include blank forms and charts, such as the U.S. Centers for Disease Control and Prevention (CDC) Growth Charts and the recent World Health Organization (WHO) Growth Standards. This book promotes the understanding and use of both conventional and international units.

Another exceptional feature of this book is that the appendices provide detailed answers to all of the exercises in Review the Information and Understand the Concepts, with step-by-step explanations to help the readers self-evaluate, make sure they understand thoroughly, and motivate them to progress at their own pace and in a self-directed manner. These answers and explanations are available online at http://thepoint.lww.com/giroux. Students should follow the directions there to access this feature.

The case studies and other learning activities are designed to incite the reader to explore diverse, well-known, and recent references, including many from the American Dietetic Association and Dietitians of Canada. An easy to use summary table entitled Quick Reference to Selected Clinical Nutrition Resources can be found on pages vii to x. In addition, an extensive up-to-date list of references and suggested resources is provided online at http://thepoint.lww.com/giroux for each section, which refers to relevant books, position papers, research articles, and Internet resources. The reader is encouraged to discover Internet resources such as the online American Dietetic Association's *Nutrition Care Manual* and the Dietitians of Canada's *Practice-based Evidence in Nutrition,* as well as multiple other credible professional and governmental web sites.

HOW TO USE THIS BOOK

There are definitely many ways to use this book, as a self-directed learning tool or to complement teaching provided by dietetic educators and course instructors.

One of the best ways to use this practical book in the university setting would be for the students to complete the different exercises in each section pro-gressively, intertwining with self-evaluation using the suggested answers provided in appendices and guidance from the educator/instructor to monitor their understanding and progress.

1. The students could Review the Information by themselves and evaluate how well they could remember the basic information on a topic, before the educator/instructor presents it as part of a lecture.
2. Using this review as grounds for building new knowledge, the educator/instructor could introduce new clinical nutrition concepts and guide the students to complete Understand the Concepts, followed by a self-evaluation of their understanding using the answers available online at http://thepoint.lww.com/giroux. Students should follow the directions at that Web site to access the answers to both Review the Information and Understand the Concepts.
3. The students could then explore the reference readings and resources on the same topic and complete the Integrate Your Learning individually as homework or possibly in class working in small groups.
4. Ultimately, the students could finish with Challenge Your Learning as indicated by their educator/instructor and with the use of diverse library resources, leading to the preparation of an assignment, an oral presentation, or a written examination.

RESOURCES FOR EDUCATORS

A separate, extensive *Instructors' Manual for Applications and Case Studies in Clinical Nutrition* is available for dietetic educators and course instructors online. It contains detailed answers to the sections Integrate Your Learning and Challenge Your Learning and other convenient teaching resources including a test bank to help instructors guide their learners in their study of clinical nutrition. Instructors may access this Instructors' Manual by following the directions online at http://thepoint.lww.com/giroux.

ACKNOWLEDGMENTS

I wish to thank all the reviewers for their constructive feedback: Dawna Torres Mughal; Valentina M. Remig; Allisha Weeden; and especially Jody Luth, RD, for her minutiae in editing; and Denise Eagan for her useful comments.

I am sincerely grateful to Mr. Paul Montgomery, managing editor, for his exceptional support, resourcefulness, guidance, and enthusiasm about the book.

Thank you very much to Mr. David Troy, acquisitions editor, for believing in this project right from the start.

Thank you also to Mr. Alain Audet, Mr. Matt Hauber, Mrs. Rebecca Kerins, and the other members of the Lippincott Williams & Wilkins team for their kind help and support.

ISABELLE GIROUX, PH.D., R.D., B.ED., P.H.EC.

Quick Reference to Selected Clinical Nutrition Resources

Selected Resources	Part 1: Dietary Constituents & Energy	Part 2.1: Anatomy of the Alimentary Tract	Part 2.2: Physiology of the Alimentary Tract	Part 3.1: Maternal Nutrition	Part 3.2: Infancy Nutrition	Part 3.3: Childhood Nutrition	Part 3.4: Nutrition in Adolescence
Pediatric Manual of Clinical Dietetics[a]				Chap. 3	Chap. 4	Chap. 5-6, 9	Chap. 7 & 9
ADA Nutrition Care Manual[b]	✓			✓	✓	✓	✓
Manual of Clinical Dietetics[c]				Chap. 7 & 8	Chap. 3	Chap. 4 & 5	Chap. 6
Nutrition Now[d]	Units 1, 4, 8, 12, 15,18, 20, 23, 25	Unit 7	Unit 7	Unit 29	Unit 29	Unit 30	Unit 30
Nutrition Through the Life Cycle[e]	Chap. 1			Chap. 2,4,6	Chap. 6 & 8	Chap. 10,12	Chap. 12, 14
Nutrition and Diet Therapy: Principles and Practice[f]	Chap. 1-4, 6, 8-9	Chap. 5	Chap. 5	Chap. 12	Chap. 12	Chap. 13	Chap. 13
Nutrition in the Prevention & Treatment of Disease[g]	Chap. 48						
PEN[h]	✓			✓	✓	✓	
Nutrition and Diagnosis-Related Care[i]	Appendix A	Section 7	Section 7	Section 1	Section 1	Section 1	Section 1
Foundations and Clinical Applications of Nutrition[j]	Chap. 1, 4-8	Chap. 3	Chap. 3	Chap. 11	Chap. 11	Chap. 12	Chap. 9 & 12
Nutrition & Diet Therapy Reviews & Rationales[k]	Chap. 1-3		Chap. 4	Chap. 5	Chap. 5	Chap. 5	Chap. 5
Nutrition and Diet Therapy: Evidence-Based Applications[l]	Chap. 1, 3-9	Chap. 10 Chap. 12	Chap. 10 Chap. 12	Chap. 11	Chap. 12		
Quick Reference to Clinical Dietetics[m]							
Krause's Food, Nutrition, & Diet Therapy[n]	Chap. 2-6	Chap. 1	Chap. 1	Chap. 7	Chap. 8	Chap. 10	Chap. 11
Nutrition Across the Life Span[o]	Chap. 1			Chap. 4 & 6	Chap. 7	Chap. 9	Chap.11 & 15
Williams' Basic Nutrition & Diet Therapy[p]	Chap. 1-4, 6-9	Chap. 5	Chap. 5	Chap. 10	Chap. 11	Chap. 11	Chap. 11
Nutrition, Diet Modifications and Meal Patterns[q]	Section 1 Module 1		Section 1 Module 1	Section 1 Module 2	Section 1 Module 2	Section 1 Module 2	Section 1 Module 2
Basic Nutrition & Diet Therapy[r]	Chap.1-8	Chap. 9	Chap. 9	Chap. 10	Chap. 11	Chap. 11	Chap. 11
Essentials of Nutrition and Diet Therapy[s]	Chap. 1, 3-8	Chap. 2	Chap. 2	Chap. 11	Chap. 12	Chap. 12	Chap. 12 & 14
Understanding Normal and Clinical Nutrition[t]	Chap. 1,4-8,10-13	Chap. 3	Chap. 3	Chap. 14	Chap. 15	Chap. 15	Chap. 15
Modern Nutrition in Health and Disease[u]	Parts I & II	Chap. 70 & 73	Chap. 70 & 73	Chap.50A,B	Chap. 51	Chap. 51	Chap. 52 &109
Nutrition Concepts and Controversies[v]	Chap. 1-2, 4-8	Chap. 3	Chap. 3	Chap. 13	Chap. 13	Chap. 14	Chap. 14
Clinical Anatomy[w]		Chap. 4, 5, 11					
Nutrition and Diet Therapy[x]	Modules 1, 3-7			Module 9	Module 9	Module 9	Module 9
Medical Physiology[y]			Part VII				
Essential Pathology[z]							
Nutrition: An Applied Approach[aa]	Chap. 1, 4-10	Chap. 3	Chap. 3	Chap. 15	Chap. 15	Chap. 16	Chap. 16
Contemporary Nutrition[bb]	Chap. 1, 4-9	Chap. 3	Chap. 3	Chap. 13	Chap. 14	Chap. 14	Chap. 14
Nutrition Throughout The Life Cycle[cc]	Chap. 1			Chap. 3-7	Chap. 8 & 9	Chap. 10	Chap. 11 & 12
Understanding Nutrition[dd]	Chap. 1,4-8,10-13	Chap. 3	Chap. 3	Chap. 15	Chap. 16	Chap. 16	Chap. 16
Nutrition for Health and Health Care[ee]	Chap. 1, 3-5, 8-9	Chap. 2	Chap. 2	Chap. 10	Chap. 11	Chap. 11	Chap. 11

Quick Reference to Selected Clinical Nutrition Resources

Selected Resources	Part 3.5: Nutrition in Adulthood	Part 3.6: Nutrition in Aging	Part 4.1: Kosher Nutrition	Part 4.2: Hispanic Nutrition	Part 4.3: Nutrition and Aboriginal People	Part 4.4: Medical Care & Records	Part 5.1: Nutrition in Care Plan
Pediatric Manual of Clinical Dietetics[a]			✓	Chap. 3	Chap. 4	Chap. 5-6, 9	Chap. 7 & 9
ADA Nutrition Care Manual[b]				✓	✓	✓	✓
Manual of Clinical Dietetics[c]		Chap. 9	Chap. 10	Chap. 70			
Nutrition Now[d]	Unit 31	Unit 31	Unit 16				
Nutrition Through the Life Cycle[e]	Chap. 16	Chap. 18	Chap.10, 16				
Nutrition and Diet Therapy: Principles and Practice[f]	Chap. 1-4, 6, 8-9	Chap. 5	Chap. 5	Chap. 12	Chap. 12	Chap. 13	Chap. 13
Nutrition in the Prevention & Treatment of Disease[g]							
PEN[h]			✓				
Nutrition and Diagnosis-Related Care[i]	Appendix A	Section 7	Section 7	Section 1	Section 1	Section 1	Section 1
Foundations and Clinical Applications of Nutrition[j]	Chap. 13	Chap. 13	Chap. 6	Appendix L	Appendix L	Appendix L	Chap. 14
Nutrition & Diet Therapy Reviews & Rationales[k]	Chap. 5	Chap. 5	Chap. 1				
Nutrition and Diet Therapy: Evidence-Based Applications[l]	Chap. 13	Chap. 13	Chap. 5	Chap. 2	Chap. 2	Chap. 2	
Quick Reference to Clinical Dietetics[m]			Chap. 7				
Krause's Food, Nutrition, & Diet Therapy[n]	Chap. 12	Chap. 13	Chap. 15	Chap. 15	Chap. 15	Chap. 15	Chap. 21
Nutrition Across the Life Span[o]	Chap. 12	Chap. 13	Chap. 11	Appendix H	Appendix H	Appendix H	
Williams' Basic Nutrition & Diet Therapy[p]	Chap. 12	Chap. 12	Chap. 4	Chap. 14	Chap. 14	Chap. 14	Chap. 17
Nutrition, Diet Modifications and Meal Patterns[q]	Section 1 Module 2	Section 1 Module 2	Section 2	Section 1 Module 2	Section 1 Module 2	Section 1 Module 2	Section 1 Module 3
Basic Nutrition & Diet Therapy[r]	Chap. 12	Chap. 12	Chap. 4	Chap. 14	Chap. 14	Chap. 14	
Essentials of Nutrition and Diet Therapy[s]	Chap. 13	Chap. 13	Chap. 5	Appendix Q	Appendix Q	Appendix Q	Chap. 15
Understanding Normal and Clinical Nutrition[t]	Chap. 16	Chap. 16	Chap. 6				
Modern Nutrition in Health and Disease[u]	Chap. 53	Chap. 54	Chap. 103				
Nutrition Concepts and Controversies[v]		Chap. 14	Chap. 6				
Clinical Anatomy[w]							
Nutrition and Diet Therapy[x]	Module 9	Module 9	Module 3	Module 2	Module 2	Module 2	
Medical Physiology[y]							
Essential Pathology[z]							
Nutrition: An Applied Approach[aa]	Chap. 16	Chap. 16	Chap. 6				
Contemporary Nutrition[bb]	Chap. 15	Chap. 15	Chap. 6				
Nutrition Throughout The Life Cycle[cc]	Chap. 13	Chap. 14					
Understanding Nutrition[dd]	Chap. 17	Chap. 17	Chap. 6				
Nutrition for Health and Health Care[ee]	Chap. 12	Chap. 12	Chap. 5		Chap. 1		Chap. 13

Quick Reference to Selected Clinical Nutrition Resources

Selected Resources	Part 5.2: Nutrition Care Plan	Part 5.3: Nutrition Inteview	Part 5.4: Nutrition Screening	Part 5.5: Complete Nutrition Assessment	Part 5.6: Dietary Assessment	Part 5.7: Nutrition Counseling and Education	Part 5.8: Jurisprudence, & Quality of care
Pediatric Manual of Clinical Dietetics[a]			Chap. 2	Chap. 10-12	Chap. 10-12	Chap. 1 & 6	
ADA Nutrition Care Manual[b]	✓		✓	✓	✓	✓	
Manual of Clinical Dietetics[c]			Chap. 9	Chap. 1 & 2	Chap. 1 & 2		
Nutrition Now[d]		Chap. 14 & 18					
Nutrition Through the Life Cycle[e]			Chap. 1	Chap. 1	Chap. 14		
Nutrition and Diet Therapy: Principles and Practice[f]	Chap. 17	Chap. 17	Chap. 16	Chap. 16	Chap. 16	Chap. 17	Chap. 28
Nutrition in the Prevention & Treatment of Disease[g]		Chap. 8	Chap. 3	Chap. 1-5	Chap. 1& 5	Chap. 6-10	
PEN[h]			✓	✓	✓	✓	✓
Nutrition and Diagnosis-Related Care[i]	Appendix B		Section 1	Appendix B	Appendix B	Appendix B	Appendix B
Foundations and Clinical Applications of Nutrition[j]	Chap. 14			Chap. 14	Chap. 14		
Nutrition & Diet Therapy Reviews & Rationales[k]				Chap. 1			
Nutrition and Diet Therapy: Evidence-Based Applications[l]			Chap. 2	Chap. 2	Chap. 2		Chap. 26
Quick Reference to Clinical Dietetics[m]			Chap. 1	Chap. 1 & 2		Chap. 5	
Krause's Food, Nutrition, & Diet Therapy[n]	Chap. 21	Chap. 22	Chap. 17	Chap. 17 & 18	Chap. 17	Chap. 22	Chap. 21
Nutrition Across the Life Span[o]			Chap. 2	Chap. 2	Chap. 2		
Williams' Basic Nutrition & Diet Therapy[p]	Chap. 17			Chap.17			
Nutrition, Diet Modifications and Meal Patterns[q]	Section 1 Module 3		Section 1 Module 3	Section 1 Module 3	Section 1 Module 3	Section 1 Module 3	Section 1 Module 3
Basic Nutrition & Diet Therapy[r]	Chap. 17			Chap. 17	Chap. 17		
Essentials of Nutrition and Diet Therapy[s]	Chap. 15	Chap. 10		Chap. 15	Chap. 15	Chap. 10	Chap. 15
Understanding Normal and Clinical Nutrition[t]	Chap. 18		Chap. 17	Chap. 17	Chap. 17	Chap. 18	Chap. 17 & 21
Modern Nutrition in Health and Disease[u]			Chap. 53 & 54	Chap. 7, 38, 49, 53, 54, 57, 71	Chap. 7 & 54		Chap. 100-101
Nutrition Concepts and Controversies[v]			Chap. 13				
Clinical Anatomy[w]		Chap. 14	Chap. 6				
Nutrition and Diet Therapy[x]		Module 9	Module 3	Module 2	Module 2	Module 2	
Medical Physiology[y]							
Essential Pathology[z]							
Nutrition: An Applied Approach[aa]				Chap. 2	Appendix E		
Contemporary Nutrition[bb]				Chap. 2	Chap. 2		
Nutrition Throughout The Life Cycle[cc]							
Understanding Nutrition[dd]							
Nutrition for Health and Health Care[ee]			Chap. 13	Chap. 13	Chap. 13	Chap. 14	Chap. 15

Quick Reference to Selected Clinical Nutrition Resources

Selected Resources	Part 6.1: Regular Diet in Health Care Institutions	Part 6.2: Modified Consistency Diets	Part 6.3: Therapeutic & Modified Mineral Diets	Part 7.1: At Risk Pregnancies	Part 7.2: Disease in Infancy and Childhood	Part 7.3: Adverse Reactions to Food	Part 7.4: Obesity & Eating Disorders
Pediatric Manual of Clinical Dietetics[a]		Ch. 35-40	Ch. 16, 23, 41-51		Ch. 13-30, 33	Ch. 19, 47, 50	Ch. 17 & 26
ADA Nutrition Care Manual[b]		✓	✓			✓	✓
Manual of Clinical Dietetics[c]		Chap. 54-57	Chap. 11,13,18, 20, 58-68	Chap. 8 & 20	Units 29 & 30	Chap. 11-13	Chap. 22-23, 45
Nutrition Now[d]				Unit 29	Units 29 & 30	Units 7 & 17	Units 10, 11, 14
Nutrition Through the Life Cycle and Practice[e]				Chap. 4-5	Chap. 8-15	Chap. 7-8 & 11	Chap. 10, 12, 15, 17
Nutrition and Diet Therapy: Principles[f]		Chap. 8	Chap. 8	Chap. 5	Chap. 5	Chap. 8	Chap. 6, 8, 10
Nutrition in the Prevention & Treatment of Disease[g]		Chap. 15	Chap. 15, 37	Chap. 30	Chap. 14, 28 & 45	Chap. 37 & 44	Chap. 12, 31-35, 43
PEN[h]		✓	✓	✓			✓
Nutrition and Diagnosis-Related Care[i]	Chap. 14 & 15	Secs. 2 & 7	Secs. 6-10, 12-16	Secs. 1, 9	Secs. 1, 3 & 5	Section 2	Section 10
Foundations and Clinical Applications of Nutrition[j]	Chap. 14	Chap. 14 & 17	Chap. 17	Chap. 11, 19	Chap. 11-12,	Chap. 17	Chap. 10 & 12
Nutrition & Diet Therapy Reviews & Rationales[k]		Chap. 8	Chap. 8	Chap. 5	Chap. 5	Chap. 8	Chap. 6, 8, 10
Nutrition and Diet Therapy: Evidence-Based Applications[l]	Chap. 14 & 15	Chap. 15	Chap. 15	Chap. 11, 19	Chap. 11-12 & 22	Chap. 10	Chap. 18
Quick Reference to Clinical Dietetics[m]	Chap. 7	Chap. 7	Chap. 7	Chap. 3	Chap. 3	Chap. 3 & 7	Chap. 3
Krause's Food, Nutrition, & Diet Therapy[n]	Chap. 21	Chap. 21 & Appendix 55	Chap. 30, 31, 37 & Appendix 53	Chap. 7, 33, 34, 41	Chap. 8-11, 32, 33, 38, 45	Chap. 30 & 32	Chap. 24-25
Nutrition Across the Life Span[o]				Chap. 5 & 6	Chap. 7-11	Chap. 9-10	Chap. 14
Williams' Basic Nutrition & Diet Therapy[p]	Chap. 17	Chap. 17	Ch.18 & App. F	Chap. 10, 20	Chap. 11 & 18	Chap. 18	Chap. 15
Nutrition, Diet Modifications and Meal Patterns[q]	Section 2	Section 2 Module 1	Section 2 Modules 2-7	Sec. 1 Mod. 2, Sec. 2 Mod. 3	Sec. 1 Mod. 2, S. 2 M. 3, 6 & 7	Section 2 Module 6	Section 2 Module 3
Basic Nutrition & Diet Therapy[r]	Chap. 17	Chap. 17	Chap. 18	Chap. 10, 20	Chap. 11 & 18	Chap. 18	Chap. 15
Essentials of Nutrition and Diet Therapy[s]	Chap. 15	Chap. 15	Chap. 15	Chap. 11, 20	Chap. 12 & 18	Chap. 18	Chap. 6
Understanding Normal and Clinical Nutrition[t]	Chap. 18	Chap. 18	Chap. 18	Chap. 14, 26	Chap. 15, 20 & 24	Chap. 24	Chap. 9
Modern Nutrition in Health and Disease[u]			Ch. 67, 68, 74, 77, 95 & App. Sec. V	Ch. 50A & 65	Ch. 51, 52, 55-61	Ch. 56, 58-59, 74, 77, 95	Ch. 60, 62-64, 87
Nutrition Concepts and Controversies[v]				Chap. 13	Chap. 13 & 14	Chap. 4 & 14	Chap. 9, 11, 13
Clinical Anatomy[w]	Mod. 13 & 14	Chap. 11		Chap. 7	Chap. 5	Chap. 5	Chap. 11
Nutrition and Diet Therapy[x]		Module 14	Module 14	Module 9	Mod. 9, 18, 23-29	Mod. 25 & 27	Mod. 17 & 22
Medical Physiology[y]				Chap. 35, 39	Chap. 27	Chap. 27	Chap. 7
Essential Pathology[z]				Chap. 18	Chap. 6	Chap. 13	Chap. 8
Nutrition: An Applied Approach[aa]				Chap. 15	Chap. 6, 15-16	Chap. 3-4	Chap. 11 & 13
Contemporary Nutrition[bb]				Chap. 13	Chap. 14	Chap. 4, 14, 16	Chap. 7, 10, 12
Nutrition Throughout The Life Cycle[cc]				Chap. 3-6	Chap. 8-12	Chap. 8	Chap. 10, 12-13
Understanding Nutrition[dd]				Chap. 15	Chap. 16	Chap. 4 & 16	Chap. 9 & 16
Nutrition for Health and Health Care[ee]	Chap. 14	Chap. 14	Chap. 14	Chap. 10, 20	Chap. 11, 17-18	Chap. 11	Chap. 7

Quick Reference to Selected Clinical Nutrition Resources

Selected Resources	Part 7.5: Cardiovascular Disease	Part 7.6: Diabetes Mellitus	Part 7.7: Gastroesophageal Reflux	Part 7.8: Peptic Ulcer Disease	Part 7.9: Inflammatory Bowel Disease	Part 7.10: Diseases of the Liver & Pancreas
Pediatric Manual of Clinical Dietetics[a]	Chap. 23	Chap. 16	Chap. 20		Chap. 20	Chap. 21 & 27
ADA Nutrition Care Manual[b]	✓	✓	✓	✓	✓	✓
Manual of Clinical Dietetics[c]	Chap. 16-19	Chap. 20-21	Chap. 26	Chap. 31	Chap. 27-28	Chap. 29, 41, 43, 45
Nutrition Now[d]	Units 18 & 19	Unit 13	Unit 7	Unit 7	Unit 7	
Nutrition Through the Life Cycle[e] and Practice[f]	Chap. 17 & 19	Chap. 3, 5, 17, 19	Chap. 8, 9, 19	Chap. 19		
Nutrition and Diet Therapy: Principles	Chap. 1-4, 6, 8-9	Chap. 5	Chap. 5	Chap. 12	Chap. 12	Chap. 13
Nutrition in the Prevention & Treatment of Disease[g]	Chap. 25	Chap. 24	Chap. 18	Chap. 18	Chap. 19	Chap. 23
PEN[h]	✓	✓				
Nutrition and Diagnosis-Related Care[i]	Section 6	Section 9	Section 7	Section 7	Section 7	Section 8
Foundations and Clinical Applications of Nutrition[j]	Chap. 20	Chap. 19	Chap. 17	Chap. 17	Chap. 17	Chap. 18
Nutrition & Diet Therapy Reviews & Rationales[k]	Chap. 6	Chap. 6	Chap. 6	Chap. 6	Chap. 6	Chap. 7
Nutrition and Diet Therapy: Evidence-Based Applications[l]	Chap. 20	Chap. 19	Chap. 22	Chap. 22	Chap. 22	Chap. 22
Quick Reference to Clinical Dietetics[m]	Chap. 3	Chap. 3	Chap. 3	Chap. 3	Chap. 3	Chap. 7
Krause's Food, Nutrition, & Diet Therapy[n]	Chap. 35-37	Chap. 33	Chap. 29	Chap. 29	Chap. 30	Chap. 31
Nutrition Across the Life Span[o]	Chap. 12	Chap. 5 & 12				
Williams' Basic Nutrition & Diet Therapy[p]	Chap. 19	Chap. 20	Chap. 18	Chap. 18	Chap. 18	Chap. 18
Nutrition, Diet Modifications and Meal Patterns[q]	Section 2 Modules 2 & 4	Section 2 Module 3	Section 2 Module 1	Section 2 Module 1	Section 2 Module 1	Section 2 Module 5
Basic Nutrition & Diet Therapy[r]	Chap. 19	Chap. 20	Chap. 18	Chap. 18	Chap. 18	Chap. 18
Essentials of Nutrition and Diet Therapy[s]	Chap. 1, 3-8	Chap. 2	Chap. 2	Chap. 11	Chap. 12	Chap. 12
Understanding Normal and Clinical Nutrition[t]	Chap. 27	Chap. 26	Chap. 23	Chap. 23	Chap. 24	Chap. 25
Modern Nutrition in Health and Disease[u]	Chap. 5, 62, 66-69	Chap. 65 & 96	Chap. 73	Chap. 73	Chap. 61 & 76	Chap. 78-79
Nutrition Concepts and Controversies[v]	Chap. 5 & 11	Chap. 4	Chap. 3	Chap. 3	Chap. 5	Chap. 3
Clinical Anatomy[w]	Chap. 3	Chap. 5	Chap. 5 & 11	Chap. 5	Chap. 5	Chap. 5
Nutrition and Diet Therapy[x]	Module 16	Module 18		Module 17	Module 17	Module 19
Medical Physiology[y]	Chap. 10-18, 28	Chap. 35	Chap. 26-27	Chap. 26-27	Chap. 26-27	Chap. 27 & 28
Essential Pathology[z]	Chap. 10-11	Chap. 22	Chap. 13	Chap. 13	Chap. 13	Chap. 14-15
Nutrition: An Applied Approach[aa]	Chap. 5-6, 8, 10	Chap. 4	Chap. 3	Chap. 3		
Contemporary Nutrition[bb]	Chap. 5 & 9	Chap. 13-14	Chap. 3	Chap. 3		Chap. 7
Nutrition Throughout The Life Cycle[cc]	Chap. 13	Chap. 13	Chap. 5			
Understanding Nutrition[dd]	Chap. 18	Chap. 18	Chap. 3	Chap. 3		Chap. 3 & 7
Nutrition for Health and Health Care[ee]	Chap. 21	Chap. 20	Chap. 17	Chap. 17	Chap. 18	Chap. 19

Quick Reference to Selected Clinical Nutrition Resources

Selected Resources	Part 7.11: Surgery & Short Bowel Syndrome	Part 7.12: Wasting Disorders	Part 7.13: Renal Disease	Part 7.14: Neurological and Psychological Disorders	Part 7.15: Nutrition Support	Part 7.16: Food/Nutrient-Drug Interactions
Pediatric Manual of Clinical Dietetics[a]	Chap. 20	Chap. 13 & 22	Chap. 28	Chap. 15 & 17	Chap. 31–34	Appendix 11
ADA Nutrition Care Manual[b]	✓	✓	✓	✓	✓	✓
Manual of Clinical Dietetics[c]	Chap. 24–25, 30	Chap. 15, 32, 61	Chap. 33–37, 67–68	Chap. 45–46	Chap. 48–53, 61	Appendix 15
Nutrition Now[d]	Unit 10	Unit 7		Units 5, 11, 14		
Nutrition Through the Life Cycle[e] and Practice[f]		Chap. 5, 7, 17, 19		Chap. 15 & 19	Chap. 9	
Nutrition and Diet Therapy: Principles	Chap. 19	Chap. 28	Chap. 26	Chap. 14 & 16	Chap. 20 & 21	Chap. 15
Nutrition in the Prevention & Treatment of Disease[g]	Chap. 38	Chap. 13, 22–26, 47	Chap. 40	Chap. 3, 41 & 43	Chap. 15–16	Chap. 17, 41
PEN[h]	✓			✓		✓
Nutrition and Diagnosis-Related Care[i]	Sections 7 & 14	Sections 13,15	Section 16	Section 4	Section 17	Appendix E
Foundations and Clinical Applications of Nutrition[j]	Chap. 17	Chap. 22	Chap. 21	Chap. 12	Chap. 14, 16	Chap. 16
Nutrition & Diet Therapy Reviews & Rationales[k]	Chap. 6	Chap. 7	Chap. 7	Chap. 6 & 7	Chap. 8	Chap. 10
Nutrition and Diet Therapy: Evidence-Based Applications[l]	Chap. 22	Chap. 23 & 25	Chap. 21	Chap. 13 & 18	Chap. 15	Chap. 17
Quick Reference to Clinical Dietetics[m]	Chap. 3	Chap. 3	Chap. 3	Chap. 3	Chap. 4	Appendix 14
Krause's Food, Nutrition, & Diet Therapy[n]	Chap. 30 & 42	Chap. 40–41	Chap. 39	Chap. 25 & 43	Chap. 3, 9 & 23, 43	Chap. 19, 43
Nutrition Across the Life Span[o]	Chap. 14	Chap. 8 & 12		Chap. 14	Chap. 8 & 10	Chap. 13
Williams' Basic Nutrition & Diet Therapy[p]	Chap. 22	Chap. 23	Chap. 21	Chap. 15	Chap. 17 & 22	Chap. 12 & 17
Nutrition, Diet Modifications and Meal Patterns[q]	Section 2 Module 1	Section 2 Module 6	Section 2 Modules 2 & 5	Section 2 Module 6	Section 1 Module 3	Section 1 Module 3
Basic Nutrition & Diet Therapy[r]	Chap. 22	Chap. 23	Chap. 21	Chap. 15	Chap. 17 & 22	Chap. 12 & 17
Essentials of Nutrition and Diet Therapy[s]	Chap. 18 & 22	Chap. 23–24	Chap. 21	Chap. 6 & 25	Chap. 17	Chap. 16
Understanding Normal and Clinical Nutrition[t]	Chap. 24	Chap. 29	Chap. 28	Chap. 9 & 29	Chap. 20–21	Chap. 19
Modern Nutrition in Health and Disease[u]	Chap. 36, 61, 64, 70, 71, 73, 75, 91	Chap. 61, 80–83	Chap. 94	Chap. 38, 87–88	Chap. 61, 83, 91, 98–99	Chap. 37, 97, 98
Nutrition Concepts and Controversies[v]		Chap. 11 & 13		Chap. 9		Chap. 14
Clinical Anatomy[w]	Chap. 5	Chap. 5 & 11	Chap. 5	Chap. 11	Chap. 1 & 5	
Nutrition and Diet Therapy[x]	Modules 15 & 17	Module 21	Module 20	Module 22	Module 14	
Medical Physiology[y]	Chap. 26–27	Chap. 1 & 11	Chap. 23–25	Chap. 7	Chap. 27	Appendix D
Essential Pathology[z]	Chap. 13	Chap. 4–5	Chap. 16	Chap. 28	Chap. 13	
Nutrition: An Applied Approach[aa]		Chap. 5 & 8	Chap. 7	Chap. 6 & 13		Chap. 16
Contemporary Nutrition[bb]		Chap. 17		Chap. 12		Chap. 15
Nutrition Throughout The Life Cycle[cc]		Chap. 13		Chap. 12		Chap. 14
Understanding Nutrition[dd]	Chap. 9	Chap. 18	Chap. 18	Chap. 9		Chap. 17
Nutrition for Health and Health Care[ee]	Chap. 18	Chap. 23	Chap. 22	Chap. 12 & 18	Chap. 15	Chap. 14

[a] American Dietetic Association. Pediatric Manual of Clinical Dietetics. 2nd Ed. Chicago: American Dietetic Association, 2003.

[b] American Dietetic Association. ADA Nutrition Care Manual. Chicago: American Dietetic Association, 2006. Online resource through www.eatright.org. Accessed June 2006.

[c] American Dietetic Association & Dietitians of Canada. Manual of Clinical Dietetics. 6th Ed. Chicago: American Dietetic Association, 2000.

[d] Brown JE. Nutrition Now. 4th Ed. Belmont, CA: Wadsworth Publishing, Thompson Learning, 2005.

[e] Brown JE, Sugarman Isaacs J, Betae Krinke U, et al. Nutrition Through the Life Cycle. 2nd Ed. Belmont, CA: Wadsworth Publishing, Thompson Learning, 2004.

[f] Cataldo CB, DeBruyne LK, Whitney EN. Nutrition and Diet Therapy: Principles and Practice. 6th Ed. Belmont, CA: Thomson/Nelson, 2003.

[g] Coulston AM, Rock CL, Monsen ER. Nutrition in the Prevention and Treatment of Disease. San Diego: Academic Press, Elsevier, 2001.

[h] Dietitians of Canada. PEN: Practice-based Evidence in Nutrition. 2006. Toronto, Ontario: Dietitians of Canada, 2006. Online electronic resource through *www.dietitians.ca.* Accessed June 2006.

[i] Escott-Stump S. Nutrition and Diagnosis-Related Care, 5th Ed. Baltimore: Lippincott, Williams & Wilkins, 2002.

[j] Grodner M, Long S, DeYoung S. Foundations and Clinical Applications of Nutrition: A Nursing Approach. 3rd Ed. St. Louis: Mosby, Elsevier, 2004.

[k] Hogan MA, Wane D. Nutrition & Diet Therapy Reviews & Rationales. Upper Saddle River, NJ: Prentice Hall, Pearson Education, 2003.

[l] Lutz CA, Przytulski KR. Nutrition and Diet Therapy: Evidence-based Applications. 4th Ed. Philadelphia: F.A. Davis Company, 2006.

[m] Lysen LK. Quick Reference to Clinical Dietetics. 2nd Ed. Sudbury, MA: Jones & Bartlett Publishers, 2006.

[n] Mahan LK, Escott-Stump S, eds. Krause's Food, Nutrition, & Diet Therapy. 11th Ed. Philadelphia: W.B. Saunders Company, 2004.

[o] Mitchell MK. Nutrition Across the Life Span. 2nd Ed. Philadelphia: Saunders, Elsevier, 2003.

[p] Nix S. Williams' Basic Nutrition & Diet Therapy. 12th Ed. St. Louis: Mosby Inc., Elsevier Science, 2005.

[q] Puckett RP, Danks SE. Nutrition, Diet Modifications and Meal Patterns. 3rd Ed. Dubuque, IA: Kendall/Hunt Publishing Company, 2002.

[r] Rodwell Williams S. Basic Nutrition & Diet Therapy. 11th Ed. St. Louis: Mosby/Elsevier Science, 2001.

[s] Rodwell Williams S, Schlenker E. Essentials of Nutrition and Diet Therapy. 8th Ed. St. Louis: Mosby, Elsevier, 2003.

[t] Rolfes SR, Pinna K, Whitney EN. Understanding Normal and Clinical Nutrition. 7th Ed. Belmont, CA: Wadsworth Publishing, Thompson Learning, 2006.

[u] Shils ME, Shike M, Ross AC, et al. Modern Nutrition in Health and Disease. 10th Ed. Baltimore: Lippincott, Williams & Wilkins, 2006.

[v] Sizer F, Whitney E. Nutrition Concepts and Controversies. 10th Ed. Belmont, CA: Wadsworth Publishing, Thompson Learning, 2006.

[w] Snell RS. Clinical Anatomy. 7th Ed. Baltimore: Lippincott, Williams & Wilkins, 2004.

[x] Stanfield PS, Hui YH. Nutrition and Diet Therapy: Self-Instructional Modules. 4th Ed. Sudbury, MA: Jones & Bartlett Publishers, 2003.

[y] Rhoades RA, Tanner GA, eds. Medical Physiology. 2nd Ed. Baltimore: Lippincott, Williams & Wilkins, 2003.

[z] Rubin E, ed. Essential Pathology. 3rd Ed. Baltimore: Lippincott, Williams & Wilkins, 2001.

[aa] Thompson J, Manore M. Nutrition: An Applied Approach. San Francisco: Pearson Education Inc., Benjamin Cummings, 2005.

[bb] Wardlaw GM, Smith AM. Contemporary Nutrition. 6th Ed. New York: McGraw-Hill Ryerson Ltd, 2007.

[cc] Worthington-Roberts BS, Rodwell Williams S. Nutrition Throughout The Life Cycle. 4th Ed. New York: McGraw-Hill, 2000.

[dd] Whitney E, Rolfes SR. Understanding Nutrition. 10th Edition. Belmont, CA: Thompson, Wadsworth, 2005.

[ee] Whitney E, DeBruyne LK, Pinna K, Rolfes SR. Nutrition for Health and Health Care. 3rd Ed. Belmont, CA: Thompson, Wadsworth, 2007.

TABLE OF CONTENTS

PART 1

Dietary Constituents and Energy

INTRODUCTION

The goal of this section is to help you build a broad understanding of the basics of human nutrition. Through a series of diverse exercises, you are invited, in a self-directed manner, to:

1) review information you have already learned on the dietary constituents and energy;
2) understand new and up-to-date concepts of fundamental nutrition;
3) integrate your previous and recently acquired knowledge; and ultimately
4) challenge your learning in practical applications and evaluate how you perform.

The basic and technical nutrition knowledge covered in this chapter will serve as a foundation to be used and built upon in all of the following chapters, as well as for the rest of your nutrition career. Therefore, it is worth making sure that you invest the effort necessary to get off to a strong start! To assist you in your learning, the answers to the exercises of the sections *Review the Information* and *Understand the Concepts* can be found in the appendix section at the end of the book.

REVIEW THE INFORMATION

Nutrients

1. What are nutrients? _____

_____

2. Fill in the blank spaces with appropriate words.

a) Some food constituents have to be part of the diet of humans to ensure growth and aid in preventing

disease. They are referred to as _____ *(1 word)* nutrients, as the body cannot synthesize them or cannot synthesize them rapidly enough in quantity sufficient to satisfy metabolic demands. This

explains the importance of consuming a _____ _____ *(2 words)* of foods to ensure that the diet provides adequate quantities of all these nutrients.

b) _____ *(1 word)* nutrients can be deleted from the diet of humans without causing specific signs of disease or growth failure.

c) A _____ _____ *(2 words)* nutrient is one that is not ordinarily required, but has to be included in the diet because of certain conditions (such as prematurity), genetic defects, or pathologic states, which impair the body's ability to synthesize nutrients.

d) Humans need the _____ (1 word) essential nutrients, but the _____ (1 word) of nutrients needed vary due to personal factors, including the stage of life, age, gender, genetic traits, body size, lifestyle habits (including physical activity, alcohol intake, and smoking), as well as the presence of a disease state or the usage of medication.

3. Which of the following are essential nutrients?

Cholesterol	Sodium	Lycopene	Biotin	Glucose
Lactose	Iron	Flavonoids	Creatine	Carnitine
Oleic acid	Calcium	Linoleic acid	Zinc	Water
Cobalamin				

Energy

4. a) Which classes of nutrients are energy-yielding?

   _____

   b) Which classes of nutrients are *not* energy-yielding?

   _____

5. How is energy stored in the human body?

   _____

6. Which of the following foods provides the most energy?

   a) A large egg
   b) A medium apple
   c) A slice (1 oz, 28 g) of whole wheat bread
   d) A cup (8 fluid oz, 237 mL) of vanilla-flavored soy milk
   e) A cup (8 fluid oz, 237 mL) of coffee with 2 tsp (10 mL) white sugar and 2 tsp (10 mL) half & half cream (10% fat)

7. Which of the following sources of carbohydrates provides the most energy per gram?

   a) White granulated sugar
   b) White powdered sugar
   c) Brown sugar (packed or unpacked)
   d) Maple sugar
   e) They all provide about 4 kcal (17 kJ/g).

8. Which of the following snacks contains the *most* energy?

   a) A medium celery stalk with a tablespoon (15 mL) of smooth regular peanut butter, and a cup (8 fluid oz, 237 mL) of vegetable juice cocktail
   b) A ¼ cup (59 mL) of sultana raisins and a cup (8 fluid oz, 237 mL) of partly skimmed (2% fat) milk
   c) A medium banana and 6¼ oz (175 g) of low-fat (1.5% fat) vanilla yogurt
   d) A small bag (1 oz, 28 g) of plain salted potato chips and a cup (8 fluid oz, 237 mL) of regular cola soft drink
   e) A medium milk chocolate candy bar (1½ oz, 42 g) and a cup (8 fluid oz, 237 mL) of lemon-lime soda pop

9. Which of the snacks in question #8 contains the *least* energy?

Macronutrients

10. Fill in the blank spaces with appropriate words.

    a) Proteins are strings of amino acids joined together by _____ (1 word) bonds.

b) The amino acids of protein differ from other energy-yielding nutrients, as their structures contain at least one _____ (1 word), in the form of a(n) _____ (1 word) group.

c) Amino acids provide _____ (1 word) for DNA and RNA synthesis.

d) Triacylglycerol or triglycerides consist of _____ _____ _____ (3 words) attached by esterification to a(n) _____ (1 word) molecule.

e) The main constituents of dietary fats are _____ _____ _____ (3 words).

f) The three most common monosaccharides are _____ (1 word), _____ (1 word), and _____ (1 word).

g) _____ (1 word) is an important source of energy and the main monosaccharide in blood.

h) Sucrose is a disaccharide composed of _____ _____ _____ (3 words) molecules.

i) Lactose is a disaccharide composed of _____ _____ _____ (3 words) molecules.

j) Maltose is a disaccharide composed of _____ _____ (2 words) molecules.

k) Starch and dextrins are digestible _____ (1 word).

l) _____ (1 word) fibers include dietary fibers and functional fibers.

m) _____ (1 word) fibers are isolated, nondigestible carbohydrates, which have beneficial physiologic effects in humans. Examples include inulin, fructan, and resistant starch. Some of them are commercially produced and added to food products.

n) Dietary fibers comprise nondigestible carbohydrates and lignin that are naturally found in plants. They are _____ (1 word) parts of plants, which are resistant to human digestive enzymes.

o) Six of the main dietary fibers are: _____, _____, _____, _____, _____, and _____ (6 words).

11. Which of these food servings has the highest **protein** content?

   a) 3 oz (84 g) steamed haddock
   b) ½ cup (118 mL) cooked medium grain white rice
   c) ½ cup (118 mL) low-fat (1% fat) cottage cheese
   d) 3 oz (84 g) broiled ground beef patty (18% fat)
   e) 1 extra large boiled egg

12. Which of these food servings has the highest **fat** content?

   a) 1 tablespoon (15 mL) chunky peanut butter
   b) 1 medium (2 oz, 56 g) butter croissant bread
   c) one link (½ oz, 14 g) of pork sausage
   d) half a medium avocado (3½ oz, 98 g)
   e) 1 extra large poached egg

13. Olive oil and _____ are the best sources of monounsaturated fatty acids, providing more than 58 g of monounsaturated fatty acids per 100 g.

   a) safflower oil
   b) canola oil
   c) soybean oil
   d) corn oil
   e) coconut oil

Water and Electrolytes

14. Fill in the blank spaces with appropriate words.

    a) Adults are approximately _____ percent *(1 word)* water by weight.

    b) Every day, individuals need enough water to replenish daily losses from _____
    (1 word), _____ *(1 word)*, and _____ *(1 word)*. Sources of water include
    water itself, beverages, and foods containing water.

    c) The total amount of body water remains relatively constant due to the homeostatic regulation of the
    _____ _____ *(2 words)*, _____ *(1 word)*, and
    _____ *(1 word)*.

    d) _____ *(1 word)* dissociate into negatively and positively charged ions when dissolved
    in _____ *(1 word)*.

15. List the main electrolytes found in the body. _____

Minerals

16. Which of these minerals are major minerals and are found in the body in amounts larger than 5 g?

Calcium	Copper	Magnesium	Phosphorus	Sodium
Chloride	Fluoride	Manganese	Potassium	Sulfur
Chromium	Iodine	Molybdenum	Selenium	Zinc
Cobalt	Iron			

17. Match these essential minerals with their primary functions in the body.
    (Note: Use each mineral only once)

Ca	P	Mg	Na	Cl	K	S	Mo
I	Fe	Zn	Cu	F	Se	Cr	Mn

    a) _____: Component of bones and tooth enamel. Helps to make teeth resistant to decay.

    b) _____: Component of teeth and bones. Part of certain enzymes and substances involved in
    energy formation. Required for maintaining body fluids at the right acid–base balance.

    c) _____: Electrolyte needed to maintain normal fluid balance and acid–base balance in the body.
    Component of the acid secreted by the stomach for digestion of food.

    d) _____: Component of teeth and bones. Involved in the transmission of nerve impulses.
    Activates enzymes involved in protein and energy formation.

    e) _____: Needed for the activation of enzymes involved in the reproduction of proteins.
    Component of many enzymes and of the hormone insulin.

    f) _____: Principal mineral of teeth and bones. Required for muscle and nerve activity, as well as
    for blood clotting.

    g) _____: Acts as an antioxidant with vitamin E to protect body cells from being damaged due to
    oxidation.

    h) _____: Part of enzymes involved in the body's utilization of oxygen and iron. Diverse functions
    in brain development, growth, and immunity, as well as cholesterol and glucose utilization.

    i) _____: Required for the formation of body fat and bones. Involved with enzymes to facilitate
    many cell processes.

    j) _____: Needed for the normal utilization of glucose and fat. Involved with insulin and needed
    for the release of energy from glucose.

k) ＿＿＿＿＿＿: Part of enzymes necessary for the transfer of oxygen from one molecule to another.

l) ＿＿＿＿＿＿: Electrolyte needed to maintain normal fluid balance and acid–base balance in the body. Required for nerve impulse transmission and muscle contraction.

m) ＿＿＿＿＿＿: Transports oxygen as a component of the protein hemoglobin found in red blood cells. Component of the muscle protein myoglobin, which makes oxygen available for muscle contraction.

n) ＿＿＿＿＿＿: Electrolyte needed to maintain normal fluid balance and acid–base balance in the body. Required for nerve impulse transmission. Assists in the contraction of muscles, including the heart.

o) ＿＿＿＿＿＿: Compound part of thyroid hormones that help to regulate growth, development, and energy production.

18. List four significant food sources of each essential mineral.

Ca: ＿＿＿＿＿＿＿＿＿＿＿＿＿＿＿＿＿＿＿＿＿＿＿＿＿＿＿＿＿＿＿＿＿＿＿

P: ＿＿＿＿＿＿＿＿＿＿＿＿＿＿＿＿＿＿＿＿＿＿＿＿＿＿＿＿＿＿＿＿＿＿＿＿

Mg: ＿＿＿＿＿＿＿＿＿＿＿＿＿＿＿＿＿＿＿＿＿＿＿＿＿＿＿＿＿＿＿＿＿＿＿

Fe: ＿＿＿＿＿＿＿＿＿＿＿＿＿＿＿＿＿＿＿＿＿＿＿＿＿＿＿＿＿＿＿＿＿＿＿

Zn: ＿＿＿＿＿＿＿＿＿＿＿＿＿＿＿＿＿＿＿＿＿＿＿＿＿＿＿＿＿＿＿＿＿＿＿

F: ＿＿＿＿＿＿＿＿＿＿＿＿＿＿＿＿＿＿＿＿＿＿＿＿＿＿＿＿＿＿＿＿＿＿＿＿

I: ＿＿＿＿＿＿＿＿＿＿＿＿＿＿＿＿＿＿＿＿＿＿＿＿＿＿＿＿＿＿＿＿＿＿＿＿＿

Se: ＿＿＿＿＿＿＿＿＿＿＿＿＿＿＿＿＿＿＿＿＿＿＿＿＿＿＿＿＿＿＿＿＿＿＿＿

Cu: ＿＿＿＿＿＿＿＿＿＿＿＿＿＿＿＿＿＿＿＿＿＿＿＿＿＿＿＿＿＿＿＿＿＿＿

Mn: ＿＿＿＿＿＿＿＿＿＿＿＿＿＿＿＿＿＿＿＿＿＿＿＿＿＿＿＿＿＿＿＿＿＿＿

Cr: ＿＿＿＿＿＿＿＿＿＿＿＿＿＿＿＿＿＿＿＿＿＿＿＿＿＿＿＿＿＿＿＿＿＿＿＿

Mo: ＿＿＿＿＿＿＿＿＿＿＿＿＿＿＿＿＿＿＿＿＿＿＿＿＿＿＿＿＿＿＿＿＿＿＿

Na: ＿＿＿＿＿＿＿＿＿＿＿＿＿＿＿＿＿＿＿＿＿＿＿＿＿＿＿＿＿＿＿＿＿＿＿

K: ＿＿＿＿＿＿＿＿＿＿＿＿＿＿＿＿＿＿＿＿＿＿＿＿＿＿＿＿＿＿＿＿＿＿＿＿＿

Cl: ＿＿＿＿＿＿＿＿＿＿＿＿＿＿＿＿＿＿＿＿＿＿＿＿＿＿＿＿＿＿＿＿＿＿＿＿

Vitamins

19. List the fat-soluble vitamins. ＿＿＿＿＿＿＿＿＿＿＿＿＿＿＿＿＿＿＿＿

20. United States and Canada fortify their refined grain products (flour, pasta, and bread) with which vitamin?

＿＿＿＿＿＿＿＿＿＿

21. Which vitamin found in dark green leafy vegetables is easily destroyed by heat? ＿＿＿＿＿＿＿

22. Which vitamin is needed for the absorption of calcium and phosphorus? ＿＿＿＿＿＿＿＿

23. Overconsumption of raw eggs can reduce the absorption of which vitamin? ＿＿＿＿＿＿＿

24. One vitamin is essential for normal blood clotting; which one? ＿＿＿＿＿＿＿

25. Give three foods fortified in vitamin D in the United States and Canada.

＿＿＿＿＿＿＿＿＿＿＿＿＿＿＿＿＿＿＿＿＿＿＿＿＿＿＿＿＿＿＿＿＿＿＿＿

26. Which vitamin present in milk is destroyed by exposure to light? ＿＿＿＿＿＿＿

27. Beta carotene is a "provitamin" or precursor of vitamin＿＿＿＿＿＿.

28. Name the vitamin produced by bacteria in our gut, that allows part of our requirements for that vitamin to be met. _____

29. Which vitamin enhances the absorption of iron? _____

30. _____ is (are) one of the richest natural sources of folate, providing more than 210 g folate per 3½ -oz (100-g) serving.

   a) Liver
   b) Raw spinach
   c) Romaine lettuce
   d) Cooked lentils
   e) Fresh orange juice

31. _____ is (are) an excellent source of vitamin E.

   a) Mushrooms
   b) Yogurt
   c) Molasses
   d) Sunflower seed kernels
   e) Grapefruit

32. _____ reduces the oxidation of lipids.

   a) Vitamin C
   b) Vitamin D
   c) Beta carotene
   d) Vitamin A
   e) Vitamin E

33. People who smoke have an increased need for which vitamin? _____

34. The intake of 1 g/day or more of vitamin _____ can cause cramps, nausea, and diarrhea, and may increase the risk of kidney stones.

35. Give six very good dietary sources of thiamin.

_____

36. Which foods are rich in niacin?

_____

37. Where can riboflavin be found in the diet?

_____

38. Which of these food servings contains the most vitamin C?

   a) 1 medium tomato
   b) 1 medium grapefruit
   c) 1 medium orange
   d) 1 medium kiwi fruit
   e) 1 medium potato

39. Which of these food servings contains the least vitamin B_{12}?

   a) 1 cup (8 fluid oz, 237 mL) skim milk
   b) 3 oz (84 g) liver
   c) 3 oz (84 g) beef
   d) 3 oz (84 g) trout
   e) 3 oz (84 g) lamb

UNDERSTAND THE CONCEPTS

Nutrients

1. What nutrient recommendations are being used for the general healthy population in both the United States and Canada? _____

2. What are the AI recommendations? _____

_____

3. What are the RDA recommendations? _____
   _____
   _____

4. What are the UL recommendations? _____
   _____
   _____

5. What are the Daily Values (DVs)? _____
   _____
   _____

Energy

6. How many kilojoules are provided by one kilocalorie? _____

7. How much energy does 1 g of each macronutrient yield?
   _____

8. Alcohol is not a nutrient, but it yields energy. How much energy is contained in 1 g of alcohol?
   _____

9. Which energy store(s) is (are) the body using in the fasting state?
   _____
   _____

10. Which source(s) of energy is (are) the body using in prolonged fasting?
    _____
    _____

11. What factors are taken into consideration when estimating the daily energy requirements of a healthy
    individual? _____
    _____

12. What are the EER recommendations? _____
    _____
    _____

13. What is TEE? _____
    _____
    _____

14. What is BEE? _____
    _____

15. What is BMR? _____
    _____

Macronutrients

16. Which of the following amino acids are essential for humans?

Glycine	Methionine	Tyrosine	Cystine	Proline
Alanine	Serine	Isoleucine	Glutamic acid	Phenylalanine
Leucine	Threonine	Arginine	Histidine	Valine
Aspartic acid	Tryptophan	Lysine		

17. Circle the essential fatty acids and provide examples of where they are found in the diet.

Arachidonic acid (20:4)   Linoleic acid (18:2)

Stearidonic acid (18:4)   Docosahexaenoic acid (22:6)

Linolenic acid (18:3)   Docosapentaenoic acid (22:5)

Eicosatrienoic acid (20:3)   Eicosapentaenoic acid (20:5)

18. According to the DRI recommendations, healthy adults should get _____ of the energy intake from fat, _____ of the energy intake from protein, and _____ of the energy intake from carbohydrate.

a) 10%–35%, 20%–40%, 45%–70%   d) 20%–35%, 10%–35%, 45%–65%
b) 25%–45%, 15%–35%, 35%–65%   e) 15%–40%, 20%–35%, 55%–70%
c) 10%–25%, 15%–40%, 40%–75%

19. What are the AMDR recommendations? _____

_____

_____

20. What are the EAR recommendations? _____

_____

_____

21. The RDA for women and men over 18 years of age is _____ of good quality protein per kilogram body weight per day.

22. Which foods are rich in saturated fats? _____

_____

23. Which foods are rich in unsaturated fats? _____

_____

24. The adequate intake of total fiber for males and females is _____ g/1000 kcal (4180 kJ) of energy intake per day.

a) 6   d) 12
b) 8   e) 14
c) 10

25. Highlight the high-fiber foods in this list. High-fiber foods provide at least 5 g of fiber per serving. Including them in the diet helps people to meet their daily fiber requirements.

Mangos (½ cup, 118 mL)   Kiwis (2)

Macaroni (1 cup, 237 mL)   Lima beans (½ cup, 118 mL)

Whole wheat pasta (1 cup, 237 mL)   Lettuce (1 cup, 237 mL)

Grapes (20)   Kidney beans (½ cup, 118 mL)

35. Identify the possible nutrient deficiencies associated with the following clinical characteristics of malnutrition.

| POSSIBLE NUTRIENT DEFICIENCIES ASSOCIATED WITH CLINICAL CHARACTERISTICS OF MALNUTRITION ||
Clinical Characteristics of Malnutrition	Possible Nutrient Deficiencies
Rickets, osteoporosis	
Anemia	
Tooth decay	
Goiter, cretinism	
Neural tube defects	
Scurvy, bleeding gums	
Impaired vision, blindness	

INTEGRATE YOUR LEARNING

1. Identify the factor(s) that may influence the need for essential nutrients.

   1- The presence in the diet of substances for which the nutrient is a precursor
   2- The presence in the diet of substances that are precursors of the nutrient
   3- The presence in the diet of substances that interfere with the absorption or utilization of the nutrient
   4- Imbalances and disproportion of other related nutrients in the diet
   5- Some genetic defects
   6- Drug–nutrient interactions

2. Which statement about the DRI recommendations is **false**?

   a) The Adequate Intake is the estimated nutrient requirement that is adequate in 50% of the population, and was used to develop the Recommended Dietary Allowances.
   b) The Recommended Dietary Allowance is the dietary intake goal for individuals, but its purpose is not to assess diets of individuals or groups.
   c) The Tolerable Upper Intake Level is the maximum nutrient intake that is not associated with adverse effects in most individuals of a healthy population.
   d) The Estimated Average Requirement is a recommendation that may be used to assess the diets of individuals or groups.
   e) The Recommended Dietary Allowance is the estimated nutrient allowance that is adequate in 97%–98% of the healthy population specific for life stage, age, and gender.

3. Refer to the *Dietary Reference Intake Recommendations* (see appendix section at the end of this book) and provide appropriate nutrient recommendations (Recommended Dietary Allowance or Adequate Intake) for the following clients considering their individual needs.

   a) Iron Recommended Dietary Allowance for a 7-month-old infant boy: _____

   b) Iron Recommended Dietary Allowance for a 25-year-old pregnant woman: _____

   c) Calcium Adequate Intake for an 18-year-old pregnant woman: _____

d) Vitamin C Recommended Dietary Allowance for a 31-year-old lactating woman: _____

e) Folate Recommended Dietary Allowance for a 20-year-old woman: _____

f) Folate Recommended Dietary Allowance for a 30-year-old pregnant woman: _____

g) Vitamin A Recommended Dietary Allowance for a 35-year-old lactating woman: _____

h) Vitamin D Adequate Intake for a 12-month-old: _____

i) Vitamin B_{12} Recommended Dietary Allowance for a 22-year-old pregnant woman: _____

4. a) Determine the energy in kilocalories (Kcal) and kilojoules (KJ) provided by a food containing 0.5 g carbohydrate, 5 g protein, and 1 g fat. _____

   b) What is the percent of the energy coming from protein in the above food? _____

5. If a slice of extra lean ham contains 39 kcal (163 kJ) and includes 2.2 g of fat, then it would have

   _____ % of the total energy from fat.

6. a) Determine the energy provided by one cup (8 fluid oz, 237 mL) of low-fat (1% fat) cow's milk, given that

   it contains 11.8 g of carbohydrates, 8.5 g of protein, and 2.6 g of fat. _____

   b) Determine the percentage of energy provided by each macronutrient in that cup (8 fluid oz, 237 mL)

   of milk. _____

7. The egg salad sandwich on whole wheat bread you just ate consisted of 11.4 g of protein, 27.6 g of fat, 31.3 g of carbohydrates, 5 g of insoluble fiber, and 176 mg of cholesterol.

   a) How many grams of available carbohydrates did it contain? _____

   b) How many kilocalories or kilojoules did it contain? _____

8. Use a *table of nutrient content of foods* (also called *food composition table*) to determine the energy and

   protein content of the following breakfast: _____

   ½ cup (4 fluid oz, 118 mL) fresh orange juice
   one small whole wheat bagel (2 oz, 56 g)
   1 Tbsp (15 mL) light plain cream cheese
   one medium hard-boiled egg (2 oz, 56 g)
   1 cup (237 mL) nonfat coffee yogurt

9. How many grams of protein represent 30% of the energy from a 2500 kcal (10,450 kJ) diet? _____

10. The following menu sample is low in which macronutrient? _____

   Breakfast
   1 cup (237 mL) oatmeal made with water
   ¼ cup (59 mL) blueberries
   1 cup (8 fluid oz, 237 mL) orange juice

   Lunch
   2 cups (474 mL) vegetable salad
   1 Tbsp (15 mL) mayonnaise
   ½ cup (118 mL) croutons
   1 pear
   1 cup (8 fluid oz, 237 mL) water

   Dinner
   1 cup (237 mL) wild rice
   ½ cup (118 mL) green peas
   ½ cup (118 mL) carrots
   1 slice apple pie

11. Match each of the following meals with the micronutrient of which they are a good source.

Calcium   Magnesium   Potassium   Iron   Zinc   Vitamin B$_{12}$ Vitamin C   Vitamin E   Folate

a) _____ Baked potato, baked fish, milk, banana

b) _____ Cooked broccoli, melted cheddar cheese, sardines, milk

c) _____ Soymilk, ready-to-eat bran cereals, plain yogurt

d) _____ Orange juice, red and green peppers, kiwi, strawberries, grapefruit

e) _____ Steamed clams, cooked spinach, beef steak, cooked navy beans

f) _____ Wheat germ, sunflower seeds, safflower oil

g) _____ Cooked lentils and pinto beans, spinach, asparagus, orange juice

h) _____ Chicken liver, sardines, cottage cheese, fortified soymilk

i) _____ Steamed crabmeat and oysters, plain yogurt

12. Here is the list of ingredients of your girlfriend's favorite brand of cereal fruit bars. She has one bar as a snack every day and is asking you if it is a healthy food choice, as she is concerned about being over-weight. Each bar (37 g, 1.3 oz) provides about 140 kcal (585 kJ).

RASPBERRY CEREAL BARS ~ INGREDIENTS

CRUST: Flour, sugar/glucose-fructose, whole oats, hydrogenated vegetable oil, water, honey, dextrose, modified milk ingredients, wheat bran, natural and artificial flavor, salt, cellulose gum, potassium bi-carbonate, soya lecithin, wheat gluten, color.

FILLING: Glucose-fructose, raspberry preserve (glucose-fructose, raspberry puree, water), glycerol, maltodextrin, sodium arginate, natural flavor, modified corn starch, citric acid [acidulant], soya lecithin, xanthan gum, calcium phosphate, malic acid, sodium citrate, color.

---

a) Which ingredient is present in the highest quantity by weight in the crust? _____

And in the filling? _____

b) Distinguish "added" versus "natural" sugars. _____

_____

_____

c) Highlight all the added sugars in the list of ingredients with a highlighter.

d) Aside from those identified using this list of ingredients, what are other sources of added sugar?

_____

_____

e) Box all the sources of dietary fiber.

f) Circle all the sources of fat in the list of ingredients.

g) What are hydrogenated oils? _____

_____

h) What are trans-fatty acids? _____

_____

i) Where are trans-fatty acids mostly found? _____

_____

_____

j) Underline all the food additives in the list of ingredients.

k) Is it a healthy food to recommend to your friend? Explain. _____

_____

_____

_____

_____

13. How can you make this lunch on-the-go healthier? Give five suggestions.

Deluxe cheeseburger with bacon
Large French fries (6½ oz, 182 g)
Large cola (3 cups, 24 fluid oz, 711 mL)
2 Chocolate glazed donuts

1) _____

2) _____

3) _____

4) _____

5) _____

14. Your grandfather is complaining about being thirsty all the time. He says he is drinking some fluids, so he does not understand why he is so thirsty. Talking with him, you realize that he drinks two cups (16 fluid oz, 474 mL) of coffee in the morning, one cup (8 fluid oz, 237 mL) of iced tea with lunch, a can (1½ cup, 12 fluid oz, 356 mL) of cola beverage in the afternoon, and a cup (8 fluid oz, 237 mL) of hot cocoa in the evening almost every day. He does not like the taste of the water from the tap, so he does not drink water. He enjoys an hour of walking after lunch.

a) What is being thirsty a sign of? _____

_____

b) Why do you think he is so thirsty? _____

_____

_____

c) What do coffee, tea, cola, and cocoa beverages have in common? _____

_____

d) What would help him solve this problem? Give five practical suggestions.

1) _____

2) _____

3) _____

4) _____

5) _____

15. Use the following DRI predictive mathematical equation to determine the Estimated Energy Requirement (EER) of a sedentary 25-year-old healthy woman, based on her estimated Total Energy Expenditure (TEE). Take into consideration that she weighs 59 kg (129.8 lb) and measures 1.65 meters (5'5"), and that the physical activity coefficient (PA) for a sedentary person is 1.00.

Estimated Energy Requirement in kcal
based on the Total Energy Expenditure for an adult woman ≥19 years old
$$= 354 - (6.91 \times \text{Age in}_{\text{years}}) + \{PA \times [(9.36 \times \text{Weight in}_{\text{kg}}) + (726 \times \text{Height in}_{\text{meters}})]\}$$

_____

16. Does going to a tanning salon increase your vitamin D status? Explain. _____

_____

17. Your 37-year-old cousin Michel had the following dinner:

Fresh Italian pork sausage, 2 links (5 oz, 140 g)
Tomato ketchup, 1 Tbsp or 15 mL
Egg noodles, 1 cup or 237 mL
Hard corn oil margarine, 2 tsp or 10 mL
Steamed broccoli, ½ cup or 118 mL
Cheddar cheese sauce, 3 Tbsp or 45 mL
Vanilla ice cream, 1 cup or 237 mL
Fresh strawberries, ½ cup or 118 mL
Peanut butter cookies, 2
Chocolate milk, 1 cup (8 fluid oz) or 237 mL

1. The energy content of this meal is
   a) low, about 400 kcal (1672 kJ)
   b) moderate, about 700 kcal (2926 kJ)
   c) high, about 1000 kcal (4180 kJ)
   d) very high, about 1300 kcal (5434 kJ)
   e) extremely high, about 1600 kcal (6688 kJ)

2. Which food contains the most energy?
   a) Pork sausages (2 links, 5 oz, 140 g)
   b) Ice cream (1 cup, 237 mL)
   c) Peanut butter cookies (2)
   d) Egg noodles (1 cup, 237 mL)
   e) Chocolate milk (1 cup, 8 fluid oz, 237 mL)

3. The fat content of this meal is
   a) low, about 20% of the energy intake
   b) moderate, about 28% of the energy intake
   c) high, about 35% of the energy intake
   d) very high, about 40% of the energy intake
   e) extremely high, about 50% of the energy intake

4. Which food contains the most fat?
   a) Pork sausages (2 links, 5 oz, 140 g)
   b) Ice cream (1 cup, 237 mL)
   c) Peanut butter cookies (2)
   d) Margarine (2 tsp, 10 mL)
   e) Chocolate milk (1 cup, 8 fluid oz, 237 mL)

5. The saturated fat content of this meal is
   a) low, about 5% of the energy intake
   b) moderate, about 10% of the energy intake
   c) high, about 14% of the energy intake
   d) very high, about 18% of the energy intake
   e) extremely high, about 25% of the energy intake

6. Which food contains the most saturated fat?
   a) Pork sausages (2 links, 5 oz, 140 g)
   b) Ice cream (1 cup, 237 mL)
   c) Peanut butter cookies (2)
   d) Egg noodles (1 cup, 237 mL)
   e) Chocolate milk (1 cup, 8 fluid oz, 237 mL)

7. The cholesterol content of this meal is
   a) low, about 10 mg of cholesterol
   b) moderate, about 70 mg of cholesterol
   c) high, about 140 mg of cholesterol
   d) very high, about 240 mg of cholesterol
   e) extremely high, about 350 mg of cholesterol

8. Which food contains the most cholesterol?
   a) Pork sausages (2 links, 5 oz, 140 g)
   b) Ice cream (1 cup, 237 mL)
   c) Peanut butter cookies (2)
   d) Egg noodles (1 cup, 237 mL)
   e) Chocolate milk (1 cup, 8 fluid oz, 237 mL)

9. Which food contains the most trans-fatty acids?
   a) Pork sausages (2 links, 5 oz, 140 g)
   b) Ice cream (1 cup, 237 mL)
   c) Peanut butter cookies (2)
   d) Hard margarine (2 tsp, 10 mL)
   e) Chocolate milk (1 cup, 8 fluid oz, 237 mL)

10. Which food is a good source of ω-6 fatty acids?
    a) Broccoli
    b) Ice cream
    c) Corn oil margarine
    d) Egg noodle
    e) Strawberries

11. The sodium content of this meal is
    a) low, about 300 mg sodium
    b) moderate, about 600 mg sodium
    c) high, about 1000 mg sodium
    d) very high, about 1600 mg sodium
    e) extremely high, about 2300 mg sodium

12. Which food contains the most sodium?
    a) Pork sausages (2 links, 5 oz, 140 g)
    b) Cheddar cheese sauce (3 Tbsp, 45 mL)
    c) Peanut butter cookies (2)
    d) Tomato ketchup (1 Tbsp, 15 mL)
    e) Chocolate milk (1 cup, 8 fluid oz, 237 mL)

18. Match these beverages with their corresponding Nutrition Facts information. Note that the nutrition information corresponds to a serving size of one cup (8 fluid oz, 237 mL) for each beverage.

a) _____ Partly skimmed (2% fat) milk

b) _____ Canned, unsweetened pure pineapple juice

c) _____ Orange soda pop

d) _____ Canned vegetable juice cocktail

e) _____ Pure fresh orange juice

f) _____ Instant breakfast prepared with partly skimmed (2% fat) milk

I

Nutrition Facts

Serving Size (248g)
Servings Per Container

Amount Per Serving

Calories 120   Calories from Fat 0

	% Daily Value*
Total Fat 0g	**0%**
Saturated Fat 0g	**0%**
Cholesterol 0mg	**0%**
Sodium 30 mg	**1%**
Total Carbohydrate 31g	**10%**
Dietary Fiber 0g	**0%**
Sugars 31g	
Protein 0g	

Vitamin A 0% · **Vitamin C 0%**
Calcium 2% · **Iron 0%**

*Percent Daily Values are based on a 2,000 calorie diet. Your daily values may be higher or lower depending on your calorie needs:

	Calories:	2,000	2,500
Total Fat	Less than	65g	80g
Saturated Fat	Less than	20g	25g
Cholesterol	Less than	300mg	300mg
Sodium	Less than	2,400mg	2,400mg
Total Carbohydrate		300g	375g
Dietary Fiber		25g	30g

Calories per gram:
Fat 9 · Carbohydrate 4 · Protein 4

II

Nutrition Facts

Serving Size (247g)
Servings Per Container

Amount Per Serving

Calories 110   Calories from Fat 0

	% Daily Value*
Total Fat 0g	**0%**
Saturated Fat 0g	**0%**
Cholesterol 0mg	**0%**
Sodium 0 mg	**0%**
Total Carbohydrate 26g	**9%**
Dietary Fiber 0g	**0%**
Sugars 22g	
Protein 1g	

Vitamin A 0% · **Vitamin C 50%**
Calcium 2% · **Iron 0%**

*Percent Daily Values are based on a 2,000 calorie diet. Your daily values may be higher or lower depending on your calorie needs:

	Calories:	2,000	2,500
Total Fat	Less than	65g	80g
Saturated Fat	Less than	20g	25g
Cholesterol	Less than	300mg	300mg
Sodium	Less than	2,400mg	2,400mg
Total Carbohydrate		300g	375g
Dietary Fiber		25g	30g

Calories per gram:
Fat 9 · Carbohydrate 4 · Protein 4

III

Nutrition Facts

Serving Size (250g)
Servings Per Container

Amount Per Serving

Calories 140   Calories from Fat 0

	% Daily Value*
Total Fat 0g	**0%**
Saturated Fat 0g	**0%**
Cholesterol 0mg	**0%**
Sodium 30 mg	**0%**
Total Carbohydrate 34g	**11%**
Dietary Fiber less than 1 gram	**2%**
Sugars 34g	
Protein 1g	

Vitamin A 0% · **Vitamin C 45%**
Calcium 4% · **Iron 4%**

*Percent Daily Values are based on a 2,000 calorie diet. Your daily values may be higher or lower depending on your calorie needs:

	Calories:	2,000	2,500
Total Fat	Less than	65g	80g
Saturated Fat	Less than	20g	25g
Cholesterol	Less than	300mg	300mg
Sodium	Less than	2,400mg	2,400mg
Total Carbohydrate		300g	375g
Dietary Fiber		25g	30g

Calories per gram:
Fat 9 · Carbohydrate 4 · Protein 4

IV

Nutrition Facts
Serving Size (281 g)
Servings Per Container

Amount Per Serving	
Calories 250 Calories from Fat 45	
	% Daily Value*
Total Fat 5g	**8%**
Saturated Fat 3g	**16%**
Cholesterol 25mg	**8%**
Sodium 260 mg	**11%**
Total Carbohydrate 36g	**12%**
Dietary Fiber 0g	**0%**
Sugars 36g	
Protein 15g	

Vitamin A 45% · **Vitamin C 50%**	
Calcium 40% · **Iron 25%**	

*Percent Daily Values are based on a 2,000 calorie diet. Your daily values may be higher or lower depending on your calorie needs:

		Calories:	2,000	2,500
Total Fat	Less than		65g	80g
Saturated Fat	Less than		20g	25g
Cholesterol	Less than		300mg	300mg
Sodium	Less than		2,400mg	2,400mg
Total Carbohydrate			300g	375g
Dietary Fiber			25g	30g

Calories per gram:
Fat 9 · Carbohydrate 4 · Protein 4

V

Nutrition Facts
Serving Size (242 g)
Servings Per Container

Amount Per Serving	
Calories 45 Calories from Fat 0	
	% Daily Value*
Total Fat 0g	**0%**
Saturated Fat 0g	**0%**
Cholesterol 0mg	**0%**
Sodium 650 mg	**27%**
Total Carbohydrate 11g	**4%**
Dietary Fiber 2g	**8%**
Sugars 5g	
Protein 2g	

Vitamin A 60% · **Vitamin C 110%**	
Calcium 2% · **Iron 6%**	

*Percent Daily Values are based on a 2,000 calorie diet. Your daily values may be higher or lower depending on your calorie needs:

		Calories:	2,000	2,500
Total Fat	Less than		65g	80g
Saturated Fat	Less than		20g	25g
Cholesterol	Less than		300mg	300mg
Sodium	Less than		2,400mg	2,400mg
Total Carbohydrate			300g	375g
Dietary Fiber			25g	30g

Calories per gram:
Fat 9 · Carbohydrate 4 · Protein 4

VI

Nutrition Facts
Serving Size (244 g)
Servings Per Container

Amount Per Serving	
Calories 120 Calories from Fat 40	
	% Daily Value*
Total Fat 4.5g	**7%**
Saturated Fat 3g	**15%**
Cholesterol 20mg	**6%**
Sodium 120 mg	**5%**
Total Carbohydrate 12g	**4%**
Dietary Fiber 0g	**0%**
Sugars 12g	
Protein 8g	

Vitamin A 10% · **Vitamin C 4%**	
Calcium 30% · **Iron 0%**	

*Percent Daily Values are based on a 2,000 calorie diet. Your daily values may be higher or lower depending on your calorie needs:

		Calories:	2,000	2,500
Total Fat	Less than		65g	80g
Saturated Fat	Less than		20g	25g
Cholesterol	Less than		300mg	300mg
Sodium	Less than		2,400mg	2,400mg
Total Carbohydrate			300g	375g
Dietary Fiber			25g	30g

Calories per gram:
Fat 9 · Carbohydrate 4 · Protein 4

CHALLENGE YOUR LEARNING

CASE STUDY

Objective:

The objective of this case is for you to apply the knowledge you have gained on dietary constituents and utilize it in a practical life situation, using your analytical and critical thinking skills.

Description:

Miss E.B. is a 19-year-old university student. She is very physically active, and is in the normal weight range for her age and sex. She says that she does not have time to eat lunch, but she seems to be meeting her daily energy and protein requirements most days.

However, Miss E.B. is very pale and has been complaining about feeling weak and irritable for months. Her mother, who convinced her to come to the medical clinic, reports that she is suffering from bouts of drowsiness, often has a headache, and is catching the flu quite easily compared to her two sisters.

Miss E.B.'s mother is convinced that her daughter is overworked and needs to slow down, but E.B. herself does not understand what is happening to her; she just feels like she is "progressively losing all her energy."

Miss E.B. tells you that her diet is very repetitive and mainly composed of the following:

Breakfast:	banana, one large
	puffed rice, 1 cup or 237 mL
	milk, 1% fat, 1⅔ cup (13.3 fluid oz) or 400 mL
Morning snack:	chocolate milk candy bar, medium
	cola soda pop or coffee, 1 cup (8 fluid oz) or 237 mL
Afternoon snack:	apple, medium, raw
	mozzarella cheese (25% fat), 1-inch cube (1 oz, 28 g)

Dinner: spaghetti noodles or mashed potatoes, 1½ cup or 356 mL
cheese or tomato sauce, ½ cup or 118 mL
slice of white bread, 1 oz or 28 g
with butter, 2 tsp or 10 mL
mixed salad greens, 2 cups or 474 mL
with balsamic vinegar dressing, 3 Tbsp or 45 mL
milk, 1% fat, 1 cup (8 fluid oz) or 237 mL
rich vanilla ice cream, ⅔ cup or 160 mL

Questions:

1. What medical condition could E.B. be suffering from?

2. What are the signs and symptoms of that medical condition?

3. Do you think E.B.'s medical condition could be related to a possible nutrient deficiency? If yes, which one?

4. How would you quantify her dietary intake of that nutrient?

5. Use a *table of nutrient contents of foods* or *food composition and diet analysis software* to quantify the content of E.B.'s diet in that nutrient.

6. What is the RDA or AI for that nutrient appropriate for a 19-year-old woman?

7. Is E.B. meeting the RDA or AI in that nutrient for her age and sex?

8. What foods could E.B. add to her diet to increase her dietary intake of that nutrient?

9. Give some specific examples of how E.B. could modify her menu to include sources of this nutrient, taking into consideration that she does not like to eat organ meats.

10. Is the RDA or AI for that nutrient the same for a man of the same age? Explain why.

11. What vitamin could help increase the absorption of that nutrient?

12. What is the RDA or AI for that vitamin for E.B.'s age and sex?

13. Is E.B. meeting her requirements in that vitamin?

14. What are sources of that vitamin?

15. Is E.B. including some sources of that vitamin in her present diet?

16. Which nutritional deficiency is most commonly found in the world today?

Case Follow-up:

The physician prescribes Miss E.B. a mineral supplement to treat her medical condition. E.B. is taking it every morning with her milk and cereal, but her medical condition is only partly solved, and now she is starting to have painful stomach cramps and constipation. She is thinking about not taking the mineral supplement anymore.

17. Why do you think that her medical condition does not seem to be completely treated with the mineral supplement?

18. Do you have any idea why she has cramps and how they can be improved?

19. What do you think is causing the constipation?

20. What can you suggest to E.B. to help reduce her constipation?

21. E.B. has been following your dietary recommendations and taking the mineral supplement prescribed by the physician, but she still feels weak. Is it possible that this medical condition also has other nutrition-related causes? Explain.

22. Use a *table of nutrient contents of foods* or *food composition and diet analysis software* to quantify the amount of energy in E.B.'s usual diet.

> banana, one large
> puffed rice, 1 cup or 237 mL
> milk, 1% fat, 1⅔ cup (13.3 fluid oz) or 400 mL
> milk chocolate candy bar, medium
> cola soda pop, 1 cup (8 fluid oz) or 237 mL
> apple, medium, raw
> mozzarella cheese (25% fat), 1-inch cube (1 oz, 28 g)
> spaghetti noodle pasta, cooked, 1½ cup or 356 mL
> cheese sauce, ½ cup or 118 mL
> slice of white bread, 1 oz or 28 g
> butter, 2 tsp or 10 mL
> mixed salad greens, 2 cups or 474 mL
> balsamic vinegar dressing, 3 Tbsp or 45 mL
> milk, 1% fat, 1 cup (8 fluid oz) or 237 mL
> rich vanilla ice cream, ⅔ cup or 160 mL

23. Use the DRI mathematical equation to determine her Estimated Energy Requirement (EER) based on her estimated Total Energy Expenditure (TEE). Note that she weighs 120 lb and is 5'7" tall, and her physical activity coefficient is 1.48 (very active).

> **Estimated Energy Requirement** in kcal
> based on the Total Energy Expenditure for an adult woman ≥19 years old
> $= 354 - (6.91 \times \text{Age}_{years}) + \{\text{PA} \times [(9.36 \times \text{Weight}_{kg}) + (726 \times \text{Height}_{meters})]\}$

24. Compare her energy intake to her Estimated Energy Requirement. Is she meeting her energy needs? Explain.

25. Would she be meeting her energy needs if she was sedentary? Explain.

26. How do you explain that she is in the normal weight range for her age and sex?

PART 2

Alimentary Tract and Nutrition

INTRODUCTION

The goal of this section is to help you review the **anatomy** and understand the **physiology** of the alimentary tract, as well as to integrate and apply your knowledge of what happens in the alimentary tract in response to a meal in a normal individual. By understanding the normal anatomy-physiology of the gastrointestinal tract, you will build the foundations to help you understand in the later chapters what happens in the gastrointestinal tract in different pathologic states, and have a better grasp of what the dietary treatment options are. Enjoy the following learning activities!

2.1 Anatomy of the Alimentary Tract

REVIEW THE INFORMATION

1. Take a pencil, and from memory, draft a sketch of the alimentary tract in the space below. Then, label the main anatomic structures involved. *Do not peek at the next page yet!*

2. Refresh your memory by looking at this diagram of the alimentary tract <u>and</u> by tracing a dotted line with arrows representing the passage of food and nutrients through its tubular structure.

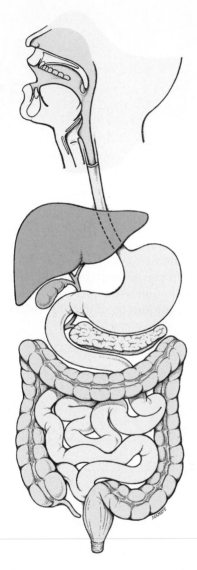

The alimentary tract. (Modified from original by Neil O. Hardy, Westport, CT.)

3. Name the four main contiguous segments forming the alimentary tract.

    1. _____

    2. _____

    3. _____

    4. _____

4. Name the sphincters and valves of the alimentary tract <u>and</u> identify their location on the diagram of question #2.

    _____

    _____

5. List the accessory organs and glands linked to the gastrointestinal tract, which are involved in the digestion of food by secreting digestive juices into the gastrointestinal tract.

_____

_____

_____

_____

6. Identify on this figure the anatomic structures of the alimentary tract using the following list.

a) Tongue
b) Pancreas
c) Esophagus
d) Ascending colon
e) Liver

f) Rectum
g) Stomach
h) Epiglottis
i) Jejunum
j) Pharynx

k) Gallbladder
l) Ileum
m) Transverse colon
n) Common bile duct

o) Ileocecal valve
p) Pyloric sphincter
q) Anal sphincter
r) Cecum
s) Oral cavity
t) Duodenum

u) Descending colon
v) Cardiac sphincter
w) Sigmoid colon
x) Salivary gland

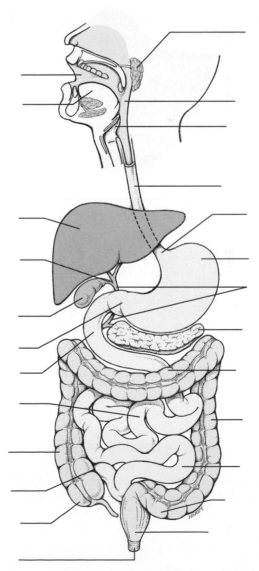

Anatomy of the alimentary tract. (From Stedman's Medical Dictionary. 27th Ed. Baltimore: Lippincott Williams & Wilkins, 2000.)

UNDERSTAND THE CONCEPTS

1. Identify the anatomic structures shown on these three figures of the oral cavity and pharynx. Note that some structures are illustrated in more than one of the figures.

____ Oral cavity	____ Hard palate	____ Palatopharyngeal arches
____ Palatine (adenoid) tonsil	____ Palatine tonsils	____ Pterygomandibular raphe
____ Vestibule or buccal cavity	____ Uvula	____ Submandibular salivary gland
____ Palatoglossal arches	____ Soft palate	____ Sublingual salivary gland
____ Parotid salivary gland	____ Epiglottis	____ Auditory (eustachian) tube

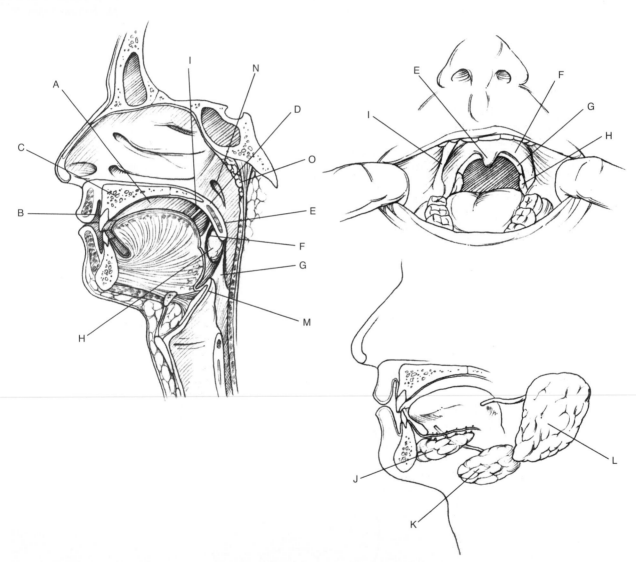

Anatomy of the oral cavity and pharynx. (Modified from Twietmeyer TA, McCracken T. Coloring Guide to Human Anatomy. 3rd Ed., New York: Lippincott Williams & Wilkins, 2001:175.)

2. What is the term for the internal area located inside the abdominopelvic cavity that contains the majority of viscera? _____

3. What is the term for the serous membrane that lines the abdominopelvic cavity walls and covers most viscera? _____

4. Identify the anatomic structures shown on these figures of the abdominal cavity (transverse section) and the stomach.

____ Fundus of stomach	____ Antrum of stomach
____ Pyloric sphincter	____ Lesser curvature
____ Mesentery	____ Cardia of stomach
____ Esophagus	____ Cardiac sphincter
____ Angulus of stomach	____ Visceral peritoneum
____ Parietal peritoneum	____ Greater curvature
____ Body of stomach	____ Duodenal bulb

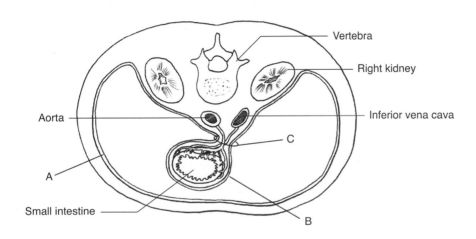

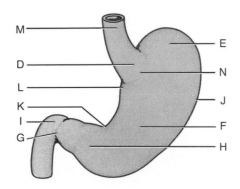

Anatomy of the abdominal cavity and stomach. (Top: From Twietmeyer TA, McCracken T. Coloring Guide to Human Anatomy. 3rd Ed. New York: Lippincott Williams & Wilkins, 2001:177. Bottom: From Shils ME, Shike M, Ross AC, et al., eds. Modern Nutrition in Health and Disease. 10th Ed. Baltimore: Lippincott Williams & Wilkins, 2006:1117.)

5. Identify the following anatomic structures on the figure of the gallbladder and biliary tree presented below.

a) Cystic duct
b) Main pancreatic duct
c) Accessory pancreatic duct
d) Major duodenal papilla
e) Minor duodenal papilla

f) Gallbladder
g) Sphincter of Oddi (or hepaticopancreatic sphincter)
h) Duodenum
i) Common hepatic duct

j) Common bile duct
k) Right hepatic duct
l) Left hepatic duct

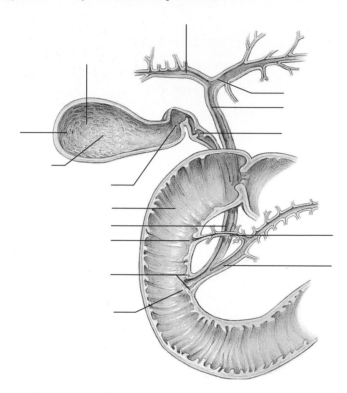

Gallbladder and biliary tree. (Modified from asset provided by Anatomical Chart Co.)

6. Identify the layers forming the wall of the gastrointestinal tract on this figure.

_____ Mucosa   _____ Epithelium   _____ Submucosa

_____ Muscularis propria   _____ Serosa or mesothelium   _____ Lamina propria

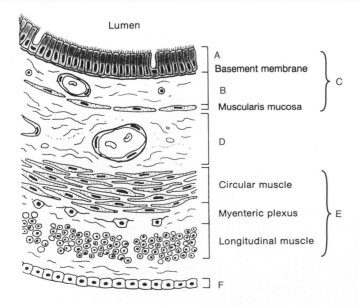

Wall of the gastrointestinal tract. (Adapted from Shils ME, Shike M, Ross AC, et al., eds. Modern Nutrition in Health and Disease. 10th Ed. Baltimore: Lippincott Williams & Wilkins, 2006:1116.)

7. Identify the anatomic structures of the small intestine and colon using these three figures.

___ Sacral flexure of rectum	___ Ileum	___ Ileocecal orifice
___ Jejunum	___ Teniae coli	___ Cecum
___ Epiploic appendages	___ Mesoappendix	___ Vermiform appendix
___ Ileocecal valve	___ Descending colon	___ Ascending colon
___ Perineal flexure of rectum	___ Transverse colon	___ Haustra
___ Transverse mesocolon	___ Splenic flexure	___ Rectum
___ Sigmoid colon	___ Anal canal	___ Hepatic flexure

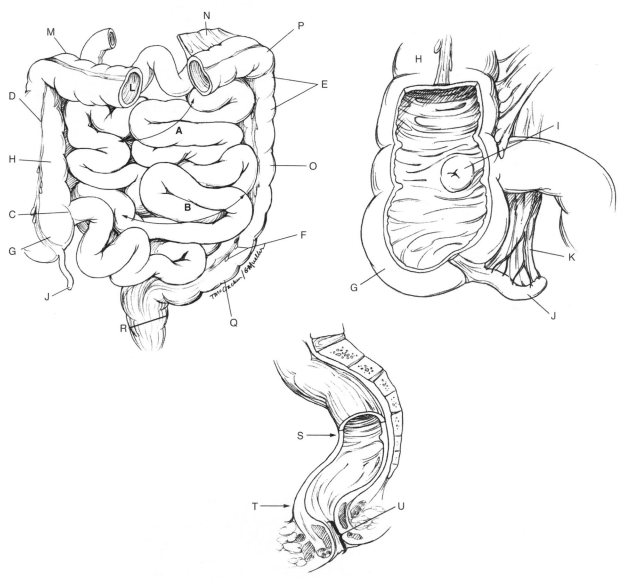

Anatomy of the small intestine and colon. (From Twietmeyer TA, McCracken T. Coloring Guide to Human Anatomy. 3rd Ed. New York: Lippincott Williams & Wilkins, 2001:179.)

8. Identify the parts of the liver and pancreas and their adjacent structures on this figure.

   a) Right lobe of liver
   b) Tail of pancreas
   c) Common bile duct
   d) Head of pancreas
   e) Body of pancreas
   f) Neck of pancreas
   g) Duodenum
   h) Ligamentum teres
   i) Left lobe of liver
   j) Diaphragm
   k) Pancreatic duct
   l) Gallbladder
   m) Common hepatic duct
   n) Falciform ligament
   o) Spleen
   p) Duodenal papilla

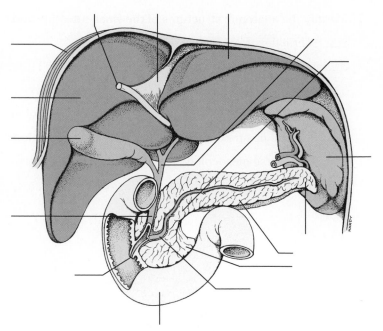

Liver, pancreas, and adjacent structures. (Modified from original by Neil O. Hardy, Westport, CT.)

INTEGRATE YOUR LEARNING

1. Label all of the anatomic structures on this figure. *(Make an effort to remember without looking at the other figures and spell the anatomic terms correctly.)*

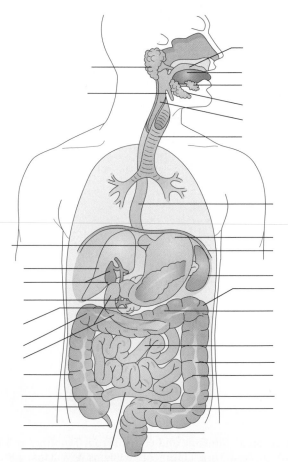

The gastrointestinal tract. (Modified from Smeltzer SC, Bare BG. Brunner & Suddarth's Textbook of Medical-Surgical Nursing. 9th Ed. Philadelphia: Lippincott Williams & Wilkins, 2000.)

2. Identify the organs and membranes shown on these sagittal sections of the abdominopelvic cavity using the following list. *(A sagittal section is a section separating the left and right portions of a three-dimensional object.)*

____ Lesser omentum	____ Rectum	____ Small intestine
____ Greater omentum	____ Transverse colon	____ Stomach
____ Pancreas	____ Duodenum	____ Abdominopelvic cavity
____ Liver	____ Peritoneum	____ Mesentery proper
____ Transverse mesentery	____ Diaphragm	____ Urinary bladder
____ Pelvic cavity	____ Abdominal cavity	____ Sigmoid mesocolon
____ Sigmoid colon		

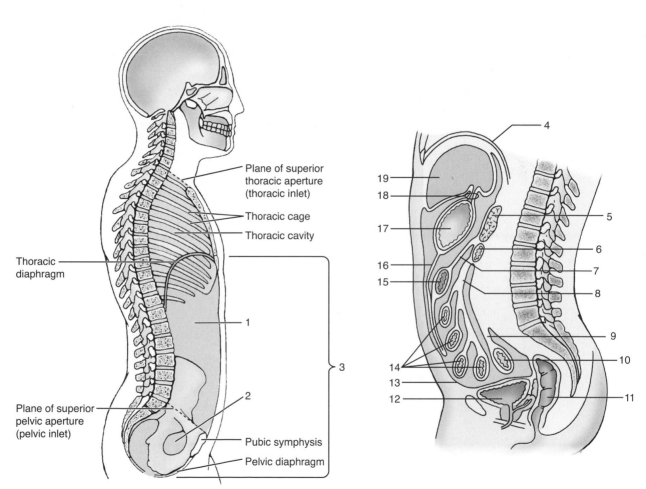

Sagittal sections of the abdominopelvic cavity. (From Moore KL, Dalley AF II. Clinical Oriented Anatomy. 4th Ed. Baltimore: Lippincott Williams & Wilkins, 1999.)

3. Clinicians often refer to the abdominopelvic quadrants to identify a specific area of the abdominal or pelvic regions, as these provide useful reference to the location of the underlying organs. Use the figure below to identify the four abdominopelvic quadrants and list the main underlying organs corresponding to each quadrant, especially those of the alimentary tract.

A Quadrant: _____

Organs: _____

_____

B Quadrant: _____

   Organs: _____

   _____

C Quadrant: _____

   Organs: _____

   _____

D Quadrant: _____

   Organs: _____

   _____

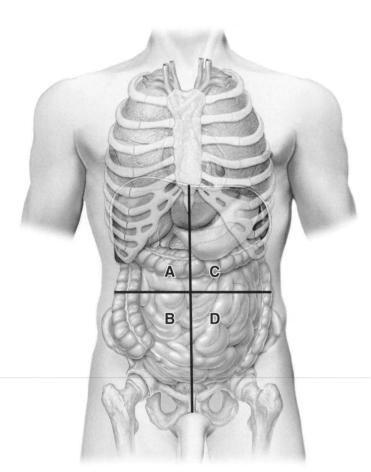

Abdominopelvic quadrants. (Modified from asset provided by Anatomical Chart Co.)

4. Fill in each blank space with the appropriate anatomy term.

   The stomach, small intestine, portions of colon, and some other organs are suspended within the

   a)_____ cavity by double sheets of b)_____, called c)_____. The latter give stability and support to the viscera, while allowing limited movement.

   The visceral d)_____ covering the outer surface of the stomach is continuous with two

   prominent e)_____, the greater and lesser f)_____.

The g)_____ is about 12 inches (30 cm) long and can be found in the retroperitoneal area. It curves around the head of the h)_____. The i)_____ is located inside the peritoneal cavity and arbitrarily starts at the ligament of Treitz. There is no change of histologic appearance at that point, but the first two-fifths of bowel beyond the ligament of Treitz forms the j)_____, while the distal three-fifths are the k)_____. The l)_____ has a larger diameter, more-prominent folds, and longer villi than the m)_____. The n)_____ bowel loops lie mostly in the left and middle upper abdomen. The proximal o)_____ is located in the middle abdominal area. The distal p)_____ is found in the right lower quadrant and joins the q)_____ at the r)_____ valve. The s)_____ and t)_____ are more mobile than the u)_____, but also attached to an extensive v)_____.

The w)_____ is about 39–59 inches (100–150 cm) in length and ends at the x)_____.

5. Identify the anatomic structures of the oral cavity and pharynx on this figure.

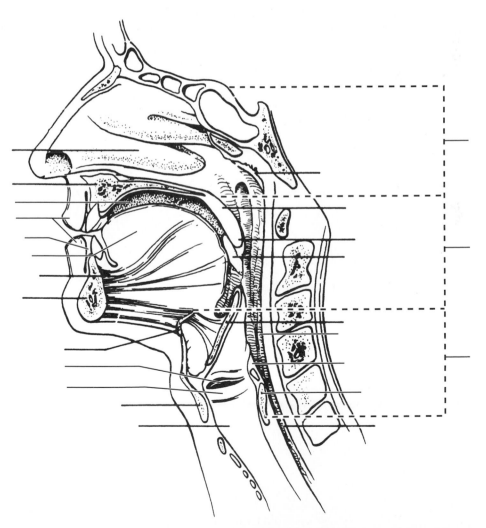

Anatomy of the oral cavity and pharynx. (From Harwood-Nuss A, Wolfson AB, et al. The Clinical Practice of Emergency Medicine. 3rd Ed. Philadelphia: Lippincott Williams & Wilkins, 2001.)

6. Identify the anatomic structures of the stomach and duodenum shown on these figures.

A = _____   M = _____

B = _____   N = _____

C = _____   O = _____

D = _____   P = _____

E = _____   Q = _____

F = _____   R = _____

G = _____   S = _____

H = _____   T = _____

I = _____   U = _____

J = _____   V = _____

K = _____   W = _____

L = _____   X = _____

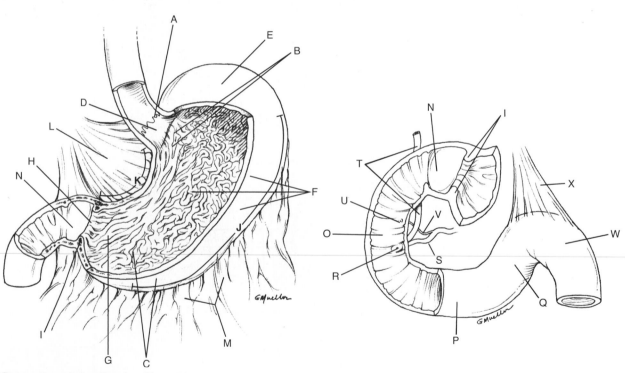

Stomach and duodenum. (From Twietmeyer TA, McCracken T. Coloring Guide to Human Anatomy. 3rd Ed. New York: Lippincott Williams & Wilkins, 2001:177.)

7. Identify the anatomic structures on this figure of the abdominal organs and vasculature.

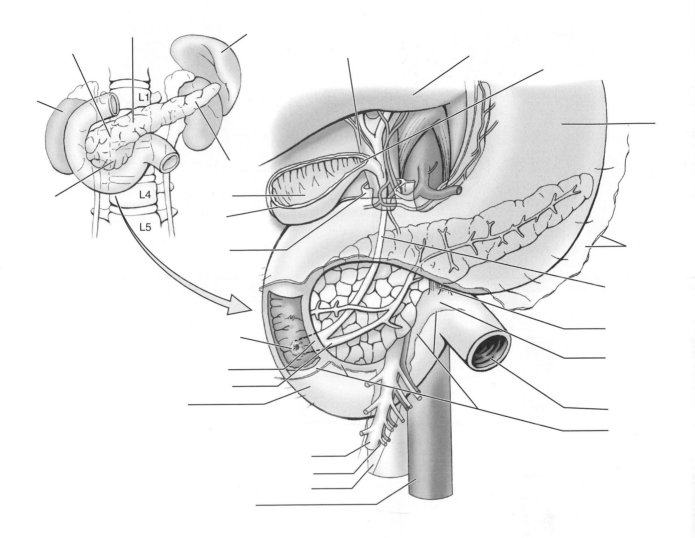

Abdominal organs and vasculature. (Modified from Moore KL, Dalley AF II. Clinical Oriented Anatomy. 4th Ed. Baltimore: Lippincott Williams & Wilkins, 1999.)

8. Identify the anatomic structures of the intestines and adjacent organs on this figure.

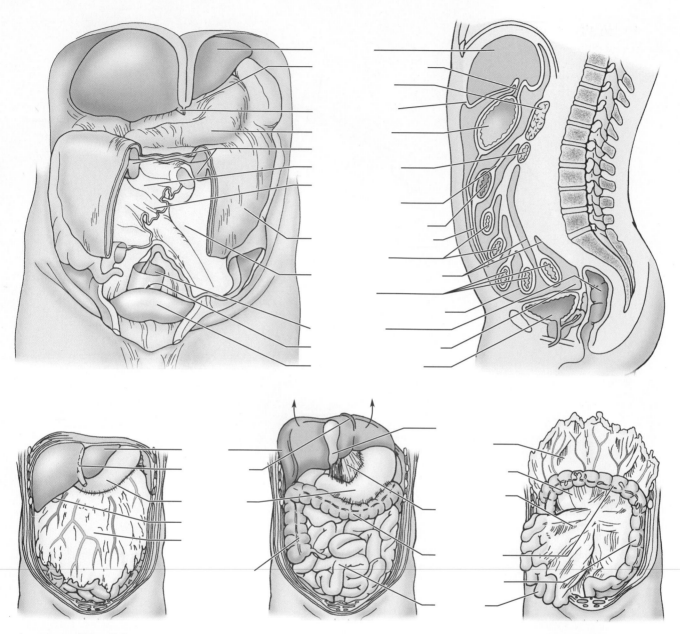

Anatomy of the abdominopelvic cavity and intestines. (Modified from Moore KL, Dalley AF II. Clinical Oriented Anatomy. 4th Ed. Baltimore: Lippincott Williams & Wilkins, 1999.)

CHALLENGE YOUR LEARNING

1. a) <u>Draw</u> a detailed diagram of the alimentary tract in the space below.
   b) <u>Identify</u> its different parts.
   c) Afterward, <u>color</u>
      - the organs forming the **tubular structure** of the alimentary tract in **red**,
      - the **accessory organs and glands** secreting digestive substances into the alimentary tract in **blue**, and
      - the **sphincters and valves** of the alimentary tract in **green**.

2. Challenge your knowledge of the anatomy of the stomach by identifying its different parts, muscular layers, mucosal lining, and glands on the following figures.

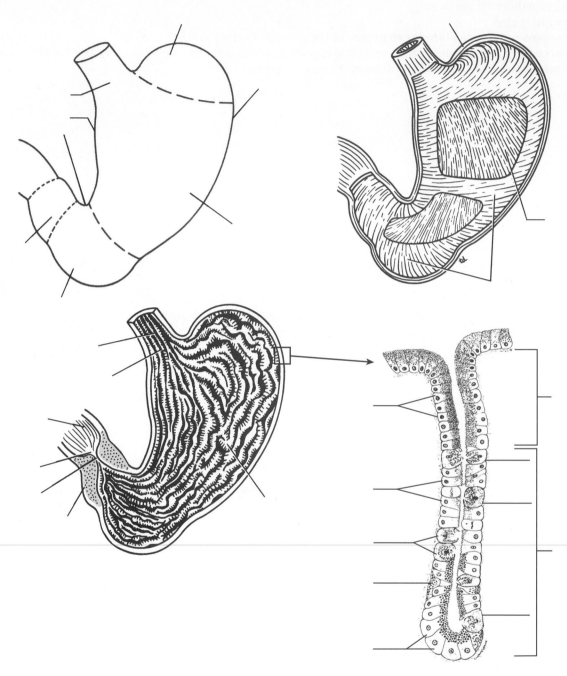

Stomach parts, muscular layers, mucosal lining, and glands. (From Snell, RS. Clinical Anatomy. 7th Ed. Baltimore: Lippincott Williams & Wilkins, 2004:235.)

3. Challenge your understanding of the anatomy of the small intestine by identifying its folds, villi, and microscopic structures on the following figures. *It is important to realize how much these components increase the surface area of the small intestine (600 times more than the surface area of a simple cylinder!).*

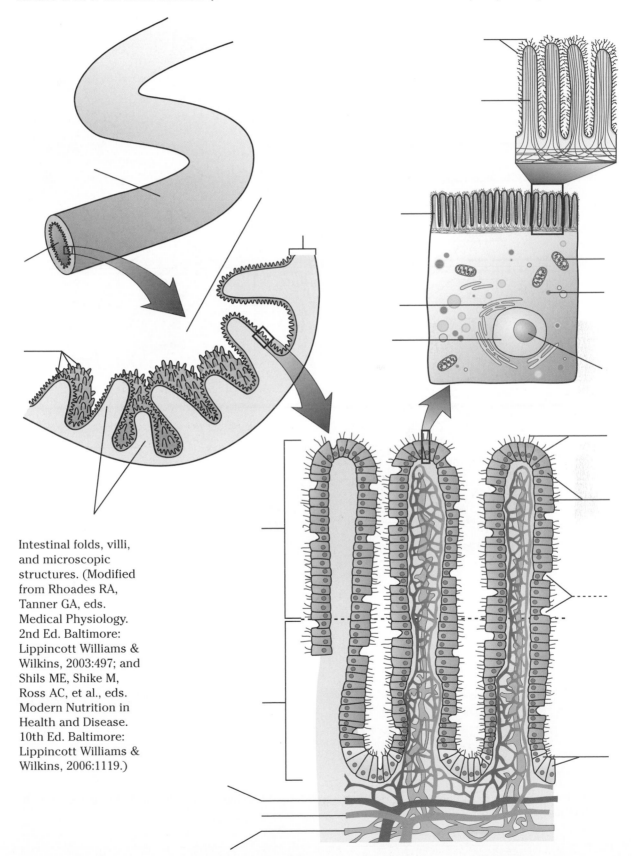

Intestinal folds, villi, and microscopic structures. (Modified from Rhoades RA, Tanner GA, eds. Medical Physiology. 2nd Ed. Baltimore: Lippincott Williams & Wilkins, 2003:497; and Shils ME, Shike M, Ross AC, et al., eds. Modern Nutrition in Health and Disease. 10th Ed. Baltimore: Lippincott Williams & Wilkins, 2006:1119.)

4. Challenge your knowledge of the anatomy of the biliary tree, duodenum, pancreas, and adjacent structures by completing these figures.

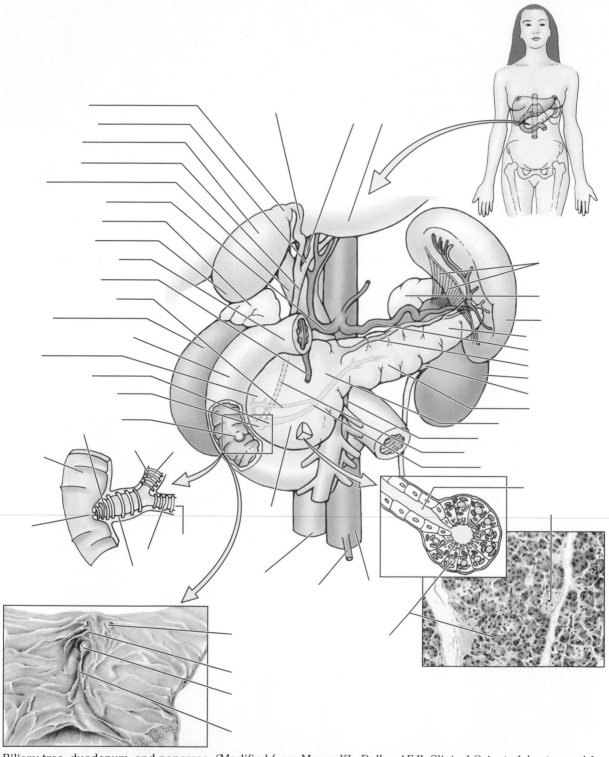

Biliary tree, duodenum. and pancreas. (Modified from Moore KL, Dalley AF II. Clinical Oriented Anatomy. 4th Ed. Baltimore: Lippincott Williams & Wilkins, 1999.)

2.2 Physiology of the Alimentary Tract

INTRODUCTION

Now that you can picture the anatomy of the alimentary tract (gastrointestinal tract), this section will help you understand what it does in action! You will discover the physiology of the alimentary tract in response to feeding. In other words, you will see how it processes the different foods you eat into their smallest components, the nutrient molecules, which can then be used by your body. You will see how the different organs and accessory glands of the alimentary tract work together as a coordinated team to fulfill two main functions: digest ingested food and absorb extracted nutrients.

REVIEW THE INFORMATION

1. Define digestion. _____
_____
_____

2. Where does the digestion of food begin? _____

3. Where does the majority of the digestion of food take place? _____

4. Explain what "motility" of the gastrointestinal tract means. _____
_____
_____

5. A masticated food morsel ready to be swallowed is called a _____

6. Fill in each blank space with an appropriate word.

    Secretion, in relation to the alimentary tract, is the process of production and *a)*_____ of

    physiologically active substances (including organic molecules, water, and *b)*_____) by

    *c)*_____ or *d)*_____, into the lumen of the alimentary tract in response to

    specific *e)*_____.

7. Define absorption in relation to the alimentary tract. _____
_____
_____

8. Distinguish between absorption by passive diffusion, facilitated diffusion, and active transport.
_____
_____
_____
_____
_____
_____

9. In what part of the alimentary tract does most of the absorption of nutrients occur?

   _____

10. How does the gastrointestinal tract absorb water?

    _____

11. Where is most of the water absorbed? _____

    _____

12. By what mechanism does the gastrointestinal tract absorb most nutrients?

    _____

13. How does the gastrointestinal tract absorb short-chain fatty acids? _____

    _____

14. What nutrient is required for the absorption of calcium by active transport in the small bowel?

    _____

15. What nutrient is required to transform ferric iron (Fe^{3+}) into ferrous iron (Fe^{2+}) in order to allow its

    absorption into the duodenum? _____

16. How does the gastrointestinal tract absorb glucose and fructose?

    _____

17. What is the term for the solution of partially digested food found in the stomach, which is later emptied

    into the intestinal lumen? _____

18. True or False.

    a) _____ The acidity of gastric juice is below a pH of 2, which is stronger than vinegar.

    b) _____ Pancreatic juice and bile both contain sodium bicarbonate and are alkaline.

    c) _____ Saliva contains a lot of sodium bicarbonate and is very alkaline.

19. To be absorbed by active transport, vitamin B_{12} must be bound to a protein known as

    a) gastric binding protein
    b) cobalamin complex
    c) pancreatic protease
    d) intestinal brush border binding protein
    e) intrinsic factor

20. a) What are hormones? _____

    _____

    b) What is the function of hormones? _____

    _____

21. Match the four mechanisms of communication used by regulatory substances (such as gastrointestinal hormones and regulatory peptides) to mediate responses in the gastrointestinal tract, with their illustration below.

    _____ Endocrine mechanism   _____ Neurocrine mechanism

    _____ Paracrine mechanism   _____ Autocrine mechanism

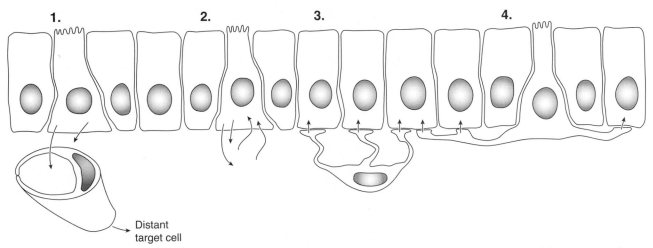

Mechanisms of communication to mediate responses. (Adapted from Yamada T, et al. Textbook of Gastroenterology. Baltimore: Lippincott Williams & Wilkins, 1999:37.)

UNDERSTAND THE CONCEPTS

1. What is the difference between mechanical, chemical, and enzymatic digestion? _____

_____

_____

_____

_____

2. You have learned in the previous section that digestion, motility, secretion, and absorption are four important processes carried out by the alimentary tract. Illustrate on this figure where these four processes take place along the alimentary tract using the following symbols:

Red "X"s	for **digestion** of food particles
Black arrows	for sections with **motility**
Blue circles	for **secretion** of digestive juices and mucus
Green diamonds	for sites of nutrient **absorption**

3. What is peristalsis? _____

_____

4. Match the parts of the alimentary tract with the corresponding type(s) of motility happening in that part of the tract.

_____ Mouth   _____ Stomach

_____ Oral cavity and pharynx _____ Small bowel

_____ Esophagus   _____ Large bowel

A) Deglutition
B) Peristalsis
C) Receptive relaxation (allowing to fill the organ)
D) Rhythmic segmentation (to allow mixing)
E) Mastication
F) Tonic contraction (to allow mixing and churning)
G) Mass movement (allowing to fill sigmoid colon)
H) Haustral churning (to allow mixing)

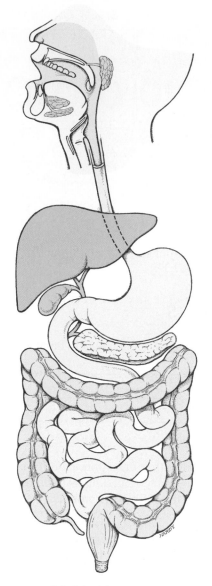

Physiology of the alimentary tract. (Modified from original by Neil O. Hardy, Westport, CT.)

I) Pendular movements (to allow mixing)
J) Defecation
K) Hunger contractions

5. Fill in the blank spaces using words from the list provided.

vagus nerve	autonomic nervous system	sensory
liver	pancreas	proximal intestine
afferents	pyloric sphincter	motor
central nervous system	sympathetic	parasympathetic

The nervous system of the gastrointestinal tract is linked to the *a)*_____ by

transmission along nerve cells (axons) in both directions, from the gastrointestinal tract to the brain and

vice versa.

The nervous connections between the gastrointestinal tract and the brain are largely due to the

*b)*_____ (or 10th cranial nerve) and to nervous pathways leaving the spinal cord. Most fibers of the vagus nerve are *c)*_____ and travel from the viscera to the spinal cord. The vagus nerve and spinal cord components comprise branches of both parts of the *d)*_____, the parasympathetic system and sympathetic system.

The activity of the *e)*_____ system increases heart rate, inhibits gastrointestinal peristalsis, and closes gastrointestinal sphincters. In contrast, the activity of the *f)*_____ system slows heart rate, increases gastrointestinal peristalsis and glandular activity, and opens gastrointestinal sphincters.

The vagus nerve supplies *g)*_____ fibers to the ear, tongue, pharynx, and larynx. It provides *h)*_____ fibers to the pharynx, larynx, and esophagus. It also provides parasympathetic and visceral afferent fibers to thoracic and abdominal viscera.

The left vagus nerve enters the abdomen on the anterior surface of the esophagus, and divides into branches that supply the anterior stomach, the *i)*_____, and the *j)*_____. The right vagus nerve enters the abdomen on the posterior surface of the esophagus, and divides into branches that supply the posterior stomach, the *k)*_____ and the *l)*_____.

6. a) Locate on this figure of the anatomy of the head and neck the food bolus, as well as the following structures:

   tongue   uvula   epiglottis   esophagus
   pharynx   larynx   soft palate   vocal cord

   interarytenoid and cricopharyngeal muscles forming the upper esophageal sphincter

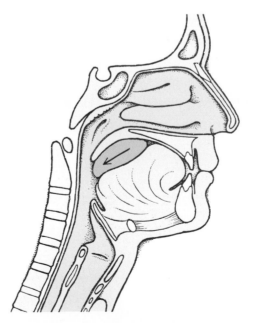

Head and neck. (From Dirckx JH, ed. Stedman's Concise Medical Dictionary for the Health Professions. Illustrated 5th Ed. New York: Lippincott Williams & Wilkins, 2005:960.)

   b) Use arrows on the previous figure to describe what happens when food is swallowed.
   c) Put in chronologic order the different steps occurring during a swallow.

   A. The larynx raises and closes the area around and between the vocal cords, keeping the bolus from entering the trachea. _____

B. Food pieces are masticated and a bolus of food particles and fluid is formed. _____

C. The upper esophageal sphincter relaxes and opens, so that the bolus can enter the esophagus. _____

D. Pressure receptors on the pharynx are stimulated by the bolus, which is then forced by the tongue into the back of the mouth, which triggers a swallow. _____

E. The tongue pushes the bolus further back into the pharynx, and the bolus tilts the epiglottis down to cover the entrance of the larynx. _____

F. A peristaltic wave carries the bolus through the esophagus toward the stomach. _____

G. As the bolus moves into the pharynx, the uvula goes up and lodges against the back wall of the pharynx, preventing food and fluid from entering the nasal cavity. _____

7. Explain the difference between exocrine and endocrine glands. _____
_____
_____
_____

8. Why does the alimentary tract secrete mucus? _____
_____
_____

9. Intestinal bacteria have important metabolic and nutritional functions, including the production of

a) biotin and vitamin K_2 c) folate and vitamin B_{12}
b) biotin and folate   d) vitamin K_2 and vitamin B_{12}

10. Name the exocrine secretions of the following organs and glands of the alimentary tract. Then, indicate the composition of these exocrine secretions.

EXOCRINE SECRETIONS OF THE ALIMENTARY TRACT		
Organs and Glands	Exocrine Secretions	Composition
Salivary glands		
Esophagus (mucosal and submucosal glands)		
Gastric glands		
Pancreas		
Liver		
Intestinal glands of duodenum		
Intestinal glands of jejunum and ileum		
Large intestine		

11. What type(s) of enzymes are involved in the digestion of proteins? _____

_____

12. What type(s) of enzymes are involved in the digestion of carbohydrates? _____

_____

13. What type(s) of enzymes are involved in the digestion of lipids? _____

_____

14. What are micelles? _____

_____

15. What is the role of bile salts? _____

_____

16. What is the enterohepatic circulation of bile salts? _____

_____

17. What is another name for salivary amylase? _____

18. What does "colonic salvage" mean? _____

_____

_____

_____

19. Fill in the blank spaces.

Adults ingest on average about 1.8 lb (0.8 kg) of food and 1.3 quarts (41 fluid oz, or 1.2 liters) of water as part of their diet each day. The exocrine secretions of the salivary glands (about

a)_____ quarts or _____ liters), b)_____ (about 0.5 quart or 0.5 liter), c)_____ (about 2.1 quarts or 2.0 liters),

d)_____ (about 1.6 quarts or 1.5 liters), and e)_____ (about 1.6 quarts or 1.5 liters) altogether represent an extra 7.4 quarts (7 liters) of fluid secreted into the alimentary tract per day. The f)_____ are very efficient at absorbing about

g)_____% of the total 8.7 quarts (2.2 gallons or 8.2 liters) of fluid entering the alimentary tract daily. Usually, only about 3.3 fluid oz (100 mL) per day are lost in

h)_____.

20. Associate the types of stomach cells with the following secretions.

_____ Surface cells   _____ Chief cells   _____ Parietal cells

A) Hydrochloric acid   B) Mucus   C) Pepsinogen   D) Gastric lipase   E) Intrinsic factor

21. Explain how the exocrine secretions of the stomach fundus, body, and antrum are different.

_____

_____

_____

22. How and where is the enzyme precursor pepsinogen activated in the enzyme pepsin?

_____

_____

_____

23. Describe the digestion process of dietary proteins by choosing the proper digestive secretion corresponding to the letters **A**, **B**, **C**, **D**, **E**, and **F**.

_____ **Carboxypeptidases** (enzymes secreted by the pancreas)

_____ **Aminopeptidase and tetrapeptidase** (enzymes secreted by brush border cells of the small intestine)

_____ **Hydrochloric acid** produced by stomach

_____ **Trypsin and chymotrypsin** (enzymes secreted by the pancreas)

_____ **Tripeptidase and dipeptidase** (enzymes secreted by brush border cells of the small intestine)

_____ Pepsinogen secreted by stomach, activated in the enzyme **pepsin** by hydrochloric acid in the stomach

Dietary proteins
↓
A
↓
Proteins of denatured structure (uncoiled)
↓
B
↓
Polypeptides
↓
C
↓
Peptides
↓
D
↓
Peptides minus terminal amino acid
↓
E
↓
Small peptides (dipeptides and tripeptides)
↓
F
↓
Amino acids

24. Describe the digestion process of long-chain triglycerides by choosing the proper digestive secretion corresponding to the letters **A**, **B**, **C**, and **D**.

_____ **Bile salts** (secreted in bile by the liver)

_____ **Intestinal lipase** (secreted by brush border intestinal cells)

_____ **Sublingual and gastric lipases**

_____ **Pancreatic lipase and colipase**

Dietary long-chain triglycerides
↓
A
↓
Diglycerides and triglycerides
↓
B
↓
Emulsified triglycerides and diglycerides
↓
C
↓
Micelles of monoglycerides and free fatty acids
↓
D
↓
Glycerol and free fatty acids

25. Describe the digestion process of complex carbohydrates by choosing the proper digestive secretion corresponding to the letters **A**, **B**, **C**, **D**, and **E**.

_____ Intestinal brush border **maltase**

_____ **Salivary amylase**

_____ Intestinal brush border **dextrinase**

_____ **Pancreatic amylase**

_____ Intestinal brush border **isomaltase**

Complex carbohydrates (starches such as amylose and amylopectin)
↓
A
↓
Dextrins and maltose
↓
A
↓
Small dextrin molecules and maltose
↓
B
↓
Very small dextrin molecules and maltose
↓
B
↓

Maltotriose   Isomaltose   Maltose
↓   ↓   ↓
C   **D**   **E**
↓   ↓   ↓
Glucose   Glucose   Glucose

26. The free fatty acids and glycerol entering the intestinal epithelial cells are resynthesized into triglycerides and incorporated into lipoproteins called _____ These lipoproteins pass into the lymphatic system and eventually enter the bloodstream to allow for distribution of triglycerides to the cells of the body.

a) very-low-density lipoproteins   c) micelles   e) high-density lipoproteins
b) low-density lipoproteins   d) chylomicrons

27. Food particles travel through the alimentary tract and stimulate or inhibit the different digestive secretions by way of regulatory substances, which are transported from one section of the alimentary tract to another by hormonal and nerve pathways. These regulatory substances or messengers are secreted by the mucosa of the alimentary tract and coordinate the response of the alimentary tract to an ingested meal.

List five of these gastrointestinal regulatory substances.

1) _____   4) _____

2) _____   5) _____

3) _____

28. Identify the three phases of stimulation of gastric hydrochloric acid secretion after ingestion of food, according to the location of the stimuli initiating the reflex.

THREE PHASES OF GASTRIC ACID SECRETION	
Phases of Gastric Acid Secretion	Stimuli
1.	Thought of food Smell, taste, chewing, swallowing of food
2.	Stomach distension Digested peptides
3.	Protein digestion products in duodenum Distension

INTEGRATE YOUR LEARNING

1. Indicate on the following summary table the digestive secretions produced by the organs of the alimentary tract, their composition, and the role of each of their digestive enzymes.

DIGESTIVE SECRETIONS PRODUCED BY THE ALIMENTARY TRACT			
Organs and Glands	Digestive Secretions	Composition of Secretion	Role of Digestive Enzymes
Salivary glands			
Stomach			
Pancreas			
Liver			
Intestine			

2. Indicate which nutrients are mostly absorbed at the sites indicated by the letters on the following diagram of the alimentary tract.

A. _____

B. _____

C. _____

D. _____

E. _____

F. _____

G. _____

H. _____

I. _____

J. _____

K. _____

L. _____

M. _____

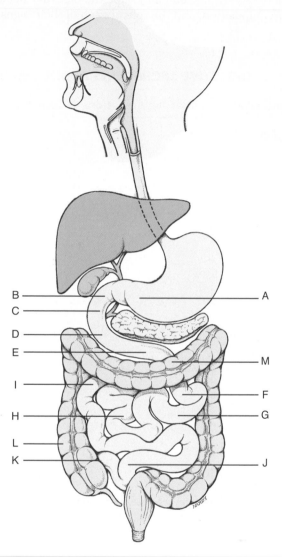

The alimentary tract and the sites of nutrient absorption. (Modified from original by Neil O. Hardy, Westport, CT.)

3. List four determinants of the capacity of fluid absorption in the intestine.

1) _____

2) _____

3) _____

4) _____

4. During what phase of the swallow does the tongue propel the bolus posteriorly?

a) Oral preparatory phase   c) Oral phase   e) Laryngeal phase
b) Esophageal phase   d) Pharyngeal phase

5. What substances are present in saliva?

    a) Bicarbonate, mucus, lipase, and alkaline phosphatase
    b) Sucrase, lipase, mucin, amylase, and water
    c) Water, lipase, mucin, amylase, and electrolytes
    d) Mucus, disaccharidases, and electrolytes
    e) Water, electrolytes, bicarbonate, mucin, and amylase

6. Which substances does the pancreas secrete into the duodenum?

    a) Enterokinase, alkaline phosphatase, lipase, insulin, and water
    b) Mucin, alkaline phosphatase, amylase, and trypsin
    c) Bicarbonate, pepsinogen, disaccharidases, lipase, amylase, and water
    d) Water, mucin, intrinsic factor, amylase, and lipase
    e) Bicarbonate, water, lipase, colipase, amylase, and trypsin

7. Which statement about the digestion of proteins is true?

    a) Most of the small peptides and amino acids are absorbed in the jejunum and ileum.
    b) Hepatic carboxypeptidases are secreted for the digestion of peptides.
    c) Trypsin, pepsin, and dipeptidases are secreted by the pancreas.
    d) Intestinal brush border dipeptidase and tripeptidase digest small peptides into amino acids.
    e) In the stomach, the enzyme pepsinogen digests proteins in polypeptides.

8. Which components are absorbed in the terminal ileum?

    a) Vitamin B_2, cholesterol, and short-chain fatty acids
    b) Vitamin B_{12}, vitamin K_2, and bile salts
    c) Soluble fibers, fatty acids, and vitamins A, D, and E
    d) Vitamin B_6, cholesterol, and bile acids
    e) Fatty acids, cholesterol, and liposoluble vitamins

9. Which statement is true about the digestion of a glass of milk and the absorption of the nutrients it contains?

    a) The digestion of lactose starts in the mouth, and then requires the action of pancreatic amylases.
    b) Calcium requires vitamin C for its absorption by passive diffusion across the jejunum.
    c) Triglycerides are hydrolyzed by gastric, pancreatic, and intestinal lipases.
    d) Riboflavin and vitamin D are absorbed by passive diffusion in the duodenum and jejunum.
    e) Cholesterol is hydrolyzed by bile salts and incorporated into micelles with fatty acids.

10. Which statement related to bowel physiology is **false**?

    a) Most of the fluid that passes through the intestine daily is absorbed, except about 3.3 fluid oz (100 mL).
    b) The maximum daily absorptive capacity of the small intestine is 12.7 quarts (12.0 liters) and that of the colon is 5.3 quarts (5.0 liters).
    c) Bacteria in the colon metabolize carbohydrate and insoluble fibers to short-chain fatty acids and gas.
    d) Of the 8.7 quarts (8.5 liters) of fluid that enters the intestine daily, usually about 2.1 quarts (2.0 liters) is derived from oral intake and the remaining amount is derived from endogenous secretions.
    e) Passive permeability in the jejunum is high, which allows rapid adjustment of the luminal osmolality in response to a meal.

11. The regulatory peptides listed on the next page are critical to accurately coordinate the numerous minute actions required for the alimentary tract to adequately handle and process ingested foods. These regulatory peptides are released by the gastrointestinal tract mucosa in response to stimuli such as the presence of protein, carbohydrate, or fat (releasers) in the gastrointestinal tract. They communicate through endocrine, neurocrine, or paracrine pathways to mediate stimulatory and/or inhibitory effects.

Use this list to complete the following table on the function of gastrointestinal regulatory peptides and hormones.

_____ Peptide YY   _____ Glucose-dependent insulinotropic peptide (GIP)

_____ Bombesin   _____ Pancreatic polypeptide

_____ Secretin   _____ Cholecystokinin (CCK)

_____ Motilin   _____ Vasoactive intestinal polypeptide (VIP)

_____ Enkephalins   _____ Gastrin

_____ Somatostatin

FUNCTION OF GASTROINTESTINAL REGULATORY PEPTIDES AND HORMONES

Regulatory Peptide	Effect	Site of Release	Releasers (or Stimulants of Release)
• ENDOCRINE			
A.	↑ gastric acid secretion	Antrum of stomach	Peptides, amino acids, distension of stomach antrum, vagal nerve
B.	↑ gallbladder contraction ↑ pancreatic enzymes and bicarbonate ↓ gastric emptying	Duodenum Jejunum	Peptides, amino acids, fatty acids
C.	↑ pancreatic and biliary bicarbonate secretion ↑ gastric pepsinogen secretion ↓ gastric acid secretion	Duodenum	Gut acidity
D.	↑ insulin release by pancreas ↓ gastric acid secretion	Duodenum Jejunum	Glucose, amino acids, fatty acids
E.	Ileal brake	Ileum	Fatty acids, glucose
F.	Stimulates gastric and duodenal motility	Duodenum Jejunum	Alkalinity in duodenum
G.	↓ pancreatic bicarbonate and enzyme secretion	Pancreas	Protein
• NEUROCRINES			
H.	Relaxes sphincters and gut circular muscles ↑ intestinal and pancreatic secretions	Mucosa and smooth muscles of gastro-intestinal tract	Stimulation of mucosal neural receptors due to the presence of food
I.	↑ gastrin release	Gastric mucosa	Stimulation of mucosal neural receptors due to the presence of food

(continued)

FUNCTION OF GASTROINTESTINAL REGULATORY PEPTIDES AND HORMONES *(continued)*

Regulatory Peptide	Effect	Site of Release	Releasers (or Stimulants of Release)
J.	↑ smooth muscle contraction ↓ intestinal secretion	Mucosa and smooth muscles of gastro-intestinal tract	Stimulation of mucosal neural receptors due to the presence of food
• *PARACRINES*			
K.	↓ gastrin release, gastric acid secretion, and pancreatic enzyme and hormone release	Gastrointestinal mucosa Pancreatic islets	Gut acidity (vagal nerve inhibits release)

Adapted from Klein S, Cohn SM, Alpers DH. Alimentary tract in nutrition. In: Shils ME, Shike M, Ross AC, et al., eds. Modern Nutrition in Health and Disease. 10th Ed. Baltimore: Lippincott Williams & Wilkins, 2006:1123(Table 70.1).

CHALLENGE YOUR LEARNING

1. Identify the gastric exocrine secretions and their main function in digestion.

GASTRIC EXOCRINE SECRETIONS		
Gastric Cell Type	**Exocrine Secretion(s) Produced**	**Function of the Product(s) Secreted**
	a_1)	a_2)
	b_1)	b_2)
	c_1)	c_2)
	d_1)	d_2)
	e_1)	e_2)

2. Which statement about the physiology of gastrointestinal regulatory peptides is true?

a) Vasoactive intestinal polypeptide relaxes sphincters and gut circular muscle.
b) Gastrin is released in the cardia and fundus of the stomach and increases gastric acid secretion.
c) Secretin is released in the jejunum and increases gastric acid secretion.
d) Cholecystokinin decreases gallbladder contraction and pancreatic enzyme secretion.
e) Motilin is released by the stomach and stimulates the motility of the jejunum.

3. Which one of these gastrointestinal substances is a neurocrine peptide?

a) Vasoactive intestinal polypeptide
b) Motilin
c) Secretin
d) Pancreatic polypeptide
e) Cholecystokinin

4. The ileal brake slows the bowel transit due to the release of _____ from the ileal mucosa.

5. Complete the following diagrams integrating your knowledge of the physiology of digestion and the absorption of macronutrients, including digestive enzymes and substances, mechanism of absorption, and absorption sites.

Digestion process

digestive enzyme(s)
and substances   *mechanism(s) of absorption*
eg, Nutrient ————————→ nutrient particles ————————————————→ absorption site(s)

DIGESTION AND ABSORPTION OF MACRONUTRIENTS

Nutrient	Digestion Process	Absorption Site
• **PROTEINS** ————	————————→ Denatured proteins	
	————————→ Polypeptides	
	————————→ Peptides	
	————————→ Peptides minus terminal amino acid	
	————————→ Small peptides (di- + tripeptides)	————→
	————————→ Amino acids	————→
• **CARBOHYDRATES** **Starches** (amylose amylopectin) ————	————————→ Dextrins and maltose	
	————————→ Small dextrins and maltose	
	————————→ Maltotriose Isomaltose Maltose	
	————————→ Glucose	————→
Sucrose ————	————————→ Glucose and fructose	————→
Lactose ————	————————→ Glucose and galactose	————→
• **TRIGLYCERIDES (TG):**		
Long-chain TG ————	————————→ Diglycerides and triglycerides	
	————————→ Emulsified diglycerides and triglycerides	
	————————→ Micelles of monoglycerides and free fatty acids	————→
	————————→ Glycerol and free fatty acids	————→
Short- or medium-chain TG (6–12 carbons) ————	————————→ Hydrosoluble hydrolyzed TG	————→

6. Complete the following diagrams integrating your knowledge of the physiology of digestion and the absorption of micronutrients and water, as well as the reabsorption of bile salts.

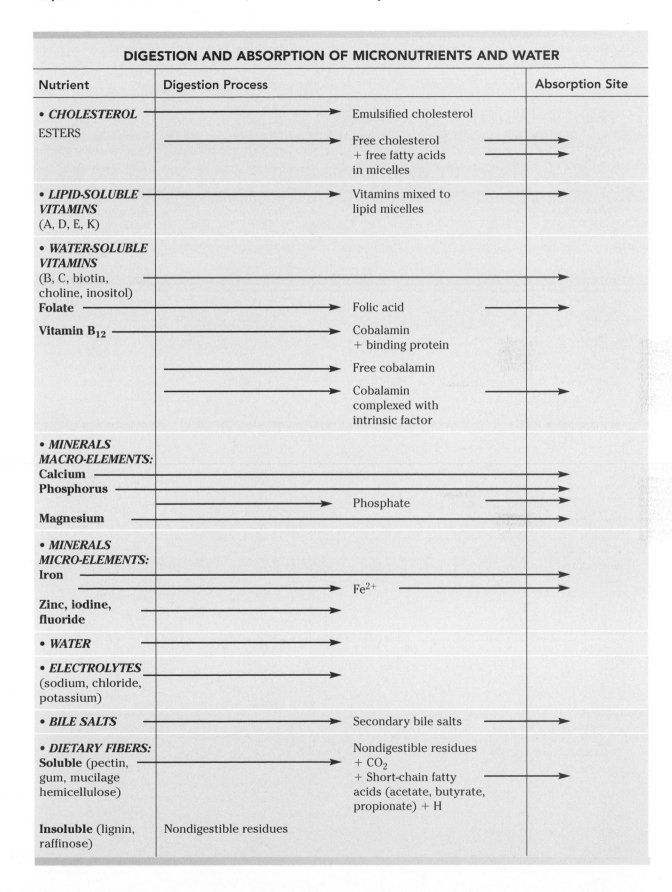

DIGESTION AND ABSORPTION OF MICRONUTRIENTS AND WATER		
Nutrient	**Digestion Process**	**Absorption Site**
• *CHOLESTEROL* ESTERS	Emulsified cholesterol	
	Free cholesterol + free fatty acids in micelles	
• *LIPID-SOLUBLE VITAMINS* (A, D, E, K)	Vitamins mixed to lipid micelles	
• *WATER-SOLUBLE VITAMINS* (B, C, biotin, choline, inositol)		
Folate	Folic acid	
Vitamin B$_{12}$	Cobalamin + binding protein	
	Free cobalamin	
	Cobalamin complexed with intrinsic factor	
• *MINERALS MACRO-ELEMENTS:* **Calcium**		
Phosphorus	Phosphate	
Magnesium		
• *MINERALS MICRO-ELEMENTS:* **Iron**	Fe^{2+}	
Zinc, iodine, fluoride		
• *WATER*		
• *ELECTROLYTES* (sodium, chloride, potassium)		
• *BILE SALTS*	Secondary bile salts	
• *DIETARY FIBERS:* **Soluble** (pectin, gum, mucilage hemicellulose)	Nondigestible residues + CO_2 + Short-chain fatty acids (acetate, butyrate, propionate) + H	
Insoluble (lignin, raffinose)	Nondigestible residues	

7. The meaning of most medical terms can be determined from their etymology (or language origin). Medical scientists borrowed words or elements from the Latin and Greek languages to describe physical features, conditions, and discoveries. Therefore, knowing elements of these languages will help you understand the language of medicine and remember the meaning of medical terms.

a) Complete this table by giving the English meaning corresponding to the Latin and/or Greek elements listed. To make it easier, look at some examples of words derived from the Latin and/or Greek elements, which are formed using the "combining forms" (prefixes or suffixes) of these elements.

MEANING OF MEDICAL TERMS FROM LATIN AND/OR GREEK ETYMOLOGY

Latin and/or Greek Elements	English Meaning	Combining Forms	Examples of Medical Terms
1. **anterior**		anter-	anterior anteroinferior anterolateral
2. **bilis**		bili-	bilious biliary biligenic bilirubin
3. **cholē**		chol(e)-	cholecyst cholecystic cholangiogram cholic choledochal
4. **derma, dermatos**		derm(at)- or -derma	dermatologist dermatology epiderm dermatitis dermatotherapy
5. **dochos**		-doch-	ductus choledochus (or common bile duct) choledochal
6. **enteron**		enter-	enteric mesentery mesenteric enterology enterosepsis
7. **gastēr, gastros**		gastr-	gastric gastrology gastrectomy gastroenterology epigastrium gastroscope
8. **hēpar, hēpatos**		hepar- or hepat-	hepatic heparin hepatocyte hepatitis hepatology hepatomegaly

(continued)

MEANING OF MEDICAL TERMS FROM LATIN AND/OR GREEK ETYMOLOGY *(continued)*

Latin and/or Greek Elements	English Meaning	Combining Forms	Examples of Medical Terms
9. **kardia**		cardi-	cardia cardiac cardiospasm cardiovascular
10. **kolon**		col- or colon-	colitis colonoscope mesocolon colonic coloscopy colostomy
11. **kystis**		-cyst(i)- or -cystis	cholecyst cholecystic cystic duct cystography
12. **latus, lateris**		later-	lateral latus lateroabdominal
13. **mesos**		mes-	mesentery mesoderm mesoappendix mesocolon mesocephalic
14. **ptyalon**		ptyal-	ptyalin ptyalism ptyalolithiasis
15. **stoma, stomatos**		stom- or stomat-	stoma stomy stomatitis
16. **vās, vasis**		vas-	vascular vasculature vasoactive vas deferens vasoparesis
17. **viscus, visceris** (plural, viscera)		viscer-or viscus-	viscera visceral viscus visceromegaly

b) Fill in this table by providing examples of words formed using the Latin and/or Greek prefixes listed.

	EXAMPLES OF MEDICAL TERMS FORMED USING A LATIN OR GREEK PREFIX	
Latin and/or Greek Prefixes	English Meaning	Examples of Medical Terms
1. **dis-** or **di-** (before v or g) or **dif-** (before f)	apart, away	
2. **epi-** or **ep-** (before a, e, o, u, or h)	upon, on, over, above	
3. **exo-**	outside, toward the outside, from the outside	
4. **peri-**	surrounding, around	
5. **retro-**	behind, in back, backward	
6. **sub-**	under	

c) Fill in this table by providing examples of words formed using the Latin and/or Greek suffixes listed.

	EXAMPLES OF MEDICAL TERMS FORMED USING A LATIN OR GREEK SUFFIX		
Latin and/or Greek Suffixes	English Meaning	Forming Adjectives or Nouns	Examples of Medical Terms
1. **–ar(y)**	pertaining to or located in	adjectives	
2. **–ase**	enzymes	nouns	
3. **-ic**	located in or pertaining to	adjectives	
4. **–ium or -um**	membranes and connective tissue, or region of the body	nouns	
5. **-ous**	full of, characterized by, or pertaining to	adjectives	

PART 3

Nutrition Throughout the Human Life Cycle

INTRODUCTION

This section focuses on **maternal** nutrition, **infancy** and **childhood** nutrition, and nutrition during **adolescence**, during **adulthood**, and in **aging**. For each stage of the life cycle, we will provide an overview of related terminology, growth and development, energy and nutrient needs, and nutrition-related topics and concerns. We will also examine some determinants of health and lifestyle choices, as well as community nutrition programs and resources. This part will focus mostly on **normalcy and health across the lifespan**, and briefly touch on nutrition assessment (which will be detailed in Part 5, Nutrition Care Process) and on disease prevention and management (which will be the topic of Part 7, Prevention and Management of Disease).

In order to assist various individuals, health care providers must understand the physiologic, psychological, social, and nutritional needs associated with each stage of the life cycle. They must also adapt their language and intervention to the needs of that particular individual.

3.1 Maternal Nutrition

REVIEW THE INFORMATION

Childbearing Years and Preconception Period

1. Listed below are some principles of meal planning, which promote good health. Match each meal planning principle with its definition.
   Adequacy   Balance   Energy control   Moderation   Variety   Nutrient density

   a) _____: To get from foods all nutrients in sufficient amounts

   b) _____: To eat a wide selection of different foods from each food group

   c) _____: To select foods that deliver abundant nutrients relative to their energy content

   d) _____: To provide foods without excess, and to follow recommended serving sizes and number of servings

   e) _____: To ensure that all food groups are represented and in the recommended proportions

   f) _____: To manage energy intake to approximately meet the body's requirements

2. What are dietary guidelines?

_____

_____

_____

_____

3. List the national dietary guidelines (2005 Dietary Guidelines for Americans <u>or</u> Canada's Guidelines for Healthy Eating).

_____

_____

_____

_____

_____

_____

4. Give the exact name of each food group in your national food guide (MyPyramid <u>or</u> Canada's Food Guide) <u>and</u> state the servings recommended daily from each group for an active pregnant woman requiring 2800 kcal (11,700 kJ)/day.

Food Group	**Daily Servings Recommended**

5. Identify the food group(s) to which each of the following foods belong.

a) Pasta: _____

b) Egg: _____

c) Ice cream: _____

d) Butter: _____

e) Oatmeal and chocolate chip cookies: _____

f) Peanut butter: _____

g) Baked beans: _____

h) Pure orange juice: _____

i) Corn on the cob: _____

j) Popcorn (air popped, unflavored): _____

k) Chocolate milk: _____

l) Plain potato chips: _____

m) French fries: _____

6. What is the size of a serving for the following foods?

   a) Milk: _____

   b) Cooked rice: _____

   c) Garden salad: _____

   d) Egg: _____

   e) Soft margarine: _____

7. What is the preconception period?

   _____

8. Some factors influencing the outcome of pregnancy cannot be changed, such as genetic factors, but others can be changed. What can mothers do to increase their chances of having a healthy pregnancy?

   _____

   _____

   _____

   _____

   _____

9. Put in chronologic order, from first (number 1) to last (number 8), the events that occur during the follicular and luteal phases of the menstrual cycle:

   a) _____: The gonadotropin-releasing hormone causes the pituitary gland to secrete some follicle-stimulating hormone and luteinizing hormone (follicular phase).

   b) _____: The rising levels of the luteinizing hormone stimulate the secretion of progesterone by the follicles (follicular phase).

   c) _____: Estrogen causes the hypothalamus to release some gonadotropin-releasing hormone (follicular phase).

   d) _____: If fertilized, the ovum signals the corpus luteum to increase its secretions, but if the ovum is not fertilized, the corpus luteum ceases its secretions and menstruation starts (luteal phase).

   e) _____: The follicle-stimulating hormone stimulates the growth of follicles on the surface of the ovary. It also increases estrogen production by the follicles and the growth of follicles (follicular phase).

   f) _____: After ovulation, the remaining follicle becomes a corpus luteum. The latter secretes progesterone and estrogen, which reduces the production of gonadotropin-releasing hormone and further stimulates the development of the endometrium (luteal phase).

   g) _____: Estrogen and progesterone stimulate the preparation of the uterine wall or endometrium (follicular phase).

   h) _____: The blood concentrations of follicle-stimulating hormone and luteinizing hormone peak and the elevation in luteinizing hormone causes the release of an ovum or ovulation (follicular phase).

10. Which women are at higher risk of having an unhealthy pregnancy? List these women.

    _____

    _____

    _____

    _____

    _____

    _____

11. When should women start adopting healthy lifestyle and eating habits to support a healthy pregnancy?

_____

_____

12. Compared to women with healthy body weights, fertility is decreased in women who are

   a) underweight   c) obese   e) a, b, and c
   b) overweight   d) b and c

13. Fill in the blank spaces with one or a few words.

   1. The health of the mother before conception influences a) _____, b) _____,
   and c) _____.

   2. Women of childbearing age are usually considered to be women between the ages of _____
   years old.

   3. a) _____ is a risk factor for low-birth-weight infants. Low birth weight is a determining factor in b) _____ of newborn deaths, and survivors have greater risk of
   serious and lifelong c) _____.

Pregnancy and Birth

14. Are the following statements TRUE or FALSE? Please explain why.

   a) _____: Healthy pregnant women can continue to be active and to participate in physical
   activity.

      Explanation: _____

      _____

   b) _____: A woman's decision to be physically active or not during pregnancy should be made
   with qualified medical advice.

      Explanation: _____

      _____

   c) _____: Conception is not a time to begin strenuous workouts and to lose weight.

      Explanation: _____

      _____

   d) _____: Body fat content influences the fertility of women.

      Explanation: _____

      _____

   e) _____: The body weight of males does not influence their fertility.

      Explanation: _____

      _____

   f) _____: Moderate exercise during lactation does not affect the quantity or composition of
   breast milk.

      Explanation: _____

      _____

15. What metabolically active organ develops inside the uterus during pregnancy, allowing for exchanges of

   nutrients and gas between the mother and the fetus? _____

16. What fluid-filled balloon-like structure houses the developing embryo/fetus? _____

17. What changes in maternal physiology occur during pregnancy?

_____

_____

18. What are common health problems during pregnancy?

_____

_____

19. Identify on the figure the terms used for stages surrounding pregnancy and birth using the following list.

_____ periconceptional   _____ postneonatal   _____ fetus

_____ postterm baby   _____ fertilization or conception _____ term baby

_____ trimester   _____ embryo   _____ perinatal

_____ newborn or neonate   _____ very preterm baby   _____ zygote

_____ infant   _____ postnatal   _____ neonatal

_____ pregnancy or gestation   _____ last menstrual period   _____ birth

_____ preterm or premature baby

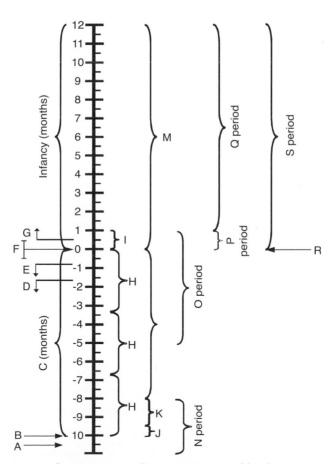

Stages surrounding pregnancy and birth.

Lactation and the Postpartum Period

20. Fill in each blank space with an appropriate word.

   a) While lactation is an automatic physiologic response, _____ is a learned behavior.

   b) An early start to breastfeeding (if possible, within the first hour after birth) is an important aspect in

   successful breastfeeding. The infant's _____ reflex is particularly strong after birth.

   c) Breastfeeding and close physical contact with the newborn facilitates _____ or affectionate attachment between the mother and her baby.

   d) Breast milk can be _____ manually or using a pump, stored in a refrigerator or freezer, and given to baby in a bottle by a family member or caregiver at the appropriate time.

21. What kind of support does a mother need to breastfeed?

   _____

   _____

22. What are the advantages to breastfeeding? List 12 advantages.

   1. _____
   2. _____
   3. _____
   4. _____
   5. _____
   6. _____
   7. _____
   8. _____
   9. _____
   10. _____
   11. _____
   12. _____

23. Breastfeeding is the optimal method of feeding infants and may continue for _____ year(s). Mothers are

   encouraged to exclusively breastfeed for at least the first _____ month(s).

   a) ≥1; 2   c) ≥3; 8   e) ≥5; 20
   b) ≥2; 6   d) ≥4; 15

24. Can women with small breasts make enough milk to successfully nurse their infant? Explain.

   _____

   _____

   _____

25. Your friend is due to have her baby any time now! Outline seven tips for successful breastfeeding that will help her.

   1. _____
   2. _____
   3. _____

4. _____

5. _____

6. _____

7. _____

UNDERSTAND THE CONCEPTS

Childbearing Years and Preconception Period

1. Body Mass Index (BMI)

   a) What is the BMI? _____

   _____

   b) Can the BMI be used with all populations and age groups? Explain. _____

   _____

   _____

   c) Give some limits of this tool. _____

   _____

   _____

   d) Complete the following table with the interpretation of the BMI ranges in adults.

BMI RANGES IN ADULTS	
BMI (kg/m^2)	Interpretation
<18.5	
18.5–24.9	
25.0–29.9	
30.0–34.9	
35.0–39.9	
≥40.0	

2. Women of childbearing age rarely have enough _____ in their diet, and unfortunately the needs for these nutrients are also increased during pregnancy.

   a) Folate and iron
   b) Cobalamin and vitamin D
   c) Vitamin A and zinc
   d) Vitamin B$_{12}$ and vitamin D
   e) Zinc and iron

3. What is the recommended maximum caffeine intake level for women of childbearing age (women who are planning to become pregnant, pregnant women, and breastfeeding mothers)?

   a) 300 mg/day
   b) 400 mg/day
   c) 500 mg/day
   d) 600 mg/day
   e) 700 mg/day

4. Women of childbearing age should limit their caffeine intake to no more than _____ mg caffeine per day

   from all sources, which represents less than _____ cup(s) (_____ mL) of percolated or filter drip coffee per day.

   a) 150; 1; 237   d) 600; 3; 711
   b) 300; 2; 474   e) 800; 3.5; 830
   c) 400; 2.5; 593

5. The following are possible side effects of taking oral contraceptives, <u>except:</u>

   a) an increase in blood cobalt concentration
   b) a reduction in serum cobalamin concentration
   c) an increased risk for venous thromboembolism
   d) a loss of weight
   e) an increase in blood triglyceride concentration

6. Associate the following terms with their description. *(Note that terms can be repeated more than once.)*

fertility	abortion	total fertility rate	teratogenic	abortion rate
fecundity	dysmenorrhea	subfertility	fertility rate	amenorrhea
infecundity	miscarriage	menarche	stillbirth	

   a) _____: A reduced level of fertility

   b) _____: Sterility or the biologic incapability to produce offspring after 12 months of unprotected intercourse

   c) _____: The number of births per thousand women of childbearing age in a population group

   d) _____: The number of live births per woman of childbearing age in a population group

   e) _____: Exposures that cause congenital abnormalities/anomalies (malformations or inborn errors of metabolism) in embryos and fetuses

   f) _____: The number of abortions per thousand childbearing age women in a population group

   g) _____: The biologic capability to generate live offspring

   h) _____: Fetal death; an infant born weighing at least 1.1 lb (500 g) or born at least 20 weeks into the pregnancy and who has no sign of life

   i) _____: The involuntary loss of a fetus within 20 weeks of pregnancy

   j) _____: A spontaneous abortion

   k) _____: The termination of a pregnancy at <20 weeks of pregnancy or before the fetus weighs 1.1 lb (500 g)

   l) _____: The absence of at least three consecutive menstrual cycles

   m) _____: Painful menstruations involving symptoms such as abdominal cramps, bloating, irritability, headache, and back pain

   n) _____: The event of the first menstrual cycle

   o) _____: The actual production of offspring

7. What is the most frequent reason why some women have a miscarriage?

   _____

8. Couples are defined subfertile if they have a delayed time to conception of _____ and/or

   _____ repeated early pregnancy losses.

   a) >6 months; ≥2   c) >18 months; ≥4   e) >12 months; ≥3
   b) >24 months; ≥5   d) >30 months; ≥6

9. Starvation diets such as in a time of famine during a war are associated with

    a) diabetes mellitus during pregnancy   d) macrosomic offspring
    b) microsomic offspring   e) sterility in women
    c) postterm births

10. In men, sperm viability and motility decrease as weight decreases to _____ below normal, and

    sperm production ceases entirely when weight loss exceeds _____ of normal weight.

    a) 10%–15%; 25%   d) 25%–30%; 40%
    b) 15%–20%; 30%   e) 30%–35%; 50%
    c) 20%–25%; 35%

11. What is the most frequent cause of infertility?

    a) Being underweight   d) Endocrine abnormalities
    b) Unknown causes   e) Endometriosis
    c) Sexually transmitted infections

12. Low _____ status contributes to infertility in men, as it is known to reduce testosterone levels and semen volume, as well as to cause hypogonadism.

    a) iron   d) β-carotene
    b) zinc   e) vitamin E
    c) selenium

13. All women who could become pregnant should take a multivitamin containing _____ of folic acid

    every day, starting at least _____ month(s) before getting pregnant and continuing through pregnancy and lactation.

    a) 0.2 mg, 1   c) 0.2 mg, 2   e) 0.6 mg, 6
    b) 0.4 mg, 3   d) 1.0 mg, 4

Pregnancy and Birth

14. Define the following terms related to pregnancy.

    a) Gravida: _____

    b) Primigravida: _____

    c) Multigravida: _____

    d) Gravid: _____

    e) Pregravid: _____

    f) Gravidity: _____

    g) Postpartum or postnatal: _____

    h) Parity: _____

    i) Nullipara: _____

    j) Primipara: _____

    k) Multipara: _____

    l) Prenatal: _____

    m) Perinatal: _____

    n) Neonatal: _____

15. Pregnancy weight gain

a) How much weight should women gain during pregnancy? Explain.

_____

_____

_____

b) Is the pattern of weight gain important? How should the weight be gained?

_____

_____

_____

c) Given that the average baby's birth weight is 7.5 lb (3.45 kg) and that healthy women usually gain about 30 lb (13.6 kg) during pregnancy, what are the other components of the pregnancy weight gain?

_____

_____

_____

16. The pregnancy Estimated Energy Requirement (EER) recommendations for women between 19 and 50 years old for the three trimesters are as follows:

First trimester EER (kcal)
= Adult women EER + Change in Total Energy Expenditure + Pregnancy Energy Deposition
= Adult women EER + 0 kcal + 0 kcal
= Adult women EER

Second trimester EER (kcal)
= Adult women EER + Change in Total Energy Expenditure + Pregnancy Energy Deposition
= Adult women EER + (8 kcal/week $\times$ 20 weeks) + 180 kcal
= Adult women EER + 160 kcal + 180 kcal
= Adult women EER + 340 kcal
or an extra 1420 kJ/day in the second trimester

Third trimester EER (kcal)
= Adult women EER + Change in Total Energy Expenditure + Pregnancy Energy Deposition
= Adult women EER + (8 kcal/week $\times$ 34 weeks) + 180 kcal
= Adult women EER + 272 kcal + 180 kcal
= Adult women EER + 452 kcal
or an extra 1890 kJ/day in the third trimester

a) Suggest four examples of different healthy snacks that a woman beginning her second trimester could include throughout the day to increase her energy intake by 340 kcal (1420 kJ) to meet her pregnancy needs?

1. _____

_____

2. _____

_____

3. _____

_____

4. _____

_____

b) Suggest four examples of different healthy snacks that a woman beginning her third trimester could include throughout the day to increase her energy intake by 452 kcal (1890 kJ) to meet her pregnancy needs?

1. _____

_____

2. _____

_____

3. _____

_____

4. _____

_____

17. The protein RDAs during pregnancy are as follows:

Adult women RDA = 0.80 g protein/kg body weight/day

All trimesters = 1.1 g protein/kg body weight/day = Adult women RDA + ~25 g/day

a) What are the protein needs of a 26-year-old pregnant woman in her second trimester weighing 160 lb?

_____

_____

_____

_____

_____

_____

b) Give an example of a breakfast that would include four food groups and meet one-third of this protein requirement.

_____

_____

_____

_____

_____

_____

18. According to current recommendations, women having a healthy diet do <u>not</u> need to augment their

_____ intake when they become pregnant, since the absorption of this nutrient is more efficient during pregnancy.

a) iron   c) vitamin A   e) vitamin C
b) calcium   d) zinc

19. Which statement is **true** about the concept of critical periods of development?

a) They are finite periods during development in which certain events may occur that will have reversible effects on later development stages.
b) They are times of slow development and cell division.
c) They occur early in development, but also throughout pregnancy.
d) Events scheduled for those times can be rescheduled at a later time.
e) An adverse influence felt early temporarily impairs development, but a full recovery is possible.

20. Which hormone produced by the placenta is detected in the urine or plasma when a pregnancy test is performed?

    a) Luteinizing hormone   d) Progesterone
    b) Placental lactogen   e) Human chorionic gonadotropin
    c) Estradiol

21. Which foods reduce the absorption of iron, and should be consumed separately from iron supplements and iron-fortified foods?

    a) Whole grain cereals   d) Unleavened whole grain breads
    b) Coffee and tea   e) All of the above
    c) Legumes

22. Use this grid to help you fill the following sentences with appropriate words pertaining to pregnancy.

	n →						a ↓					
							← m		d ↓			
	b →							e ↓				
p →												
							← h					
						← k						
	j → g ↑											
									← i			
l →										c ↑		
	f →											
	o ↑											

Words Pertaining to Pregnancy

a) _____ (word of 7 letters) is the main energy source during the fetal period.

b) Blood concentration of most minerals and vitamins is lower during pregnancy due to

_____ (word of 12 letters).

c) A certain degree of edema is normal during pregnancy and is due to lower _____ (word of 7 letters) concentration of the blood.

d) During pregnancy, iron, folate, and _____ (word of 9 letters) are especially important to allow for the increase in the number of erythrocytes.

e) _____ (word of 4 letters) and folate supplements are usually indicated for pregnant women.

f) Preformed vitamin A (retinol) is _____ (word of 11 letters) if taken in overdose by pregnant women.

g) Health care professionals advise women not to take any _____ (word of 7 letters) during pregnancy.

h) Enriched wheat flour and refined grain products are fortified in _____ (word of 6 letters) in the United States and Canada to help pregnant women and women in their childbearing years to have an adequate intake of that vitamin.

i) The newborn of an obese mother is more likely to be _____ (word of 10 letters) and the risk is increased if both parents are obese.

j) Problems more frequently faced by _____ (word of 10 letters) mothers include perinatal mortality, lengthened delivery, low-birth-weight infant, delivery before 37 weeks of pregnancy, and increased need for neonatal intensive care.

k) _____ (word of 7 letters) mothers are at increased risk of having a spontaneous abortion, birth complications, placenta problems, vaginal bleeding, a low-birth-weight infant, or an infant suffering from sudden infant death syndrome.

l) Women in their third trimester of pregnancy should not take _____ (word of 7 letters), as this medication may lead to excess hemorrhage when giving birth.

m) A sign of excess _____ (word of 5 letters) retention is a high or sudden pregnancy weight increase.

n) The _____ (word of 8 letters) disabilities frequently seen in infants with alcohol-related neurodevelopmental disorders can be avoided when women are reminded to abstain from drinking alcohol during pregnancy and lactation.

o) Not skipping meals, having many small meals throughout the day, and drinking fluids between meals

help control _____ (word of 6 letters) of pregnancy.

p) Pregnant women and those lactating should use _____ (word of 7 letters) salt to prevent goiter and cretinism in offspring. Deficiency in that mineral is the most frequent preventable factor in the etiology of mental retardation worldwide.

23. According to the latest RDAs, the adequate folate intake from the diet is _____ μg/day during

pregnancy and _____ μg/day during lactation.

a) 200; 100   b) 400; 300   c) 600; 500   d) 800; 700   e) 1000; 900

24. An underweight pregnant teenager should strive for a weight gain of about _____ lb (_____ kg) during pregnancy.

a) 20; 9.1   b) 25; 11.4   c) 30; 13.6   d) 35; 15.9   e) 40; 18.2

25. Which factor(s) contribute to a high-risk pregnancy?

    a) Age ≤18 years old   d) Low socioeconomic status

    b) Drug usage   e) All of the above

    c) Pregnant mother still breastfeeding a previous child

26. These problems are associated with pregnancy in older women, <u>except</u>

    a) higher incidence of cesarean deliveries

    b) higher incidence of genetic abnormalities in the infant, such as Down syndrome

    c) higher incidence of chronic conditions accompanying aging in the mother, such as hypertension and diabetes mellitus

    d) higher risk of growth retardation and birth defects

    e) higher incidence of postterm births

27. Women tend to modify their eating pattern and food choices when they become pregnant. Explain why <u>and</u> give some examples.

_____

_____

_____

28. Food aversions and cravings are frequent during pregnancy.

    1. What are the most common food cravings?

_____

_____

    2. What are the most common food aversions?

_____

_____

    3. What are the most common abnormal nonfood cravings?

_____

_____

    4. Fill in each blank space with the appropriate word.

        a) _____ is an abnormal compulsion to ingest substances of little or no nutritional value over a sustained period of time. This eating disorder presents many *b)* _____ for the fetus and mother. It is sometimes linked to *c)* _____ deficiency. *d)* _____ specifically defines the obsessive ingestion of dirt or clay, whereas *e)* _____ refers to compulsive ingestion of ice or freezer frost. Women are often *f)* _____ of their abnormal or irrational cravings.

29. Determine if these statements about herbal products and botanical supplements are TRUE or FALSE, and justify your answers.

    a) _____ Herbal products and botanical supplements are natural and safe during pregnancy.

        Justification: _____

        _____

    b) _____ Herbal and botanical remedies are a healthy alternative to over-the-counter medications during pregnancy.

        Justification: _____

        _____

30. Artificial sweeteners

   a) Which artificial sweeteners are <u>not</u> considered safe during pregnancy? _____

   _____

   b) Which artificial sweeteners are generally recognized as safe (GRAS) to be used in moderation during

   pregnancy? _____

   _____

31. Avoidance of food contamination and food-borne illness

   1. Fill in each blank space with the appropriate word.

   Women are at *a)* _____ risk of food-borne illness during pregnancy. Some of the most

   frequent causes of *b)* _____ in pregnant women are many food- or water-borne pathogens

   (bacteria, *c)* _____, or protozoa). They include *d)* _____, *Listeria monocytogenes*,

   Toxoplasma gondii, *Campylobacter*, *Shigella*, *Helicobacter pylori*, *Cryptosporidium*, *e)*_____, and
   hepatitis A.

   The *f)* _____ *Listeria monocytogenes* causes *g)*_____, which can result in
   miscarriage, premature delivery, infection in the newborn, or stillbirth. *Listeria monocytogenes* can even

   survive and grow on foods stored in the *h)* _____. It can contaminate meat and fish products,

   *i)*_____ products, and leafy vegetables.

   The *j)* _____ *Toxoplasma gondii* causes *k)* _____, which can result in mental

   retardation or death of the fetus. It can be found in *l)* _____ foods, like meat, vegetables, and

   fruits. Cats are *m)* _____ for *Toxoplasma gondii*, so garden soil and cat litter containing cat
   feces are sources of contamination.

   Therefore, pregnant women who have *n)* _____-like symptoms should bear in mind all
   potential causes, including a food-borne illness.

   2. Give 10 practical ways in which pregnant women can avoid food-borne illnesses caused by harmful
   microorganisms.

   1. _____

   _____

   2. _____

   _____

   3. _____

   _____

   4. _____

   _____

   5. _____

   _____

   6. _____

   _____

   7. _____

   _____

8. _____

_____

9. _____

_____

10. _____

_____

3. Chemical contamination of water and food is also a concern for pregnant women and their fetuses. How can pregnant women avoid ingesting harmful heavy metals?

_____

_____

_____

_____

_____

_____

32. Which should **not** be recommended to a constipated pregnant woman?

a) Try eating prunes or drinking prune juice.
b) Increase your fiber intake to 1 oz (28 g)/day.
c) Walk and be active.
d) Increase your fluid intake to 13 cups (3.2 quarts or 3.0 liters) per day.
e) Take an over-the-counter laxative.

33. What is the incidence of nausea and vomiting during pregnancy?

a) One out of 10 women suffer from nausea and vomiting.
b) Three out of 10 women have nausea, and one out of 10 vomits.
c) Five out of 10 women have nausea, and two out of 10 vomit.
d) Seven out of 10 women have nausea, and four out of 10 vomit.
e) All women suffer from nausea and vomiting at some point during their pregnancies.

34. Which statement is **false** about heartburn during pregnancy?

a) It is recommended to avoid eating just before bed.
b) It is recommended to avoid carbonated beverages.
c) There is reflux of the stomach contents into the esophagus.
d) It is primarily due to estrogen.
e) There is relaxation of the cardiac sphincter.

Lactation and the Postpartum Period

35. Which statement about breastfeeding and postpartum body weight is **incorrect**?

a) Breastfeeding facilitates mobilization of body fat stored during pregnancy.
b) Breastfeeding does not promote rapid weight loss, but all breastfeeding women do lose weight.
c) Most breastfeeding women lose 1–2 lb (0.45–0.9 kg)/month for the first 4–6 months.
d) Breastfeeding women are recommended to eat at least 1800 kcal (7520 kJ)/day.
e) Breastfeeding women are recommended not to lose more than about 1.5 lb (0.7 kg)/week.

36. *Breast milk best meets the nutrient needs of infants*. Explain why.

_____

_____

_____

37. Link each hormone of lactation with its physiologic effects.

Hormones of Lactation	Physiologic Effects
Prolactin	• Promotes uterine contraction
	• Stimulates milk ejection from the nipples
	• Inhibits ovulation
Oxytocin	• Stimulates milk production by the breasts
	• Minimizes maternal postpartum blood loss

38. **The release of milk during a breastfeeding session**

1. What is the foremilk?

_____

2. What is the hindmilk?

_____

3. What is the draught reflex? _____

_____

4. What is the letdown reflex? _____

_____

39. **Carbohydrate content of breast milk**

1. What is the percent of energy from carbohydrate in human milk? _____

2. Does the carbohydrate content of breast milk change depending on the mother's diet?

_____

3. a) What is the main carbohydrate of breast milk? _____

   b) Why is that an advantage for infants? _____

_____

4. Why do oligosaccharides, a type of carbohydrates found in breast milk, have a protective role?

_____

5. a) What are bifidus factors? _____

_____

   b) Why are bifidus factors an advantage to breastfed infants? _____

_____

6. Another advantage to breast milk is that it contains an enzyme to help older infants digest infant

cereals. What enzyme is it? _____

40. **Protein content of breast milk**

1. a) What is the percent of energy from protein in human milk? _____

   b) Why is that an advantage for infants? _____

2. Does the protein content of breast milk change depending on the mother's diet? _____

3. a) What is the main protein of breast milk? _____

   b) Why is consumption of this protein an advantage for infants? _____

_____

4. a) What is the main immunoglobulin found in breast milk? _____

   b) How does it help reduce intestinal infections in infants? _____

_____

41. **Lipid content of breast milk**

   1. a) What is the percent of energy from fat in breast milk? _____

      b) Why is this percent of energy from fat an advantage for infants? _____

      _____

   2. Does the lipid content of breast milk change depending on the mother's diet? Explain.

      _____

      _____

   3. a) What is the main lipid in breast milk? _____

      b) Why is consuming this lipid an advantage for infants? _____

      _____

   4. What component of breast milk aids in the digestion of the lipids it contains?

      _____

   5. a) What other lipid components are found in breast milk? _____

      _____

      b) Which of these lipid components is not added to commercial infant formulas?

      _____

42. An advantage of human milk is that it is *isosmotic* or isotonic.

   1. What does this mean?

      _____

      _____

   2. Explain why this is an advantage.

      _____

      _____

   3. Do you need to give extra water to your young infant when he or she is hot if you are exclusively breastfeeding? Explain.

      _____

      _____

      _____

43. **The onset of lactation**
   Fill in each blank space with one word from the following list.

   | laxative | energy | transition | lysozyme | water | immunity | colostrum | lactoferrin |
   | antibodies | yellowish | fat | mature | lactose | true | factor | progesterone |

   Estrogen and a) _____ cause the growth of mammary glands in pregnant women.

   b) _____ is the first milk (or premilk) secreted by the mother's breasts, before the onset of

   c) _____ lactation. It is produced during the first three days of lactation. This d) _____

   translucent fluid is especially rich in e) _____ and helpful in protecting the infant from

   infections against which the mother has f) _____. Compared to g)_____

   breast milk, it contains more proteins, immunoglobulins, h)_____-soluble vitamins, and minerals like sodium, potassium, and chloride. It also acts as a natural *i)* _____ to help newborns pass their first stool. Newborns start by taking in 0.07–0.34 fluid oz (2–10 mL) per nursing session.

Between the third and the 10th day of lactation, the breasts become fuller and produce a *j)* _____ milk, which becomes denser in *k)* _____, *l)* _____, fat, and *m)* _____-soluble vitamins. After about 2 weeks, the breasts produce mature milk.

Besides antibodies, breast milk contains other antibacterial factors protecting infants against gastroin-testinal infections. *n)* _____ inhibits gastrointestinal bacterial growth by breaking down bacterial cell walls. *o)* _____ is an iron-binding protein, which does not support intestinal bacterial growth, but rather increases iron bioavailability for absorption. Furthermore, breast milk contains an intestinal growth *p)* _____, which increases the intestinal epidermal cell growth and increases its resistance to infection.

44. Breast milk has a higher proportion of energy from _____ than what is recommended for adults.

    a) fat   b) carbohydrate   c) protein   d) glucose   e) a and c

45. Since the milk of mothers contains only low amounts of _____, the recommendation for adequate intake of this micronutrient is the same for breastfeeding or nonbreastfeeding women.

    a) riboflavin   b) potassium   c) vitamin E   d) vitamin D   e) ascorbic acid

46. Are the following statements TRUE or FALSE?

    a) _____: When breastfeeding mothers drink alcohol, the milk consumption of their infants is lower.

    b) _____: Since HIV can be transmitted by breast milk, HIV-infected mothers who have access to proper infant formula should not breastfeed their infants.

    c) _____: Cigarette smoking reduces the amount of milk produced by breastfeeding mothers.

    d) _____: The quantity of water mothers drink daily does not influence the amount of breast milk they generate.

    e) _____: Mothers with large breasts are more successful at breastfeeding their infants than mothers with small breasts.

    f) _____: Exclusive breastfeeding up to 6 months of age can help reduce the incidence of obesity in the offspring.

    g) _____: Regular or intense physical activity reduces milk production in lactating women.

47. **Nutritional needs during lactation**

    1. a) What is the daily energy cost of breastfeeding? _____

       b) What are the daily energy needs of breastfeeding mothers?

       _____

       _____

       _____

       _____

    2. a) What is the daily protein need of breastfeeding mothers?

       _____

       b) How does it compare to the protein need during pregnancy?

       _____

3. a) What is the daily carbohydrate need of breastfeeding mothers?

    _____

    b) How does it compare to the carbohydrate need during pregnancy?

    _____

4. Which micronutrients do women have increased need for during lactation?

    _____

    _____

48. What are some of the problems commonly encountered by women when breastfeeding?

    _____

    _____

INTEGRATE YOUR LEARNING

1. What is the term for "the absence, temporary or permanent, of menstrual periods," which can be observed,

    for example, in young women who are starving themselves for the sake of fashion? _____

2. _____ means painful menstruation due to signs and symptoms such as lower abdomi-
    nal cramps, headache, back pain, bloating, irritability, etc.

3. Women who are pregnant or breastfeeding need to have a) _____ servings of milk prod-
    ucts per day to meet their calcium needs. One serving of milk products can be b) _____
    of milk, c) _____ of yogurt, or d) _____ of natural cheddar or
    American cheese.

4. What does it means if the nurse tells you that this woman is G5P3?

    _____

5. Give five possible causes of miscarriage:

    1) _____

    2) _____

    3) _____

    4) _____

    5) _____

6. A term infant is an infant born between the _____ weeks of gestation.

    a) 36th and 38th   b) 36th and 40th   c) 42nd and 44th   d) 38th and 40th   e) 38th and 42nd

7. The developing organism, from 2 to 8 weeks of pregnancy, is called the _____.

    a) zygote   b) neonate   c) blastocyst   d) embryo   e) fetus

8. Basic organ structures appear in which one of the following developmental periods?

    a) Fetal period   c) Perinatal period   e) Zygote period
    b) Embryonic period   d) Blastocyst period

9. You are explaining to a young woman in her early 20s the importance of optimal health and nutritional sta-
    tus **before** conception and she says: "Why is this so important? I will just have to be more careful about
    what I eat when I find out that I am pregnant!"

What do you say to convince her? Give a detailed answer including examples.

_____

_____

_____

_____

_____

_____

10. Why should all women who could become pregnant be taking folic acid?

_____

_____

_____

_____

_____

11. Explain how intense physical activity can impact fertility in women.

_____

_____

_____

_____

12. Explain how the following factors can reduce fertility in men.

a) Alcohol intake: _____

_____

b) Heat: _____

_____

c) Environmental contaminants: _____

_____

d) Steroid abuse: _____

_____

13. According to the current recommendations for pregnancy, women with a healthy pre-pregnancy body

weight should gain _____ lb (_____ kg) during pregnancy.

a) 30–40; 13.6–18.0   c) 20–30; 9.1–13.6   e) 15–25; 7.0–11.5
b) 20–35; 9.1–16.0   d) 25–35; 11.5–16.0

14. Explain why the Body Mass Index is **not** a tool to use **during** pregnancy?

_____

_____

_____

_____

_____

15. How many grams of protein should a woman add to her diet per day in the first, second, and third trimesters of pregnancy, according to the RDAs?

   a) No need to increase protein intake during pregnancy anymore
   b) 25 g/day
   c) 5 g in the first trimester, 20 g in the second trimester, and 24 g in the third trimester
   d) 10 g in the first trimester, 20 g in the second trimester, and 25 g in the third trimester
   e) 15 g in the first trimester and 25 g in the second and third trimesters

16. Which statement is **false** about the pregnancy Estimated Energy Requirement (EER)?

   a) It is the dietary energy intake recommendation predicted to meet the needs of 97% to 98% of pregnant women in a population group.
   b) Predictive mathematical equations have been used to determine the EER from estimated total energy expenditure data.
   c) It is equal to the adult EER for women for the first trimester.
   d) It includes the energy needs associated with deposition of tissue needed during pregnancy.
   e) It includes the change in total energy expenditure with the weeks of pregnancy.

17. In the second and third trimesters, women with a healthy pre-pregnancy body weight should gain an

   average of _____ lb (_____ kg)/week.

   a) 0.5; 0.2   b) 0.75; 0.3   c) 1.0; 0.5   d) 1.25; 0.6   e) 1.5; 0.7

18. Pregnant women who were obese before pregnancy are recommended to gain about _____ lb

   (_____ kg) weekly after the first trimester.

   a) 0.15; 0.07   b) 0.25; 0.1   c) 0.5; 0.2   d) 0.75; 0.3   e) 1.0; 0.5

19. Which of the following nutrients have **higher** adequate dietary intake recommendations for pregnancy than for lactation?

   a) Calcium and iron   d) Vitamin D and folate
   b) Phosphorus and vitamin D   e) Iron and folate
   c) Calcium and phosphorus

20. Women who are underweight at conception should

   a) gain 2.5 lb (1.1 kg) weekly during the whole pregnancy
   b) eat a high-fat, low carbohydrate diet
   c) gain 0.7 lb (0.3 kg) weekly during the whole pregnancy
   d) gain a minimum of 1.0 lb (0.5 kg) weekly after the first trimester
   e) avoid breastfeeding

21. Women who have a pre-pregnancy BMI of less than _____ kg/m^2 are considered underweight

   according to U.S. guidelines. It is recommended that these women gain _____ lb (_____ kg) throughout pregnancy.

   a) 23.8; 20–32; 9.1–14.5   d) 20.8; 26–38; 11.8–17.3
   b) 22.8; 22–34; 10.0–15.5   e) 19.8; 28–40; 12.5–18.0
   c) 21.8; 24–36; 10.9–16.4

22. A teenage girl is referred to you at the beginning of her pregnancy. She is 16 years old, she measures 5'7" tall, and her pre-pregnancy body weight was 116 lb. The physician explicitly asked her not to start the Accutane treatment she was about to start and not to drink alcohol.

   a) What was her pre-pregnancy BMI?

   _____

   _____

   _____

b) What is your interpretation of her BMI? _____

c) How much weight do you recommend she gain during her pregnancy? Explain why.

_____

_____

_____

_____

d) Why did the physician explicitly ask her not to start the Accutane treatment?

_____

_____

_____

e) What cluster of signs and symptoms is seen in infants of mothers who consumed alcohol during pregnancy?

_____

_____

_____

f) Explain the following statement concerning alcohol intake during pregnancy: "Less is better, none is best!"

_____

_____

_____

g) What about breastfeeding mothers—should they take a glass of wine to relax before breastfeeding? Explain your position.

_____

_____

23. Using the EER equation for adult women, estimate the pregnancy EER of an active 32-year-old healthy pregnant woman in her 22nd week of pregnancy, knowing that she measures 6′ and weighed 171 lb pre-pregnancy. *(Note: Physical Activity coefficient = 1.25 for active adult women.)*

> Adult women EER
> $= 354 - (6.91 \times \text{Age in years}) + \{PA \times [(9.36 \times \text{Weight in kg}) + (726 \times \text{Height in meters})]\}$

24. Are the following statements TRUE or FALSE? Please explain why.

a) _____: Nausea and vomiting during pregnancy are referred to as morning sickness, because they only occur after waking up.

Explanation: _____

_____

b) _____: Nausea and vomiting during pregnancy tend to appear a month after conception and usually disappear around 2.5 months of pregnancy.

Explanation: _____

_____

c) _____: Pregnant women who are constipated should take an over-the-counter laxative pill.

Explanation: _____

_____

d) _____: Relaxed gastrointestinal muscle tone during pregnancy contributes to the increased incidence of heartburn and constipation.

Explanation: _____

_____

e) _____: Women should not eat or drink during labor.

Explanation: _____

_____

25. What nutritional recommendations would you give to pregnant women suffering the following common health problems during pregnancy?

a) **Nausea and vomiting**

Recommendations: _____

_____

_____

_____

_____

_____

_____

b) **Constipation**

Recommendations: _____

_____

_____

_____

_____

_____

_____

c) **Heartburn (gastroesophageal reflux)**

Recommendations: _____

_____

_____

_____

_____

_____

26. Complete this table with possible micronutrient deficiency(ies) in mothers associated with clinical characteristics of malnutrition in newborns.

INFANT MALNUTRITION RESULTING FROM MALNUTRITION IN MOTHERS	
Clinical Characteristics of Malnutrition in <u>Infants</u>	Possible Micronutrient Deficiency(ies) in <u>Mothers</u>
a) Congenital rickets	
b) Infantile beriberi, brain lesions	
c) Goiter, cretinism	
d) Spina bifida	
e) Scurvy, bleeding gums	
f) Impaired vision, night blindness	
g) Anemia	

27. Nutrient toxicities can also cause adverse pregnancy outcomes. What complications are associated with too much intake of the following nutrients during pregnancy?

   a) Iodine: _____

   b) Vitamin D: _____

   c) Vitamin A (retinol): _____

28. Subfertility can be due to

   a) infrequent ovulation delaying the time to conception
   b) sperm abnormality delaying the time to conception
   c) repeated early pregnancy losses
   d) a and b
   e) a, b, and c

29. In what circumstances would a multivitamin and mineral supplement be recommended during pregnancy?

   _____

   _____

   _____

30. Fill in this summary table of the DRI recommendations for some key nutrients preconception, during pregnancy, and during lactation. *(You can refer to the DRI recommendation tables in the appendix.)*

KEY DRI RECOMMENDATIONS FOR WOMEN OF CHILDBEARING AGE							
	Protein RDA (g/kg/day)	Carbohydrate RDA (g/day)	Water AI (L/day)	Iron RDA (mg/day)	Calcium AI (mg/day)	Folate RDA (μg/day)§	Vitamin D AI (μg/day)§
Preconception*							
Pregnancy*							
Lactation*							

* For women 19–50 years old.
§ Micrograms (mcg) per day.

31. The government and other agencies or coalitions sponsor community nutrition programs throughout the country to help people in need.

    a) Name some of the federal, state/provincial, and local programs available to provide food and nutrition services targeted to women and families in your area.
    b) Identify the main activities that each community nutrition program provides.

  1. Federal program: _____

    Activities: _____

  2. Federal program: _____

    Activities: _____

  3. State/provincial program: _____

    Activities: _____

  4. State/provincial program: _____

    Activities: _____

  5. Local program: _____

    Activities: _____

  6. Local program: _____

    Activities: _____

32. Outline 10 tips for healthy lifestyle and weight control in the postpartum period.

  1. _____

  2. _____

  3. _____

  4. _____

  5. _____

  6. _____

  7. _____

  8. _____

  9. _____

  10. _____

33. Select an appropriate term from this list to complete the sentences below. *(Half of the terms will remain unmatched.)*

protein	oligosaccharides	carbohydrate	isosmotic	A	folate
let-down	lipases	hypotonic	energy	fat	lactose
lactobacillus bifidus	cobalamin	secretory	T	draught	

a) The _____ reflex is when the milk at the back of the breast moves toward the nipple after the milk at the front of the breast has been drawn off.

b) _____ are a type of carbohydrates found in breast milk, which reduce the binding of pathogenic bacteria and toxins to the intestine of the infant.

c) _____ is a characteristic of breast milk.

d) Modifications in the food intake of mothers can influence the _____ content of the milk they produce.

e) The presence of _____ in breast milk facilitates the digestion of milk fat by the infant.

f) Colostrum contains more _____ per volume than mature breast milk.

g) Human milk's secretory immunoglobulins _____ help protect breastfed offspring against intestinal infection and diarrhea.

h) Breastfeeding mothers not eating any animal foods tend to have a lower intake of the following nutrients: _____ , iron, vitamin D, iron, zinc, protein, and calcium.

CHALLENGE YOUR LEARNING

CASE STUDY

Objective

This case is an opportunity to challenge your understanding of the maternal nutrition recommendations and principles you have learned, and to show you how to use them in real situations to help pregnant, lactating, and postpartum women.

Description

B.B., a 38-year-old pregnant Italian American woman, came to consult you, the dietitian, at the prenatal health clinic. She is 5′3″ tall. This is her third pregnancy. She is currently G3P1 and her first child is 2 years old. Before this pregnancy, she weighed 193 lb and her pants' waist size was about 37″. She gained 18 lb during the first 18 weeks of pregnancy. She is coming to ask for your help, as she "does not want to gain any more weight." She is actually restricting her sodium intake in order to lose weight. She tells you "I gained 50 lb with my first two pregnancies and I did not lose any weight even though my first child weighed 11 lb and I breastfed him for 1 complete month." You also find out that she is taking ½ oz (15 g) of cod liver oil every day as a self-prescribed natural product.

1. Underline the significant pieces of information from the case.

2. What was B.B.'s pre-pregnancy BMI?

3. What is the interpretation of her pre-pregnancy BMI?

4. What does her pants' waist size before pregnancy tell us?

5. What chronic diseases are associated with obesity and excess abdominal body fat deposition?

6. What is the recommended pregnancy weight gain for her pre-pregnancy BMI?

7. What is the pregnancy weight gain recommended for the first trimester?

8. What pregnancy weight gain is recommended for B.B. in the second and third trimesters according to her pre-pregnancy BMI?

9. Ideally, what would have been her desirable body weight at 18 weeks of pregnancy, given that she weighed 193 lb before pregnancy?

10. What should you tell her about the weight she gained and the rest of her pregnancy?

11. What will be her overall pregnancy weight gain if she follows your recommendations (reflecting the current weight gain guidelines)?

12. Why is it not recommended to lose weight during pregnancy?

13. Estimate B.B.'s Pregnancy EER at 18 weeks of pregnancy, keeping in mind that she is sedentary.

> Adult women EER
> $= 354 - (6.91 \times \text{Age in years}) + \{PA \times [(9.36 \times \text{Weight in kg}) + (726 \times \text{Height in meters})]\}$

14. What factors should you keep in mind when estimating the energy requirement of a pregnant woman?

15. What are B.B.'s daily protein needs at 18 weeks of pregnancy?

16. Give B.B. an example of a 1-day menu that she could follow, based on the energy and protein needs you estimated for her. Make sure that this 1-day menu is well balanced and includes a variety of foods from all food groups, as well as helps B.B. to meet her other pregnancy nutrient requirements (including iron, folate, calcium, vitamin D, etc.). Keep in mind that B.B. is an American of Italian descent.

    Double-check the energy and nutrient composition of your 1-day menu using a nutrient analysis software program (e.g., ESHA Food Processor).

17. What is the recommendation for sodium intake during pregnancy?

18. Why is sodium especially important during pregnancy?

19. Why is sodium restriction not a good idea during pregnancy?

20. If she is currently G3P1 and her first child is 2 years old, what can be assumed?

21. Why is this woman at risk for complications during pregnancy?

22. What is a macrosomic baby?

23. What usually causes a macrosomic baby to be born?

24. What screening test is performed between the 24th and 28th weeks of pregnancy?

25. Cod liver oil is a concentrated source of which nutrient?

    a) What is the pregnancy UL for the above nutrient?

    b) Is B.B. exceeding the UL?

    c) What is the toxicity risk?

26. How long is it recommended for women to breastfeed?

27. What kind of weight loss should women expect when breastfeeding?

28. Explain why B.B. did not lose weight while breastfeeding.

Case Follow-up

B.B. comes back to visit you after 2 weeks and you can see that she is worried. She has gained 4 lb over the last 2 days. She is complaining of having sore swollen feet and of not being able to put on her shoes anymore. She says that she did not eat much in the last few days and does not understand why she gained all that weight.

29. What kind of weight do you think she has gained?

30. What is to be done about this abrupt weight gain?

31. Why does she have sore swollen feet and why is she not able to put on her shoes?

32. Is edema normal during pregnancy?

33. What is preeclampsia?

34. Define proteinuria.

Case Follow-up

The physician prescribes B.B. an antihypertensive drug that she should take for the remainder of her pregnancy to control her blood pressure and prevent pedal edema. With the physician's care and your healthy eating advice, she delivers a healthy and beautiful baby girl at 41 weeks of pregnancy. She comes back to see you at 1 month postpartum, she is breastfeeding, and she is eager to lose weight. Her current body weight is 213 lb. She explains that before she had children, her usual body weight was 136 lb and that is the weight she is hoping to return to.

35. What are the guidelines for weight loss in the postpartum period and while breastfeeding?

36. What was her BMI when she was 136 lb? Was it in the BMI range associated with good health?

37. Using the BMI formula, determine what would be an ideal body weight range for B.B.'s height.

38. If she loses about 1 lb/week, how long will it take her to reach her usual body weight?

3.2 Infancy Nutrition

REVIEW THE INFORMATION

1. Fill in the blank spaces with one choice from the following list.

composition	head circumference	gestational age	eight
seven	2500	skin color	7¾–10 (3500–4500)
weaning	birth weight	Apgar score	42

1) _____ is the strongest predictor of an infant's probable future health status.

2) Newborns weighing _____ lb (_____ g) at birth are more likely to survive the first 12 months of life.

3) The weight of a newborn is influenced by many factors, including the a) _____. Healthy term infants generally weigh more than those born preterm and less than those born postterm

(after b) _____ weeks of pregnancy).

4) Low-birth-weight infants weigh <5 lb a) _____ oz or b) _____ g at birth.

5) The a)_____ is a quick assessment method to determine the overall health of

newborns. The muscle tone, heart rate, breathing, reflexes, and b)_____of the infants are

rated on a scale of one to 10, at 1 and 5 minutes after birth. A score over c)_____ at 5
minutes predicts a healthy infant.

6) Body parameters used to assess the growth of infants and toddlers over time include their weight,

length, and _____.

7) Commercial infant formulas try to match the _____, digestibility, and performance of
breast milk.

8) _____ is the progressive transition from nursing or bottle-feeding to drinking from a
cup, with the parallel introduction of other foods to the infant's or toddler's diet to replace the breast milk
or infant formula.

2. The growth of children is the most rapid

a) during infancy (first year of life)
b) during the toddler years (1–3 years old)
c) in preschoolers (3–5 years old)

d) in school-age children (5–10 years old)
e) in the preteen years (9–12 years old)

3. The average birth weight in both the United States and Canada is about _____

a) 5½ lb (2500 g)
b) 6 lb (2720 g)

c) 6½ lb (2910 g)
d) 7¼ lb (3290 g)

e) 7¾ lb (3520 g)

4. Which source of energy does the brain almost exclusively rely on, which also represents approximately
38% of the energy in breast milk?

a) Fat
b) Protein

c) Carbohydrate
d) Cholesterol

e) Amino acids

5. _____ is the main source of carbohydrate for breastfed infants and infants given a cow's
milk–based infant formula.

a) Sucrose
b) Oligosaccharide

c) Galactose
d) Lactose

e) Glucose

6. What food should newborns be given?

_____

7. Do formula-fed infants need a vitamin D supplement? Explain why.

_____

8. What enzyme present in breast milk helps infants with the digestion of dietary starches once they start

eating their first solid food? _____

9. All newborns in the United States and Canada receive a single supplemental injection dose of

_____ at birth to prevent deficiency.

a) vitamin D
b) vitamin A

c) iron
d) vitamin K

e) vitamin E

10. What is the main protein of cow's milk, and therefore the main source of protein in cow's milk–based infant
formulas?

a) Whey
b) Lactalbumin

c) Casein
d) Albumin

e) Avidin

11. The energy and nutrient needs of infants, based on pounds or kilograms of body weight per day, are higher than for _____.

   a) toddlers
   b) school-age children
   c) teenagers
   d) adults
   e) all of the above

12. At 12 months old, infants can ingest and digest more complex foods. By this time, they should be eating

   a) milk products, including yogurt and cheese
   b) bread, cereal, rice, and pasta
   c) vegetables and fruits
   d) meat, poultry, fish, beans, and eggs
   e) a variety of foods from all food groups

UNDERSTAND THE CONCEPTS

1. The growth of infants is influenced by

   a) their gestational age and birth weight
   b) the type of feeding (breastfed or formula fed)
   c) the stature of their parents
   d) their environment
   e) all of the above

2. Very-low-birth-weight (VLBW) babies weigh less than _____ lb

   (_____ g) at birth.

   a) 2.2 (or 2¼); 1000   b) 3.3 (or 3⅓); 1500   c) 4.4; 2000   d) 5.5 (or 5½); 2500   e) 6.6; 3000

3. A newborn of weight for gestational age between the 10th and 90th percentiles on growth charts born at 40 weeks of pregnancy is

   a) a term infant, who is small for gestational age
   b) a preterm infant, who is large for gestational age
   c) a term infant, who is normal for gestational age
   d) a postterm infant, who is normal for gestational age
   e) a preterm infant, who is normal for gestational age

4. A newborn of weight for gestational age under the third percentile on growth charts born at 39 weeks of pregnancy is

   a) a term infant, who is small for gestational age
   b) a preterm infant, who is normal for gestational age
   c) a preterm infant, who is small for gestational age
   d) a term infant, who is normal for gestational age
   e) a postterm infant, who is small for gestational age

5. A newborn of weight for gestational age under the third percentile on growth charts born at 36 weeks of pregnancy is

   a) a term infant, who is small for gestational age
   b) a term infant, who is normal for gestational age
   c) a preterm infant, who is normal for gestational age
   d) a preterm infant, who is small for gestational age
   e) a very preterm infant, who is normal for gestational age

6. A newborn of weight for gestational age over the 95th percentile on growth charts born at 43 weeks of pregnancy is

   a) a postterm infant, who is normal for gestational age
   b) a term infant, who is normal for gestational age
   c) a postterm infant, who is small for gestational age
   d) a postterm infant, who is large for gestational age
   e) a term infant, who is large for gestational age

7. Which statement is true about the body weight of babies in their first days of life?

   a) Infants may lose up to 10% of their birth weight during the first few days of life without cause for alarm.
   b) Health care providers become concerned when weight loss continues beyond 3 days of life.
   c) Health care providers become concerned when the lost weight is not regained to achieve birth weight by 10 days of life.
   d) Health care providers become concerned when the newborn has not gained 1 lb (454 g) in the first 10 days of life.
   e) Health care providers become concerned when weight loss continues beyond 10 days of life.

8. Infants' birth weight usually _____ by about 5 months and _____ by 1 year.

   a) doubles; triples   d) triples; quintuples
   b) doubles; quadruples   e) quadruples; quintuples
   c) triples; quadruples

9. Infants' length usually increases by about _____% in the first year.

   a) 50   d) 125
   b) 75   e) 150
   c) 100

10. An infant's stage of motor development influences his or her nutritional needs and his or her ability to feed.

    1- Put in chronologic order the stages of motor skills development listed below.
    2- Indicate (in parentheses) at what month infants usually acquire these gross motor skills.
       (However, remember that infants will learn at their own pace.)

       a) _____ Crawl/creep (_____ month[s])

       b) _____ Stand alone without support (_____ month[s])

       c) _____ Lift chin up when lying on the stomach (_____ month[s])

       d) _____ Sit with support (_____ month[s])

       e) _____ Walk alone without support (_____ month[s])

       f) _____ Lift chest up when lying on the stomach (_____ month[s])

       g) _____ Walk when led by holding a hand (_____ month[s])

       h) _____ Pull himself or herself up to stand holding furniture (_____ month[s])

       i) _____ Sit alone without support (_____ month[s])

       j) _____ Sit in a high chair (_____ month[s])

       k) _____ Stand with help (_____ month[s])

       l) _____ Grasp an object with the palm of his or her hand (_____ month[s])

       m) _____ Reach to grasp an object and miss (_____ month[s])

       n) _____ Crawl up stairs (_____ month[s])

       o) _____ Stand holding on to furniture (_____ month[s])

11. Between _____ months, infants learn to drink from a "sippy" cup, which is a cup with a lid and spout, sometimes with handles and an antileak valve.

    a) 2 and 5   d) 8 and 11
    b) 4 and 7   e) 10 and 13
    c) 6 and 9

12. By _____ months of age, infants usually sit in a chair, self-feed finger foods using the pincer grasp technique, drink from an open cup, and say a few words.

    a) 6   d) 10
    b) 7   e) 12
    c) 8

13. Which food remains the main food (main source of energy and nutrients) up to 12 months of age?

    a) Breast milk   d) Iron-fortified infant cereals
    b) Infant formula (iron fortified)   e) a and/or b
    c) Infant cereals

14. It is necessary to bring all water for feeding infants (including that to prepare infant formula) under _____ months of age to a rolling boil for at least _____ minutes to ensure that it is pathogen free.

    a) 1; 5   d) 4; 2
    b) 2; 4   e) 5; 1
    c) 3; 3

15. What is the energy density of mature breast milk?

    a) 8 kcal/fluid oz (111 kJ/100 mL)   d) 20 kcal/fluid oz (284 kJ/100 mL)
    b) 12 kcal/fluid oz (167 kJ/100 mL)   e) 24 kcal/fluid oz (334 kJ/100 mL)
    c) 16 kcal/fluid oz (217 kJ/100 mL)

16. Infants exclusively breastfed have a daily energy intake of about _____ kcal (_____ kJ) in the first 4 to 6 months.

    a) 250; 1045   d) 1500; 6270
    b) 500; 2090   e) 2000; 8360
    c) 1000; 4180

17. What is the Estimated Energy Requirement (EER) of an 8-month-old boy weighing 18 lb 8 oz?

    Note: EER for 7 to 12 months $= TEE + Energy\ deposition$
    $= ((89 \times weight_{(kg)}) - 100) + 22\ kcal$

18. Which statement about the estimated energy requirements per pound or kilogram body weight of infants is <u>incorrect</u>?

    a) The proportion of energy needed to support basal metabolism, growth, and activity changes throughout the first year of life.
    b) An infant's daily energy needs for growth are greatest between 6 and 12 months of life.
    c) During the first 2 months of life an infant's thermoregulatory system requires extra energy to adapt from womb temperature to room temperature.
    d) The basal metabolic energy needs are about the same during the first 12 months.
    e) The basal energy requirement of infants is more than that of adults per pound or kilogram body weight.

19. The DRI micronutrient recommendations for young infants are _____, which are based on the mean intake of healthy breastfed infants.

    a) RDAs   d) AIs
    b) EERs   e) ULs
    c) EARs

20. What is the adequate intake of protein for younger infants aged 0–6 months old?

   a) 0.62 g/kg/day (about 0.3 g/lb/day)   d) 1.52 g/kg/day (about 0.7 g/lb/day)
   b) 0.92 g/kg/day (about 0.4 g/lb/day)   e) 1.82 g/kg/day (about 0.8 g/lb/day)
   c) 1.22 g/kg/day (about 0.6 g/lb/day)

21. What is the protein RDA of an 8-month-old boy weighing 18.5 lb?

   _____

22. What provides the main energy supply for infants? _____

23. Which of the following fatty acids is(are) present in significant quantities in breast milk?

   a) Linolenic acid   d) Eicosapentaenoic acid (EPA)
   b) Docosahexaenoic acid (DHA)   e) All of the above
   c) Linoleic acid

24. Which long-chain omega-3 fatty acid, synthesized from linoleic acid, promotes optimal development of the central nervous system, and is found abundantly in the retina of breastfed infants?

   a) Linolenic acid   d) Eicosapentaenoic acid (EPA)
   b) Docosahexaenoic acid (DHA)   e) Oleic acid
   c) Arachidonic acid

25. The fact that breast milk contains _____ is especially an advantage for infants born before 37 weeks of pregnancy.

   a) Linolenic acid   d) Linoleic acid
   b) Docosahexaenoic acid (DHA)   e) Oleic acid
   c) Cholesterol

26. If an infant is partially breastfed, it is recommended to give

   a) iron-fortified soy-based infant formula up to 12 months of age
   b) follow-up iron-fortified cow's milk–based infant formula up to 12 months
   c) fortified soy beverage
   d) iron-fortified cow's milk–based infant formula up to 12 months
   e) pasteurized whole cow's milk up to 24 months

27. Indicate whether the following are TRUE or FALSE, and justify your answer.

   1- _____: Breast milk is more economical than commercial powder, concentrate, or ready-to-feed human milk substitutes.

   Justification: _____
   _____

   2- _____: Follow-up commercial infant formulas contain more calcium and protein than starter infant formulas and are designed for older infants (6–18 months old).

   Justification: _____
   _____

   3- _____: Breastfed babies have softer stools than most formula-fed babies.

   Justification: _____
   _____

   4- _____: When infant formula is introduced at birth, it does not have to be iron-fortified until 6 months of age.

   Justification: _____
   _____

5- _____: When solids are introduced into the infant's diet, whole milk should become their main milk source.

    Justification: _____

_____

6- _____: Commercial infant formulas are as good as breast milk.

    Justification: _____

_____

7- _____: Babies exclusively breastfed can be weaned directly to drinking from a cup.

    Justification: _____

_____

28. How is the alimentary tract of newborns different from that of older children? Explain.

_____

_____

_____

_____

_____

_____

_____

_____

29. **Introduction of the first complementary foods**

    1- What should be the first solid food introduced into the diet of infants?

_____

    2- How is this first solid food prepared and served?

_____

_____

    3- At what age is this first solid food introduced?

_____

_____

    4- How much of this food is given at a time?

_____

_____

    5- How can a parent determine if an infant is ready for the introduction of this first solid food? Explain.

_____

_____

_____

_____

6- Give five reasons why it is advantageous to introduce this food as the first solid food in the diet of infants.

I. _____

II. _____

III. _____

IV. _____

V. _____

7- What time of the day is it better to introduce and offer this first solid food? Explain why.

_____

_____

_____

8- What should a parent do if baby does not like this solid food? Give six practical suggestions.

I. _____

II. _____

III. _____

IV. _____

V. _____

VI. _____

9- Can this first solid food be introduced even earlier? Why?

_____

_____

_____

_____

_____

10- How can allergic reactions to the first solid foods be prevented?

_____

_____

_____

_____

_____

11- Can the introduction of solid foods be delayed? Why?

_____

_____

_____

_____

_____

30. What other categories of food can progressively be introduced between 6 and 12 months of age? Indicate how and why these foods are introduced.

_____

_____

_____

_____

_____

_____

_____

_____

31. A food allergy

a) can be infection related
b) is not associated with an immune system reaction
c) is more common than food intolerance
d) can be caused by a toxic response
e) to milk often resolves by 3 years of age

32. Which of the following is **not** one of the most common food allergens in infants and children?

a) Fish
b) Eggs
c) Wheat
d) Rice
e) Soy

33. Which statement about the U.S. Centers for Disease Control and Prevention (CDC) growth charts is **incorrect**?

a) They are based on comparative data from large-scale studies of healthy infants and are one of the most useful nutrition assessment tools used in pediatrics.
b) They allow for assessment of growth trends from birth to 20 years old for each sex.
c) They help to assess the past and present growth of infants and children.
d) They help to predict future or expected growth patterns of infants and children.
e) They range from the fifth to the 95th percentiles.

34. Which statement is **false** about the Centers for Disease Control and Prevention (CDC) growth charts?

a) Successive length and weight measurements over time are required to more accurately estimate an infant's growth pattern.
b) Length-for-age measurements of less than the third percentile are a nutritional indicator that the infant may be stunted or short because his or her parents are short.
c) Weight-for-length measurements of less than the third percentile may indicate dehydration, recent malnutrition, or a genetic disorder.
d) The head circumference of infants is an indicator of the size of their brain, and it is used to screen for possible health, developmental, and nutritional abnormalities.
e) When successive measures plotted on a growth chart over time result in an unanticipated crossing of at least two percentile lines upward, it is believed to be an indication of growth failure or failure to thrive.

35. What does the 50th percentile curve represent on the head circumference-for-age growth chart?

_____

36. An infant with a weight on the 85th percentile curve of the weight-for-age growth chart

_____ infants of same age and sex in the reference population.

a) weighs <15% of the
b) weighs <85% of 100
c) weighs <15% of 1000
d) weighs >15% of the
e) weighs >15% of 100

37. The World Health Organization (WHO) published new growth standards, including growth charts, for infants and children in April 2006. *(See the appendix section at the end of this book.)*

a) List the types of growth standards for infants published by the WHO in 2006.

_____

_____

_____

_____

_____

_____

b) What is innovative about the 2006 WHO growth standards?

_____

_____

_____

_____

_____

_____

c) How are the WHO growth standards (2006) different from the Centers for Disease Control and Prevention (CDC) growth charts (revised in 2002)?

_____

_____

_____

_____

_____

_____

38. These are indications of dietary protein overload in an infant, which can happen when the infant formula is not diluted enough during its preparation, <u>except</u>

a) dehydration   c) elevated blood urea   e) acidosis
b) fever   d) constipation

39. Which of these statements about the importance of fat in the diet of infants is **false**?

a) Fat imparts flavor and satiety.
b) It protects their internal organs and keeps them warm.
c) Fat is a concentrated source of energy.
d) It supplies essential amino acids.
e) It promotes the growth of their brain and nervous system.

40. Infants living in far north communities and being exclusively breastfed should receive, from birth, a daily vitamin D supplement of _____ μg/day, which is usually given in the form of oral drops.

a) 5   b) 10   c) 15   d) 20   e) 25

41. About _____ % of the energy provided by breast milk comes from fat.

a) 40   c) 50   e) 60
b) 45   d) 55

42. _____ deficiency is the leading cause of anemia in infants.

    a) Folate   b) Vitamin B_{12} c) Iron   d) Protein   e) None of the above

43. Fruit juices

    a) can be introduced at about 7 months of age
    b) should be pure juice diluted 1:1 with water and given in a cup
    c) should be limited to about 4 fluid oz (125 mL)/day
    d) should not replace breast milk, infant formula, or other nutrient-dense foods, like infant cereals
    e) all of the above

44. Of the following foods, which would be the best choice to offer to a 7-month-old infant?

    a) Very ripe mashed banana   d) Sliced cucumber
    b) Diced cooked ham   e) Grated cheddar cheese
    c) Scrambled egg

45. The most prevalent nutrient deficiency among Canadian and U.S. infants is a deficiency in which

    micronutrient? _____

46. "A condition of inadequate weight or height gain thought to result from an energy intake deficit, whether

    or not the cause can be identified as a health problem" is the definition for _____. It can
    be organic (caused by a disease state) and/or inorganic (possibly the result of parental neglect) in nature.

47. The infant formula used in case of intolerance to both cow's milk– and soy-based infant formulas contains
    amino acids and small peptides instead of whole proteins. What is the term for this special formula?

    _____ formula.

INTEGRATE YOUR LEARNING

1. Complete this figure summarizing feeding options for healthy term infants.

    ┌─────────────────────┐
    │   **Breast Milk**   │
    └─────────────────────┘

         <u>**OR**</u>

    ┌─────────────────────┐   ┌─────────────────────┐
    │   │ (→ Then →)│   │
    └─────────────────────┘   └─────────────────────┘

    <u>**OR**</u> **IF protein allergy** → ┌─────────────────┐
                                              │   │
                                              └─────────────────┘

    <u>**OR**</u> **IF lactose intolerance** → ┌─────────────────┐
                                                  │   │
                                                  └─────────────────┘

    <u>**OR**</u> **IF milk-free formula** → ┌─────────────────┐
          required or preferred   │   │
                                               └─────────────────┘

Feeding Options for Term Infants

2. Between 4 and 6 months, infants learn to

   a) swallow nonliquids and chew
   b) sit in a high-chair
   c) control and turn their head
   d) grasp an object with the palm of their hand
   e) all of the above

3. Which is **not** a sign that an infant is ready to eat solid foods?

   a) The infant is able to sit with support and to control his or her head.
   b) The infant indicates a desire for food or signs of satiety/disinterest.
   c) The infant is reaching his or her mouth with his or her hands.
   d) The infant sticks out his or her tongue when fed.
   e) The infant is grasping objects with his or her hands.

4. The daily Recommended Dietary Allowance for _____ for 5- to 12-month-old infants is more than that of an adult man.

   a) folate
   b) iron
   c) calcium
   d) vitamin D
   e) vitamin K

5. What are the many reasons why cow's milk is **not** appropriate as the first milk for newborns and young infants?

   _____

   _____

   _____

   _____

   _____

   _____

   _____

   _____

   _____

   _____

6. Indicate when foods should be introduced in the diet of infants and how they should be fed using this summary table. (*Note: Foods from different cultures and ethnicities can be integrated in the diet of infants using this progression model. There are numerous successful ways to feed healthy infants. The order in which the different foods within a main food group are introduced is not rigid.*)

FOODS INTRODUCED IN THE DIET OF INFANTS

Foods	0–4 months	4–6 months	6–9 months	9–12 months
Breast milk OR iron-fortified infant formula				
Pasteurized whole cow's milk				
Iron-fortified infant cereal				
Other grain products				
Vegetables				
Fruit				
Meat and alternatives				
Milk products				
Added sugars, salt, spices, and fat				
Soy or rice beverages, and herbal teas				
Texture(s)				

7. Explain why it is important for parents and caregivers **not** to restrict the diet of their infants according to their own food choices, likes, and dislikes.

_____

_____

_____

_____

_____

8. What are five feeding practices contributing to a low iron intake in healthy infants?

   1) _____

   2) _____

   3) _____

   4) _____

   5) _____

9. What are nine main safety issues when feeding infants?

   1) _____

   2) _____

   3) _____

   4) _____

   5) _____

   6) _____

   7) _____

   8) _____

   9) _____

10. a) Which vitamin is given as one preventive intramuscular dose to infants at birth?

    _____

    b) Why is supplementation of this vitamin required?

    _____

    _____

11. Fill in each blank space with one or a few appropriate words.

    The stomach of a newborn is smaller and has a more a)_____shape than that of an older

    child. The stomach of a newborn secretes less b)_____ and c)_____,

    and the gastric emptying time is d)_____. Consequently, it is not recommended to give
    solids to a newborn, as their digestion would be inefficient. When solids are introduced before

    e)_____ months of age, they can cause digestive problems or f)_____.

12. What is the term for the nutrient deficiency that can occur in infants fed exclusively cow's milk for the first
    6–12 months of life, and that is characterized by hemorrhages under the skin, bent legs, and thighs rotated

    open? _____

13. Fill in this summary table of the DRI recommendations for some key nutrients in infancy. *(You can refer to the DRI recommendation tables in the appendix section at the end of the book.)*

KEY DRI RECOMMENDATIONS FOR INFANTS									
Months of age	Protein (g/day)	Iron (mg/day)	Calcium AI (mg/day)	Fluoride AI (mg/day)	Vitamin D AI (μg/day)§	Vitamin K AI (μg/day)§	Vitamin A AI (μg/day)§	Vitamin C AI (mg/day)	Folate AI (μg/day)§
0–6	AI =	AI =							
7–12	RDA =	RDA =							

§ Micrograms (mcg) per day.

14. Take a look at each of the four simplified weight-for-length growth chart sketches provided below and explain whether each infant is growing normally based on his or her pattern of measurements over time. *(Note: The dots represent measurements plotted over time, every 3 months, and the full line represents the 50th percentile curve. You can also refer to the Centers for Disease Control and Prevention [CDC] growth charts in the appendix section at the end of the book.)*

1- Infant A: _____

_____

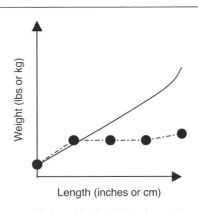

"Infant A" Weight-for-Length
A.   **Growth Curve**

2- Infant B: _____

_____

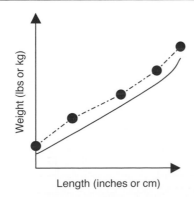

"Infant B" Weight-for-Length
B.   **Growth Curve**

3- Infant C: _____

_____

_____

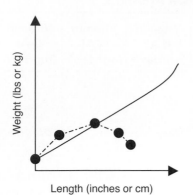

"Infant C" Weight-for-Length
C.   **Growth Curve**

4- Infant D: _____

_____

_____

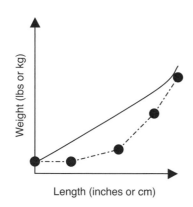

"Infant D" Weight-for-Length
D.   **Growth Curve**

CHALLENGE YOUR LEARNING

1. **Food intolerance and hypersensitivity**

   1) What is milk intolerance?

   _____

   2) What causes milk intolerance?

   _____

   _____

   3) What is lactase deficiency?

   _____

   _____

4) What is milk hypersensitivity?

_____

_____

5) Explain the difference between "milk intolerance" and "milk hypersensitivity."

_____

_____

6) Use this table to distinguish between the possible symptoms of lactose intolerance and milk/food allergy.

SYMPTOMS OF LACTOSE INTOLERANCE AND FOOD ALLERGY		
Possible Symptoms	Lactose Intolerance	Milk/Food Allergy
Skin rash, eczema, hives, swelling of tissues		
Vomiting, spitting, regurgitation		
Sleep disruption, sleeplessness, irritability		
Increased mucus production, nasal congestion and infection		
Coughing and wheezing		
Blood in stool		
Constipation		
Diarrhea		
Stomach bloating		
Gas		
Abdominal pain and cramps, colic		
Anaphylaxis*		
Failure to thrive		

* Anaphylaxis can result in an anaphylactic shock, which is a severe and often fatal form of shock due to a strong immunoglobulin E (IgE) antibody reaction causing a violent smooth muscle contraction and capillary dilatation.

7) Indicate whether the following statements are TRUE or FALSE, and justify your answer.

a) _____: Family history is a weak indicator of the risk of food allergy in infants.

Justification: _____

_____

b) _____: Milk allergy affects 20% of young infants and is very rare among adults.

Justification: _____

_____

c) _____: Milk allergy does not usually last past 3 years of age.

Justification: _____

_____

d) _____: Lactose intolerance is more common in children than adults.

Justification: _____

_____

e) _____: A large proportion of infants allergic to cow's milk protein are also allergic to other animals' milk (e.g., goat) protein, and to soy protein.

Justification: _____

_____

f) _____: Infants with a milk allergy tend to also have allergies to other foods like eggs, fish, and nuts.

Justification: _____

_____

8) Can milk allergy cause lactose intolerance and vice versa? Explain your answer.

_____

_____

_____

_____

_____

_____

9) What are the most common food allergens in infants and young children?

_____

_____

10) Which foods have a low allergenicity, and would be good to start with when following the progression of the introduction of solids?

a) Types of milks: _____

b) Types of cereals: _____

c) Types of vegetables: _____

d) Types of fruit: _____

e) Types of meats: _____

11) What can be done if a formula-fed infant has lactose intolerance due to a gastrointestinal infection?

_____

_____

_____

_____

12) What can be done if a breastfed infant has lactose intolerance due to a gastrointestinal infection?

_____

_____

_____

_____

13) What can be done if a formula-fed infant has an allergy to cow's milk protein?

_____

_____

_____

_____

14) What is used instead of lactose in the preparation of lactose-free infant formula?

_____

15) What type of fat is sometimes used in the preparation of hydrolysate formulas? Why?

_____

_____

CASE STUDY

Objectives

This case will help you to apply the theoretic knowledge you have gained on infant nutrition and enable you to use your judgment to help this mother appropriately meet the needs of her baby within her environmental resources and constraints.

Like any real-life situation, this case will help you realize that there is often a gulf between the theoretic and professional recommendations of health care professionals and their implementation. This gulf is complex and is shaped by a multitude of factors, including cultural beliefs and levels of knowledge. One of the roles of health care professionals is to assess and assist their clients as individuals and to guide them in the application of theory. This does not mean that the theory is only true in books, but rather that to be useful, theory has to be translated by the health care professional into simple everyday terms that individuals will understand and be able to employ in their own lives.

Description

A young mono-parental mother is asking you if her infant, M.N., is developing normally. The mother is wondering if her 11-month-old girl has developmental delays. According to her mother, little M.N. does not seem to explore the world around her and appears less active than her peers.

M.N. is her mother's first baby and was born after 41 weeks of a healthy pregnancy. Her mother was 18 years old, just out of high school, and still living with her parents when she became pregnant. M.N.'s mother is 5'7" tall and weighed about 138 pounds before pregnancy. She gained 28 pounds over the pregnancy, while working at a gas station.

Her mother presently takes care of little M.N. in a one-room apartment near town, where she moved when M.N. was 30 days old. The mother does not work, lives alone, and has slim financial support from her older brother. She tells you that M.N. was a beautiful, healthy, and content newborn. According to her baby book, M.N. weighed 7.5 lb (3.4 kg) at birth, measured 20.1 inches (51 cm) long, and had a head circumference of 13¾ inches (34.9 cm).

You find out from the nurse that she presently weighs 14.5 lb (6.6 kg), she measures 26.4 inches (67 cm) long, and her head circumference is now 16¾ inches (42.5 cm). The nurse also gives you additional information about M.N.'s growth history, which was provided by the family physician:

GROWTH DATA FOR M.N.			
Age (Months)	Weight (lb) [kg]	Length (inches) [cm]	Head Circumference (inches) [cm]
1	9.0 [4.1]	21.7 [55]	14½ [36.8]
4	11.9 [5.4]	24.2 [61.5]	16 [40.6]
6	13.0 [5.9]	24.8 [63]	16¼ [41.3]
9	14.5 [6.6]	26.0 [66]	16 ⅜ [42.2]

When you ask the mother how she fed her infant, this is what she tells you: "I breastfed M.N. for the first month and she liked it, but I was really tired when we moved and I stopped. I gave her whole cow's milk as I could not afford to buy the expensive baby milk." You find out that M.N. has been receiving whole cow's milk in a bottle since about 1 month of age, and the only other foods that she presently eats on a regular basis are rice, oatmeal, applesauce, mashed potatoes, and puréed sweet potatoes.

Her mother says that M.N. lacks an appetite at mealtime, but she drinks milk throughout the day and night. You take a close look at M.N. and find her pale, weak, and dehydrated. Her mother insists that M.N. has colic and is constipated, and that it is making her very irritable, even during the night.

When checking for developmental milestones, here is what you find out. M.N. smiled at 1 month, laughed at 3 months, clapped her hands at 9 months, and she can now say "mama." She sat by herself at 6 months, stood with help at 9 months, and crawled at 10 months, but is not yet using the pincer grasp technique to pick things up. M.N. turns when called by name. She has not been offered a sipper cup yet.

1. What was M.N.'s mother's pre-pregnancy BMI?

2. Did M.N.'s mother gain the recommended amount of weight during pregnancy? Explain.

3. Plot all of the weight, length, and head circumference data on the following Centers for Disease Control and Prevention (CDC) growth charts provided in the appendix section at the end of the book.

   • Weight-for-age percentiles: Girls, birth to 36 months
   • Length-for-age percentiles: Girls, birth to 36 months
   • Head circumference-for-age percentiles: Girls, birth to 36 months
   • Weight-for-length percentiles: Girls, birth to 36 months

4. Why are growth charts useful?

5. What was the *weight-for-age* percentile of M.N. at birth? Give your interpretation.

6. What was the *length-for-age* percentile of M.N. at birth? Give your interpretation.

7. What was the *head circumference-for-age* percentile of M.N. at birth? Give your interpretation.

8. What was the *weight-for-length* percentile of M.N. at birth? Give your interpretation.

9. What do you conclude about the size of M.N. at birth? Justify your answer.

10. What is the present *weight-for-age* percentile of the little girl? Give your interpretation.

11. What is the average weight for an 11-month-old girl according to the weight-for-age Centers for Disease Control and Prevention (CDC) growth chart?

12. What is M.N.'s percent ideal body weight (% IBW)? Give your interpretation.

13. What happened to M.N.'s *weight-for-age* percentile from birth to 11 months of age? Give your interpretation.

14. Did M.N. have a normal pattern of weight gain over time for her age? Explain why.

15. What is the present *length-for-age* percentile of the little girl? Give your interpretation.

16. What is the average length for an 11-month-old girl according the length-for-age Centers for Disease Control and Prevention (CDC) growth chart?

17. What happened to M.N.'s *length-for-age* percentile from birth to 11 months of age? Give your interpretation.

18. Did M.N. have a normal pattern of length increase over time for her age? Explain why.

19. What is head circumference an indicator of?

20. What is the present *head circumference-for-age* percentile for the little girl? Give your interpretation.

21. What is the average head circumference for an 11-month-old girl according to the head circumference-for-age Centers for Disease Control and Prevention (CDC) growth chart?

22. What happened to M.N.'s *head circumference-for-age* percentile from birth to 11 months of age? Give your interpretation.

23. Did M.N. have a normal pattern of head circumference enlargement over time for her age? Explain why.

24. What are the possible long-term implications of M.N.'s head circumference pattern over time?

25. What is the present *weight-for-length* percentile for the little girl? Give your interpretation.

26. What happened to M.N.'s *weight-for-length* percentile from birth to 11 months of age? Give your interpretation.

27. Did M.N. have a normal pattern of weight gain for her length over time? Explain why.

28. What do you conclude about M.N.'s overall growth in her first 11 months of life, based on the weight, length, and head circumference data provided? (Is she growing well? Why?)

29. How often should infants be measured and weighed ideally?

30. What are the physical signs and symptoms that little M.N. is **not** healthy?

31. What condition could explain these physical signs and symptoms?

32. What are possible complications of this condition?

33. **Are there any problems in the way the mother has fed her infant**, which most likely have a role to play in the resulting growth pattern and present health condition of the infant? Explain.

34. You explain to the mother that she and M.N. are eligible for some help through a local maternal and early childhood community support program. Give the mother six practical suggestions to help her meet M.N.'s nutritional needs and have a positive impact on her health status.

    1) _____

    2) _____

    3) _____

    4) _____

    5) _____

    6) _____

35. Did M.N. achieve the normal motor and mental developmental milestones for her age? Explain.

36. Is M.N. having delays in her motor and mental development for her age? Explain.

37. Explain why iron is added to the diet of infants with the introduction of solid foods between 4 and 6 months of age.

Case Follow-up

The young mother is relieved and thankful for your help and that of the pediatric clinic. You can see that she wants to do her best to offer M.N. everything she needs to grow healthy. She has started to participate in educational activities organized by the maternal and early childhood community support program on a weekly basis. In addition, the program is providing her with free iron-fortified follow-up infant formula, infant cereals, and diapers for M.N.

Convinced to help M.N. catch up and grow even better, the mother decides to give M.N. more concentrated infant formula by putting less water in the preparation of the infant formula. After a week, M.N. develops fever and diarrhea and needs to be hospitalized.

When asking the mother how she prepares the infant formula, the mother also tells you that she has taken the habit of preparing the infant formula for her baby with boiling hot water. She says that she found out that the powder mixes and dissolves much better with boiling water.

38. What is a possible cause of the infant's fever and diarrhea in this situation?

39. What are consequences of preparing commercial infant formula with boiling hot water?

3.3 Childhood Nutrition

REVIEW THE INFORMATION

1. Fill in each blank space with an appropriate word from the following list.

five	help	girls	three	peers	routine	families
others	three	self	run	language	slower	why
eaters	ten	dislikes	centimeters	social	centimeters	pounds
imitating	inches	one	self	five	inches	choices
no	boys	variable	limits	teeth	kilograms	

1- **Toddlers** are a) _____ to b) _____ year(s) old. Their growth is c) _____ than that of infants, which results in a decreased appetite. Toddlers grow by an average of 5 d) _____ (or 13 e) _____) during their second year of life. Toddlers learn to walk independently, f) _____, and jump. By that time, they have most of their primary g) _____ and want to feed themselves. Toddlers like to explore their environment and are usually willing to try new foods. They need h) _____ in their life and regular meals and snacks. They can have sudden changes in likes and i) _____, and they show their independence by saying j) "_____." Toddlers learn principally by k) _____ their parents and caregivers.

2- **Preschoolers** are a) _____ to b) _____ year(s) old. They are curious and often ask c) "_____?" for explanations in order to understand their environment. As they develop their independence, they try to control their environment, but still need their parents to set d) _____ for them. They have a broader e) _____ circle and learn to interact, play, and cooperate with others. Preschool children like to f) _____ with meal preparation activities and at the grocery store. Their appetite can be g) _____ and the amount of food they eat may change from meal to meal and day to day. They have their favorite foods and can become picky h)_____. A way to avoid power struggles over food is to offer them i)_____. Their j)_____ develops quickly and they learn to make complete sentences.

3- **School-age or middle-age children** are a) _____ to b)_____ years old. School-age children grow an average of 2½ c)_____ (or about 6 d)_____) in height and 7 e)_____ (or 3.2 f)_____) in weight each year. They become g) _____-efficient, as they learn what to do and how to do it. They begin to understand many aspects of a situation and the point of view of

h)_____. Their lifestyle is still mostly influenced by their immediate i)_____, but external factors begin to have more impact on their health choices. School-age children develop a sense of

j) _____ and learn their role as part of their family, school, and community.

4- **Preteenagers or preadolescents** are 9–12 years old: 9–11 years old for a) _____ and 10–12 years old for b)_____. c) _____ are increasingly important for preteenagers, and they spend more time and eat more meals away from their family and home environment.

2. Aside from the strong influence exerted by parents and siblings, which external influences have a growing impact on the health habits and food choices of school-age children and preadolescents?

_____

_____

3. The growth pattern of children informs us about their

   a) bone mass and density
   b) health and nutritional status
   c) future adult weight and stature
   d) appetite and activity level
   e) intelligence and motor skills

4. Optimal growth hinges on

   a) adequate nutrition
   b) a nurturing environment
   c) the absence of chronic disease and a normal endocrine function
   d) the child's genetic constitution
   e) all of the above

5. Overall, the growth of _____ is slow and gradual.

   a) infants and toddlers
   b) preschoolers and early school-age children
   c) school-age children and preteenagers
   d) preteenagers and teenagers
   e) teenagers

6. Which of the following foods provide(s) at least 200 mg calcium? Circle them.

   a. 1 cup (8 fluid oz, 237 mL) milk (whole, partly skimmed, or skimmed)
   b. 2 oz (56 g) dry roasted almonds
   c. 1 cup (237 mL) bok choy (cooked or fresh)
   d. ½ cup (118 mL) plain yogurt
   e. 1 cup (237 mL) broccoli (fresh or cooked)
   f. 1 cup (8 fluid oz, 237 mL) orange juice with added calcium
   g. 2 oz (56 g) cheddar cheese
   h. 1 cup (237 mL) fruit yogurt (partly skimmed)
   i. ½ cup (118 mL) tofu made with calcium
   j. 1 cup (237 mL) boiled white beans
   k. 1 cup (237 mL) frozen yogurt (whole, partly skimmed, or skimmed)
   l. 1 cup (237 mL) cooked soybeans
   m. 1 cup (8 fluid oz, 237 mL) soy beverage with added calcium
   n. 1 slice of white bread

7. Use this grid to find 16 good food sources of iron for children.

S	N	A	E	B	Y	O	S	C	S
E	A	B	R	E	A	D	S	E	U
N	K	E	N	I	S	I	A	R	G
E	R	E	V	I	L	O	E	E	A
K	O	F	I	S	H	E	P	A	R
C	P	R	U	N	E	A	E	L	A
I	L	E	G	U	M	E	S	S	P
H	U	S	P	I	N	A	C	H	S
C	M	T	O	C	I	R	P	A	A

Food Sources of Iron

1-_____   9-_____

2-_____   10-_____

3-_____   11-_____

4-_____   12-_____

5-_____   13-_____

6-_____   14-_____

7-_____   15-_____

8-_____   16-_____

8. _____ increases the absorption of nonheme iron.

   a) Vitamin A   c) Vitamin C   e) Vitamin E
   b) Vitamin B_{12} d) Vitamin D

9. _____ is required for the absorption of calcium by active transport in the small intestine.

   a) Vitamin A   c) Vitamin C   e) Vitamin E
   b) Vitamin B_{12} d) Vitamin D

UNDERSTAND THE CONCEPTS

1. The Centers for Disease Control and Prevention (CDC) growth charts allow using the Body Mass Index (BMI) to screen children of _____ for possible excess fat accumulation.

   a) 1 year and older
   b) 2 years and older
   c) 3 years and older
   d) 4 years and older
   e) 5 years and older

2. When using the Centers for Disease Control and Prevention (CDC) growth charts, a BMI-for-age between the _____ is an indication that the child may be **overweight**, and that further investigation is necessary.

   a) 70th to <80th percentiles
   b) 75th to <85th percentiles
   c) 80th to <90th percentiles
   d) 85th to <95th percentiles
   e) 90th to <97th percentiles

3. When using the Centers for Disease Control and Prevention (CDC) growth charts, a BMI-for-age at the _____ percentile or more is an indication that the child may be **obese**, and that further investigation is necessary.

   a) 80th
   b) 85th
   c) 90th
   d) 95th
   e) 97th

4. What measurements can be done to determine if a child with a high BMI-for-age has excess body fat?

   _____

5. When using the Centers for Disease Control and Prevention (CDC) growth charts, a BMI-for-age below the _____ percentile is used as an indication that the child may be **underweight**, and that further investigation is necessary.

   a) 3rd
   b) 5th
   c) 10th
   d) 15th
   e) 20th

6. Indicate whether the following statements are TRUE or FALSE, and justify your answer.

   1- _____: The reference range of BMI for children is different from that of adults.

   Justification: _____
   _____
   _____

   2- _____: The BMI of children is fairly constant throughout childhood.

   Justification: _____
   _____
   _____

   3- _____: The reference range of BMI-for-age in children is different for girls and boys.

   Justification: _____
   _____
   _____

   4- _____: It is normal for young children to have a decrease in BMI between 2 and 5 years of age.

   Justification: _____
   _____
   _____

7. Pedro is a 4½-year-old boy. He presently weighs 42 lb (19.1 kg) and is 41.5 inches (105.5 cm) tall. Use the 2006 World Health Organization (WHO) growth standards to determine the following anthropometric information about Pedro. *(WHO growth charts can be found in the appendix section at the end of this book or online at www.who.int/childgrowth.)*

a) Height-for-age and sex

a- What is Pedro's height-for-age z score? _____

b- What is your interpretation of Pedro's height-for-age z score?

_____

c- What is Pedro's height-for-age percentile? _____

d- What is your interpretation of Pedro's height-for-age?

_____

b) Weight-for-age and sex

a- What is Pedro's weight-for-age z score? _____

b- What is your interpretation of Pedro's weight-for-age z score?

_____

c- What is Pedro's weight-for-age percentile? _____

d- What is your interpretation of Pedro's weight-for-age?

_____

c) Weight-for-length and sex

a- What is Pedro's weight-for-length z score? _____

b- What is your interpretation of Pedro's weight-for-length z score?

_____

c- What is Pedro's weight-for-length percentile? _____

d- What is your interpretation of Pedro's weight-for-length?

_____

d) BMI-for-age and sex

a- What is Pedro's BMI? _____

b- What is Pedro's BMI-for-age z score? _____

c- What is your interpretation of Pedro's BMI-for-age z score?

_____

d- What is Pedro's BMI-for-age percentile? _____

e- What is your interpretation of Pedro's BMI-for-age and sex?

_____

8. These healthy eating recommendations are appropriate for active 9-year-old boys requiring about 1800 kcal (7520 kJ)/day, <u>except</u>

a) Eat 6 oz (168 g) of grain products every day.
b) Eat 2½ cups (590 mL) of vegetables daily.
c) Eat 10 oz of meat, poultry, fish, eggs, dry beans, or nuts.
d) Enjoy 1½ cups (355 mL) of fruits each day.
e) Include 3 cups (24 fluid oz, 710 mL) of milk and milk products in your diet daily.

9. Toddlers can bite for many reasons. List six of them.

1) _____

2) _____

3) _____

4) _____

5) _____

6) _____

10. What kinds of food characteristics, preparation, or serving styles do toddlers like?

_____

_____

_____

_____

11. Indicate whether the following statements are TRUE or FALSE, and justify your answers.

1- _____: Parents and caregivers should offer nutritious foods and children should decide the amount to eat.

Justification: _____

_____

_____

2- _____: Parents should not force their child to eat or restrict the amount of food they eat.

Justification: _____

_____

_____

3- _____: Children who eat breakfast perform better at school.

Justification: _____

_____

_____

4- _____: Snacks are an important part of a child's daily food intake.

Justification: _____

_____

_____

5- _____: Snacks are unnecessary treats for school-age children.

Justification: _____

_____

_____

6- _____: Infants and children instinctively prefer sweet or slightly salty foods.

Justification: _____

_____

_____

7- _____: To help them lose weight, parents should not give overweight children snacks.

Justification: _____

_____

_____

12. Feeding children and the development of eating habits

1- Indicate if the following parental strategies are GOOD or NOT recommended to help children develop healthy eating habits for a lifetime.

2- For each strategy that is NOT recommended, indicate in parenthesis what eating problem this parental strategy may lead to.

a) _____ Offering two or three snacks a day to children (_____)

b) _____ Ensuring that children have a regular meal pattern, including breakfast, lunch, and dinner (_____)

c) _____ Making time to enjoy family meals with children at home (_____)

d) _____ Giving a snack before or instead of a meal (_____)

e) _____ Having a television in the dining room for children to watch during mealtime, so they stay longer at the table (_____)

f) _____ Rewarding children with candies and junk food when they are good

(_____)

g) _____ Offering again a food that was rejected at the first attempt (_____)

h) _____ Forcing children to clean their plate because food is expensive (_____)

i) _____ Giving for dinner only what a child has refused to eat for lunch that day

(_____)

j) _____ Giving children small servings and letting them ask for more (_____)

k) _____ Giving children snacks when they are watching television programs

(_____)

l) _____ Letting children eat indiscriminately between meals and snacks (_____)

m) _____ Telling children that they will not have a favor or treat if they do not eat their vegetables (_____)

n) _____ Severe restriction of high-fat and high-sugar foods, like candies, to prevent chronic disease and cavities (_____)

o) _____ Punishing a toddler for being messy when self-feeding (_____)

p) _____ Asking children if they are hungry before offering them an afternoon snack

(_____)

q) _____ Preparing and serving differently a food that your child dislikes (_____)

r) _____ Using food as a comfort when a child is sad or as a distraction when a child is lonely

(_____)

s) _____ Asking children to take only four bites when they are not hungry (_____)

t) _____ Offering a food you dislike so that children have a chance to discover it

(_____)

u) _____ Eating slowly with your children and respecting their satiety signals

(_____)

v) _____ Not letting children touch, explore, and play with new foods (_____)

w) _____ Involving children in the planning and preparation of nutritious and safe lunch box

meals for themselves (_____)

13. Use the Estimated Energy Requirement (EER) formula to estimate the energy needs of a 6-year-old boy, who is 46 inches tall, weighs 46 lb, and is lightly active.

Note: EER (kcal) for boys 3–8 years

$= TEE + Energy\ deposition$

$= 88.5 - [61.9 \times Age_{(yrs)}] + \{PA \times ([26.7 \times Wt_{(kg)}] + [903 \times Ht_{(m)}])\} + 20\ kcal$

PA = 1.00 if physical activity level is sedentary
PA = 1.13 if physical activity level is lightly active
PA = 1.26 if physical activity level is active
PA = 1.42 if physical activity level is very active

_____

_____

_____

_____

_____

_____

_____

_____

14. Indicate the appropriate protein Recommended Dietary Allowance (RDA) for each age group by choosing the corresponding dot in each of the three columns and by joining them. *(Note: A choice may be used more than once or not be used)*

Age groups (males & females)	Protein RDAs (g/kg/day)	(g/day)
1–3 years old •	• 0.80	• 34
4–8 years old •	• 0.95	• 13
9–13 years old •	• 1.10	• 19

15. What are the Acceptable Macronutrient Distribution Ranges recommended for children?

_____

_____

_____

_____

_____

_____

16. What are six ways for parents and caregivers to include milk in the diet of children?

1) _____

2) _____

3) _____

4) _____

5) _____

6) _____

17. Toddlers like to have a regular schedule for eating meals and snacks, and prefer eating familiar foods in familiar surroundings. This helps them to meet their need for

   a) control   c) security   e) socialization
   b) attention   d) autonomy

18. A child's weight usually increases by about _____ kg (_____ lb) yearly until adolescence.

   a) 0.5–0.9; 1–2   c) 3.6–4.1; 8–9   e) 6.4–6.8; 14–15
   b) 2.3–2.7; 5–6   d) 5.0–5.5; 11–12

19. Energy and protein requirements per pound or kilogram body weight

   a) decrease gradually between 1 and 18 years of age
   b) stay similar during all childhood
   c) augment gradually between 1 and 18 years of age
   d) decrease in toddler years, and augment afterward
   e) augment in toddler years, and decrease afterward

20. Children suffering from chronic protein-energy malnutrition

   a) have faster catch-up growth than those with acute malnutrition
   b) are wasted and thinner than normal
   c) had temporary lack of dietary intake
   d) are stunted
   e) are thin for their height

21. High _____ intake in toddlers is a frequent reason for not having enough iron in the diet.

   a) milk or juice   c) fruit and vegetable   e) rice or soy beverage
   b) cereal   d) snack

22. These are consequences of iron overdose, <u>except</u>

   a) gastrointestinal bleeding   c) toxic shock   e) nausea and vomiting
   b) hair loss   d) coma

23. Health professionals recommend parents and caregivers limit the caffeine intake of 4- to 6-year-old children to no more than _____ mg caffeine per day from all sources, which represents about _____ can(s) of cola beverage per day (a can being 12 fluid oz or 355 mL).

   a) 15; ⅛   c) 35; ½   e) 55; 2
   b) 25; ¼   d) 45; 1

24. Which nutrient is used to make neurotransmitters, and most notably, those that regulate the ability to pay attention, which is crucial to learning?

   a) Vitamin C   c) Vitamin K   e) Iron
   b) Vitamin D   d) Magnesium

25. Which statement related to the effect of obesity on growth of children is **false**?

   a) Obese children begin puberty earlier than children of normal weight.
   b) Obese girls have an earlier age of menarche than girls of normal weight.
   c) Obese children grow taller at first, but then stop growing at a shorter height, compared to children of normal weight.
   d) Obese children have a slower metabolic rate than children of normal weight.
   e) Obese children have a greater bone mass and appear "stocky" compared to children of normal weight.

26. According to the Dietary Reference Intake guidelines, the Recommended Dietary Allowances for iron are _____ mg/day for children between 1 and 3 years, _____ mg/day for children between 4 and 8 years, and _____ mg/day for children between 9 and 13 years of age.

    a) 5; 7; 10   b) 7; 10; 8   c) 6; 10; 13   d) 11; 14; 15   e) 12; 10; 8

27. The Tolerable Upper Intake Level for iron for children up to 13 years old is _____ mg/day.

    a) 30   b) 40   c) 50   d) 60   e) 70

28. Short-answer questions

    1- According to the national food guide (My Pyramid for Kids <u>or</u> Canada's Food Guide to Healthy Eating), how much milk product is recommended per day for children between 6 and 8 years old?

    _____

    2- The most prevalent nutrient deficiency among North American children is a deficiency in which micronutrient? _____

    3- The intake of four micronutrients tends to be especially low in children from vegan families and should be assessed. Which micronutrients are they?

    _____

    4- *a)* What is the term for the apparent hyperactivity caused in a child by the combination of lack of sleep, overstimulation, and anxiety?

    _____

    b) What is your main <u>dietary</u> recommendation for a child with that problem?

    _____

    5- _____ intake is often overlooked as a source of "hyper" behavior in children.

INTEGRATE YOUR LEARNING

1. Indicate some developmental characteristics for each age group in this table.

DEVELOPMENTAL CHARACTERISTICS OF DIFFERENT AGE GROUPS				
Developmental Characteristics	Toddlers	Preschoolers	School-Age Children	Preteenagers
Age (years)				
Physical growth and development				
Appetite, feeding skills, and behavior				
Language and motor skills development				
Cognitive development, behavior, and special needs				

2. Parents are asking you which beverages they should offer their healthy 20-month-old daughter and 7-year-old son.

1- Which beverages do you recommend or not recommend for each child from the following list?

Coffee	Wine or beer	Chocolate milk	Enriched soy or rice beverage
Soda pop	Iced tea	Milkshake	Fruit-flavored drink
Water	Diet cola	Whole cow's milk	Herbal tea
Sport drink	Pure fruit juice	Partly skimmed cow's milk	

a) For their daughter:

_____

_____

_____

_____

_____

b) For their son:

_____

_____

_____

_____

2- What are the five bone-building micronutrients found in enriched cow's milk?

_____

3- Compare cow's milk to other beverages (including soda pop, cola, coffee, fruit-flavored drinks, and sport drinks) in terms of their nutritional value.

_____

_____

_____

_____

_____

4- Convince these parents that milk is important to include in children's diets. Explain your arguments.

_____

_____

_____

_____

_____

_____

_____

_____

3. Fill in this summary table of the DRI recommendations for some key nutrients for children. *(DRI recommendation tables can be found in the appendix section at the end of this book.)*

DRI RECOMMENDATIONS FOR CHILDREN AND DIETARY SOURCES OF NUTRIENTS

Nutrients	DRIs	1–3 years old	4–8 years old	9–13 years old Females	9–13 years old Males	Good Dietary Sources for Children
Protein	RDA (g/kg/day)					
Total Fiber	AI (g/day)					
Water	AI (L/day)					
Vitamin D	AI (μg/day)[§]					
Vitamin C	RDA (mg/day)					
Fluoride	AI (mg/day)					
Zinc	RDA (mg/day)					
Vitamin A	RDA (μg/day)[§]					
Vitamin E	RDA (mg/day)					
Folate	RDA (μg/day)[§]					
Vitamin B$_{12}$	RDA (μg/day)[§]					

§ Micrograms (mcg) per day.

4. Your friend has healthy school-age children and she tells you: "Many parents I talked to give nutrient supplements to their children. Do you think I should give some to my children? What kind would you recommend giving them?"

   Explain what you would tell her.

   _____

   _____

   _____

   _____

   _____

   _____

   _____

5. Are low-carbohydrate diets recommended for children? Explain your answer.

   _____

   _____

   _____

   _____

   _____

   _____

   _____

CHALLENGE YOUR LEARNING

CASE STUDY

Objectives

The case of P.B. will help you understand what the nutritional needs of toddlers are and how challenging it can be for new parents to offer the best diet to favor the growth of their young child, especially when it is the first child in the family. Toddlers are not mini-adults and they do have special needs. Keep that in mind as you are trying to help the parents.

Description

P.B., an 18-month-old toddler, is growing on the slow side of normal. P.B. is the only child in his family and both his parents are quite tall. The pediatrician refers him to you for a nutritional assessment. In planning the first visit, you ask P.B.'s parents to prepare a detailed record of their son's food intake over 3 days, including a weekend day. At the visit, the parents give you the food record illustrated in the table below. They tell you that this food record is representative of their son's food intake in the last few months. The mother explains that P.B. is hungry for breakfast, but that he does not eat much for the other meals and ends up playing with his food a lot. When asking parents questions, you find out that P.B. really likes juice and regularly asks for it throughout the day. You also realize that P.B.'s parents are giving him a children's chewable multivitamin and mineral supplement tablet with breakfast.

	RECORD OF P.B.'s FOOD INTAKE OVER 3 DAYS		
Food Intake	**Thursday, March 25, 2007**	**Friday, March 26, 2007**	**Saturday, March 27, 2007**
Breakfast (around 7:00 a.m., at home)	Rice ready-to-eat breakfast cereal, ⅓ cup (79 mL) Honey, 1 tsp (5 mL) Milk 1% fat, ⅓ cup (79 mL)	Rice ready-to-eat breakfast cereal, ⅓ cup (79 mL) Honey, 1 tsp (5 mL) Milk 1% fat, ⅓ cup (79 mL)	Rice ready-to-eat breakfast cereal, ⅓ cup (79 mL) Honey, 1 tsp (mL) Milk 1% fat, ⅓ cup (79 mL)
Morning Snack (time varied, at home)	Hard cheese curds, 2 small pieces Fruit beverage, ½ cup (4 fluid oz, 118 mL) in a baby bottle	4 Green grapes Fruit beverage, ½ cup (4 fluid oz, 118 mL) in a baby bottle	½ Mini box of raisins Fruit beverage, ½ cup (4 fluid oz, 118 mL) in a baby bottle
Lunch (time and place varied)	White bread, ½ slice Peanut butter, 1 Tbsp (15 mL) Grape jelly, 1 tsp (5 mL) Apple juice, ½ cup (4 fluid oz, 118 mL)	White bread, ½ slice Light cream cheese, 1 Tbsp (15 mL) 1 Small carrot stick Chocolate milk 1% fat, ⅓ cup (79 mL)	5 French fries, with salt and ketchup ¼ Plain child-size restaurant hamburger Orange soda pop, ⅓ cup (79 mL)
Early Afternoon Snack (before dinner place varied)	Red popsicle (at aunt's house)	Green popsicle (at aunt's house)	10 Jellybeans (at home)

(continued)

RECORD OF P.B.'s FOOD INTAKE OVER 3 DAYS   *(continued)*

Food Intake	Thursday, March 25, 2007	Friday, March 26, 2007	Saturday, March 27, 2007
Late Afternoon Snack (before dinner, place varied)	Apple juice, ½ cup (4 fluid oz, 118 mL) in a baby bottle	Apple juice, ½ cup (4 fluid oz, 118 mL) in a baby bottle	Apple juice, ½ cup (4 fluid oz, 118 mL) in a baby bottle
Dinner (time and place varied)	¼ Plain hot dog, with ketchup Applesauce, 2 Tbsp (30 mL) Milk 1% fat, ⅓ cup (79 mL)	¼ Slice pizza, pepperoni and cheese 1 Glazed mini-doughnut Cola beverage, ⅓ cup (79 mL)	Basmati rice, ¼ cup (59 mL) Soy sauce, 1 tsp (5 mL) Cooked frozen peas, 2 Tbsp (30 mL) Milk 1% fat, ⅓ cup (79 mL)
Evening Snack (time varied, at home)	½ cup (118 mL) popcorn, with butter and salt	1 Glazed mini-doughnut	Mini ice-cream cone, with 2 Tbsp (30 mL) low-fat vanilla ice-cream
Bedtime Snack (around 8 p.m., at home)	Fruit beverage, ⅓ cup (79 mL) in a baby bottle	Milk 1% fat, ⅓ cup (79 mL) in a baby bottle	Apple juice, ⅓ cup (79 mL) in a baby bottle

1. What important principles of diet planning are used to promote health in toddlers? List eight of them.

   Principle #1: _____

   Principle #2: _____

   Principle #3: _____

   Principle #4: _____

   Principle #5: _____

   Principle #6: _____

   Principle #7: _____

   Principle #8: _____

2. Analyze P.B.'s diet.

   1- Identify 13 **problems** with the current dietary intake of P.B. according to the food record table provided above. *(Note: Try to prioritize your list, starting with the most critical problems.)*

   2- Indicate in brackets which **principle** of diet planning promoting health (from Q 1.) is not followed.

   3- For each problem, make a practical **suggestion** in line with the principles of diet planning promoting good health, so that P.B.'s parents can modify and improve the dietary intake of their toddler. *(Note: Explain your suggestion and provide some concrete examples.)*

   Problem 1: _____

   [**Principle #**_____]

   Suggestion: _____

   Problem 2: _____

   [**Principle #**_____]

   Suggestion: _____

Problem 3: _____

[Principle #_____]

Suggestion: _____

Problem 4: _____

[Principle #_____]

Suggestion: _____

Problem 5: _____

[Principle #_____]

Suggestion: _____

Problem 6: _____

[Principle #_____]

Suggestion: _____

Problem 7: _____

[Principle #_____]

Suggestion: _____

Problem 8: _____

[Principle #_____]

Suggestion: _____

Problem 9: _____

[Principle #_____]

Suggestion: _____

Problem 10: _____

[Principle #_____]

Suggestion: _____

Problem 11: _____

[Principle #_____]

Suggestion: _____

Problem 12: _____

[Principle #_____]

Suggestion: _____

Problem 13: _____

[Principle #_____]

Suggestion: _____

3. Use the following table to propose a realistic 3-day toddler menu appropriate for P.B. This sample menu illustrating how to integrate your suggestions will be helpful to explain to P.B.'s parents how to progressively implement the dietary changes you are recommending for their toddler.

SUGGESTED 3-DAY TODDLER MENU FOR P.B.

Food Intake	Day 1	Day 2	Day 3
Breakfast			
Midmorning Snack			
Lunch			
Midafternoon Snack			
Dinner			
Midevening Snack			

4. Is the 3-day sample menu you prepared for P.B. meeting daily food group servings recommended for toddlers? Use the following table to find out and readjust your menu if necessary.

FOOD GROUP SERVINGS RECOMMENDED DAILY AND SERVING SIZES FOR TODDLERS

	Approximate Number of Toddler-Size Servings Recommended Daily	Approximate Size of One Serving for Toddlers	Day 1 (number of servings) and [total amount]	Day 2 (number of servings) and [total amount]	Day 3 (number of servings) and [total amount]
Grains	5–6	• ½ slice bread • ⅓–½ cup (79–118 mL) rice, pasta, cereal			
Meat and alternatives	2–3	• One egg • 2–4 Tbsp (30–60 mL) meat, beans, poultry or fish			

FOOD GROUP SERVINGS RECOMMENDED DAILY AND SERVING SIZES FOR TODDLERS   *(continued)*

	Approximate Number of Toddler-Size Servings Recommended Daily	Approximate Size of One Serving for Toddlers	Day 1 (number of servings) and [total amount]	Day 2 (number of servings) and [total amount]	Day 3 (number of servings) and [total amount]
Milk products	4	• ⅓–½ cup (79–118 mL) milk • 2–4 Tbsp (30–60 mL) cottage cheese • 1 oz (1 inch cube, 28 g) hard cheese			
Vegetables	3–4	• 2–4 Tbsp vegetable (30–60 mL or ⅛–¼ cup)			
Fruits	3–4	• ⅓–½ cup (79–118 mL) fruit juice* • 2–4 Tbsp fruit (30–60 mL or ⅛–¼ cup) • ½ small fruit			

* Limit juice to a maximum of ½ cup (4 fluid oz, 118 mL) per day.

5. Analyze your 3-day sample menu with diet analysis software to see if your sample menu will meet P.B.'s daily energy and nutrient needs.

NUTRIENT ANALYSIS OF 3-DAY MENU FOR P.B.

Energy and Nutrients	DRIs	Daily Needs of Toddlers (1–3 years old)	Content of Day 1	Content of Day 2	Content of Day 3	3-Day Average
Energy	**Average EER for males (kcal/day) [kJ/day]**					
Protein	RDA (g/day)					
Carbohydrate	RDA (g/day)					
Total fiber	AI (g/day)					
Iron	RDA (mg/day)					
Calcium	AI (mg/day)					
Vitamin D	AI (μg/day)					
Vitamin C	RDA (mg/day)					

(continued)

NUTRIENT ANALYSIS OF 3-DAY MENU FOR P.B. *(continued)*

Energy and Nutrients	DRIs	Daily Needs of Toddlers (1–3 years old)	Content of Day 1	Content of Day 2	Content of Day 3	3-Day Average
Zinc	RDA (mg/day)					
Vitamin A	RDA (µg/day)					
Vitamin E	RDA (mg/day)					
Folate	RDA (µg/day)					
Vitamin B$_{12}$	RDA (µg/day)					

Case Follow-Up

The mother phones in a panic at the clinic 5 days later to ask you what to do with P.B., who has just accidentally ingested about three animal-shaped children's chewable multivitamin and mineral supplement tablets while she was answering the door. The composition of each chewable multivitamin and mineral supplement tablet is described in the table below.

COMPOSITION OF A TABLET OF P.B.'S CHEWABLE MULTIVITAMIN AND MINERAL SUPPLEMENT

Nutrient	Amount per Tablet
Vitamin A	5000 IU
Vitamin B$_1$ (thiamin)	1.5 mg
Vitamin B$_2$ (riboflavin)	1.5 mg
Vitamin B$_6$ (pyridoxine)	1.0 mg
Vitamin B$_{12}$ (cobalamin)	3 µg
Biotin	30 µg
Vitamin C	50 mg
Vitamin D	400 IU
Vitamin E	10 IU
Folic acid	0.1 mg
Niacin	15 mg
Pantothenic acid	10 mg
Calcium	160 mg
Iron (ferrous fumarate)	4 mg
Phosphorus	125 mg
Copper	1 mg

6. What is your advice to the worried mother?

7. Why should parents and caregivers be warned that children's multivitamin mineral supplements represent a poisoning danger for children?

8. Determine if the total amount of nutrients P.B. accidentally ingested exceed the Tolerable Upper Intake Levels (UL) for vitamins and minerals. Also indicate the signs and symptoms of nutrient overdose and toxicity.

AMOUNT OF NUTRIENTS INGESTED BY P.B. IN COMPARISON WITH TOLERABLE UPPER INTAKE LEVELS

Nutrient	Amount Ingested in Three Supplement Tablets	Comparison of Amount Ingested versus UL ($>$, $<$, $=$)	UL for Toddlers (1–3 years old)	Overdose and Toxicity Signs and Symptoms
Vitamin A				
Vitamin B$_1$ (thiamin)				
Vitamin B$_2$ (riboflavin)				
Vitamin B$_6$ (pyridoxine)				
Vitamin B$_{12}$ (cobalamin)				
Biotin				
Vitamin C				
Vitamin D				
Vitamin E				
Folate				
Niacin				
Pantothenic acid				
Calcium				
Iron				
Phosphorus				
Copper				

9. How many micrograms of vitamin A (as Retinol Equivalents) did P.B. ingest, supposing that he accidentally ingested three supplement tablets? *(Note that 1 μg Retinol Equivalent [RE] equals 3.33 IU of retinol.)*

10. How many micrograms of vitamin D (as cholecalciferol) did P.B. ingest, supposing that he accidentally ingested three supplement tablets? *(Note that 1 μg vitamin D [as cholecalciferol] equals 40 IU of vitamin D.)*

11. How many milligrams of vitamin E (as α-tocopherol) did P.B. ingest, supposing that he accidentally ingested three supplement tablets? *(Note that 1 IU of vitamin E equals 0.67 mg α-tocopherol.)*

12. Which nutrient(s) did P.B take in overdose that could harm him, supposing that he accidentally ingested three supplement tablets?

13. Which nutrient contained in multivitamin mineral supplements is the most often involved in poisoning deaths of children under 6 years old?

14. Define hemochromatosis.

3.4 Nutrition in Adolescence

REVIEW THE INFORMATION

1. Use this grid to help you fill the text with appropriate words related to the teenage period.

The Teenage Period

Adolescence is the period of intense a) _____ (word of 8 letters), intellectual, emotional, and social b) _____ (word of 7 letters) and development occurring between c) _____ (word of 6 letters) and 21 years of age. Physically, adolescents rapidly transform from a child to a young adult's body as they go through d) _____ (word of 7 letters) at the beginning of adolescence. Puberty is characterized by sexual maturation, the adolescent growth e)_____ (word of 5 letters), and changes in body composition. The teenage growth pattern is f) _____ (word of 9 letters) for males and females. Females generally mature earlier and deposit more g) _____ (word of 3 letters) tissue than males, who develop more muscle tissue. As adolescents adjust to their fast-growing bodies, they become self-conscious and sometimes awkward and worried about their changing size, h)_____ (word of 5 letters), abilities, and emerging sexuality. Emotionally, they need to be reassured by parents and other significant adults that this is a i) _____ (word of 6 letters), desirable, and important phase of their maturation to adulthood. This way they can develop a positive personal j) _____ (word of 8 letters) and be confident in their ability to take on responsibilities and become self-sufficient. Adolescents need k)_____ (word of 7 letters) and encouragement from their families as they develop their potential, establish their own value system, create their life vision, and struggle to become socially l) _____ (word of 10 letters). Acceptance by m)_____ (word of 5 letters) is very important for adolescents, who spend a lot of time n) _____ (word of 4 letters) from home as they strive to become independent. However, sooner or later, adolescents follow their occupational aspirations and find their o)_____ (word of 4 letters). Generally, adolescents are energetic, p) _____ (word of 6 letters), idealistic, sensitive, and curious individuals, who are eager to learn and try q)_____ (word of 3 letters) ways of doing things.

2. Malnutrition can result from

   a) inadequate energy intake   d) excess nutrient intake
   b) inadequate nutrient intake   e) all of the above
   c) excess energy intake

3. Which chemical form of iron is more easily absorbed?   _____

UNDERSTAND THE CONCEPTS

1. Fill in each blank space with the appropriate word.

   The teenage growth spurt starts in preadolescence and consists of 2–3 years of a) _____ growth, followed by a few years of b) _____ growth. It generally starts at 10–11 years old and peaks at about c) _____ years old for females. For males, it usually starts at 12–13 years old and peaks at about d) _____ years of age. The early stage of the growth spurt is characterized by rapid e) _____ growth, during which females grow about 6¾ inches (17 cm) and males about 8¾ inches (22 cm) taller. This growth ends with the closure of the f) _____ or extremities of bones. The later stage of the growth spurt consists mainly of g) _____ growth. Females gain an average of h) _____ lb or i) _____ kg. Their hips widen and fat deposition favors the development of breasts, as well as the onset of menses or *j)* _____.

Males gain about *k)* _____ lb or *l)* _____ kg during this period, principally in

lean body mass. *m)* _____ changes influence the growth, state of mind, and sexual awareness and maturation of adolescents. In males, sexual maturation is characterized by an enlargement of the

testicles and the penis, changes in the *n)* _____ causing deepening of the voice, and the

appearance of body hair in the *o)* _____, underarm, chest, and genital areas. In females,

secondary sexual changes include the maturation of *p)* _____ and breasts, and appearance

of body hair in the genital areas. *q)* _____, a skin condition, may develop during this period.

2. How does the growth spurt of puberty affect nutritional needs during adolescence?

   _____

3. The _____ of puberty varies between adolescents.

   a) starting age   c) overall duration   e) a, c, and d
   b) sequence of changes   d) pace of each change

4. What is the implication of the last question on the way a group of teenagers of the same age look physically?

   _____

   _____

   _____

   _____

5. What body part(s) grow(s) first during the adolescent growth spurt?

   a) Trunk   c) Hips and chest   e) Feet and hands
   b) Shoulders   d) Calves and forearms

6. Youth gain nearly _____% of their adult bone mass during their teenage growth.

   a) 10   c) 30   e) 50
   b) 20   d) 40

7. Throughout adolescence, teens gain as much as _____% of their healthy adult body weight.

   a) 10   c) 30   e) 50
   b) 20   d) 40

8. The lean body mass of males increases by _____% from ages 10–17 years old.

   a) 10   c) 30   e) 50
   b) 20   d) 40

9. The average percent body fat of teenage girls increases from 16% to _____% over the period of adolescence.

   a) 17   c) 27   e) 37
   b) 20   d) 30

10. After the occurrence of menarche, females need to have a minimum of _____% body fat to sustain a regular cycle of ovulation.

    a) 16   c) 25   e) 33
    b) 19   d) 29

11. The start of menses can range between _____ and _____ years of age.

    a) 7; 15   c) 11; 19   e) 15; 23
    b) 9; 17   d) 13; 21

12. The mean age for menarche is about _____ years of age.

    a) 10–11   c) 14–15 e) 18–19
    b) 12–13   d) 16–17

13. Indicate whether the following statements are TRUE or FALSE, and justify your answer.

    1- _____: Adolescents often change the way they eat, but the eating habits they adopt as late adolescents are usually maintained in adulthood.

    Justification: _____

    _____

    _____

    2- _____: Females limiting their energy intake can have delayed menarche.

    Justification: _____

    _____

    _____

    3- _____: Teenagers' folate intake is usually adequate.

    Justification: _____

    _____

    _____

    4- _____: Adolescents have higher calcium and phosphorus needs than adults.

    Justification: _____

    _____

    _____

    5- _____: Teenagers' calcium intake is often inadequate.

    Justification: _____

    _____

    _____

    6- _____: Milk products are fattening and can cause acne.

    Justification: _____

    _____

    _____

    7- _____: Vitamin A supplementation helps to reduce acne.

    Justification: _____

    _____

    _____

    8- _____: Teenagers can easily get the iron they need from vegetables and legumes.

    Justification: _____

    _____

    _____

9- _____: Teenage boys aged 14 years and older have higher iron needs than teenage girls.

Justification: _____

_____

_____

10- _____: Teenage girls usually have a low iron intake.

Justification: _____

_____

_____

14. What is the vitamin A tolerable upper intake level (UL) for teenagers?

_____

_____

_____

15. Why are iron needs increased during adolescence? Explain.

_____

_____

_____

16. What is the term for the abnormal absence of monthly menstruations, which can occur after menarche?

_____

17. What can cause monthly menstruations to stop in a teenager?

_____

_____

_____

_____

18. Based on the DRI recommendations, are there any nutrients for which the RDA or AI are not increased in the transition from childhood to adulthood?

_____

_____

_____

19. What <u>general</u> eating and food-related behaviors characterize the adolescent population?

_____

_____

_____

_____

_____

20. Give examples of <u>healthy</u> eating and food-related behaviors found in adolescents.

_____

_____

_____

_____

_____

_____

_____

_____

_____

_____

_____

21. Give examples of <u>unhealthy</u> eating and food-related behaviors found in adolescents.

_____

_____

_____

_____

_____

_____

_____

_____

_____

_____

_____

_____

_____

22. Which nutrients are often inadequate in the diet of teenagers?

_____

_____

_____

23. Which nutrients are often found in excess in the diet of teenagers?

_____

24. Because of their active nature, teens are often on the go. Give 12 concrete tips to help teens eat healthy on the go.

_____

_____

_____

_____

_____

_____

_____

_____

_____

_____

_____

_____

_____

25. The aspect having the least effect on the macronutrient requirements of teenagers is their

   a) age
   b) physical activity level
   c) degree of biologic and sexual maturation
   d) age at start of puberty
   e) rate of growth

26. What factors affect bone growth and development?

_____

_____

_____

27. What are the calcium Adequate Intakes (AI) for boys and girls between 9 and 18 years of age?

   a) 1000 mg/day for girls and 1200 mg/day for boys between 9 and 18 years old
   b) 1000 mg/day for girls and boys between 9 and 13 years old, and 1200 mg/day for girls and boys between 14 and 18 years old
   c) 1200 mg/day for girls and boys between 9 and 13 years old, and 1300 mg/day for girls and boys between 14 and 18 years old
   d) 1000 mg/day for boys and 1300 mg/day for girls between 9 and 18 years old
   e) 1300 mg/day for boys and girls between 9 and 18 years old

28. Calcium bioavailability

Complete each space with an appropriate choice from the lists provided in parentheses.

One cup (8 fluid oz) or 237 mL of a) _____ (skim, 1% fat, 2% fat, whole, or all of these

answers) milk provides b) _____ (15, 115, 215, 315, or 415) mg of calcium, of which

c) _____ (32, 42, 52, 62, or 72) % is absorbed. Therefore, a cup (8 fluid oz, 237 mL) of milk

provides d) _____ (10, 93, 98, 101, or none of these answers) mg of bioavailable calcium.

One cup (8 fluid oz, 237 mL) of white beans contains e) _____ (7, 70, 170, 270, or 370) mg of

calcium, of which f) _____ (7, 17, 27, 37, or 47) is absorbed, providing about

g) _____ (3, 6, 29, 59, or none of these answers) mg of bioavailable calcium.

29. Explain the nutritional and health consequences of the following practices.

a) Drinking alcohol

_____

_____

_____

_____

_____

b) Cigarette smoking

_____

_____

_____

_____

_____

c) Marijuana smoking

_____

_____

_____

_____

_____

_____

d) Using cocaine

_____

_____

_____

_____

_____

30. What are eating disorders?

_____

_____

_____

_____

_____

31. Give some examples of eating disorders teenagers may have.

_____

_____

_____

_____

_____

INTEGRATE YOUR LEARNING

1. Determine if the following statements characterize _male_ or _female_ adolescents.

    a) They start their growth spurt earlier. _____

    b) They generally grow at a faster rate. _____

    c) Their energy needs peak sooner. _____

    d) They have higher lean body mass. _____

    e) They attain lower height and weight. _____

    f) They have higher iron needs. _____

    g) They tend to control their body weight by increasing their physical activity. _____

    h) They tend to control their body weight by restricting their dietary intake. _____

2. Adolescents, even of the same age, are at different stages of sexual and biologic maturation. What is the impact of this statement on the nutritional needs of the adolescent population?

    _____

    _____

3. What should be taken into consideration when determining the nutritional needs of adolescents?

    _____

    _____

    _____

4. Describe how physical and sexual maturation in teenage girls can affect them psychologically and emotionally, especially for those starting puberty early.

    _____

    _____

    _____

    _____

    _____

5. Describe how a late physical and sexual maturation in teenage boys can affect them psychologically and emotionally.

    _____

    _____

    _____

6. What factors influence iron absorption?

7. What factors increase iron absorption?

8. What factors decrease iron absorption?

9. What are the three stages of development of iron depletion leading to iron deficiency anemia, which can be detected by laboratory measurements?

1-

2-

3-

10. Is anemia always due to iron deficiency? Explain.

11. What are the effects of malnutrition due to the <u>lack</u> of food intake during adolescence?

_____
_____
_____
_____
_____
_____

12. What are the consequences of malnutrition due to <u>excess</u> food intake during adolescence?

_____
_____
_____
_____
_____
_____

13. What factors are promoting overweight and obesity in our adolescent populations? Explain five of them.

1- _____
_____

2- _____
_____

3- _____
_____

4- _____
_____

5- _____
_____

14. What are the dangers of vitamin A supplementation by misinformed teenagers?

_____
_____
_____
_____
_____
_____

15. Which statement is true about addictive substances?

    a) People abusing alcohol are often said to have "the munchies" as they snack all the time.
    b) Smoking marijuana increases the risk of lung cancer, similar to smoking tobacco.
    c) Cocaine abusers have an increased enjoyment of eating, especially of sweets.
    d) Weight loss is common in those who stop tobacco smoking.
    e) Cocaine abuse frequently leads to eating disorders.

16. Teenagers think short term and sometimes have unrealistic perceptions about their health, which prevents them from seeing the consequences of their actions in the longer term. Give some examples illustrating this.

_____

_____

_____

_____

_____

_____

17. Fill in this summary table of the DRI recommendations for some key nutrients for youth. *(DRI recommendation tables can be found in the appendix section at the end of this book.)*

DRI RECOMMENDATIONS FOR KEY NUTRIENTS FOR MALE AND FEMALE YOUTH

Nutrients	DRIs	12–13 years old Males	12–13 years old Females	14–18 years old Males	14–18 years old Females	Tolerable Upper Intake Level (UL)
Protein	AMDR (% of energy)					
Carbohydrate	AMDR (% of energy)					
Fat	AMDR (% of energy)					
Protein	RDA (g/day)					
Carbohydrate	RDA (g/day)					
Total fiber	AI (g/day)					
Total water	AI (L/day)					
Iron	RDA (mg/day)					
Calcium	AI (mg/day)					
Vitamin D	AI (μg/day)[§]					
Vitamin C	RDA (mg/day)					
Zinc	RDA (mg/day)					
Vitamin A	RDA (μg/day)[§]					
Vitamin E	RDA (mg/day)					
Folate	RDA (μg/day)[§]					
Vitamin B_{12}	RDA (μg/day)[§]					

[§] Micrograms (mcg) per day.

CHALLENGE YOUR LEARNING

CASE STUDY

Objectives

With this case you will see how active some teenagers can be and what aspects need to be taken into consideration to help them meet their nutritional and growth needs so they become healthy adults. Teenage girls especially might have a harder time acquiring a healthy nutritional status due to social and peer pressures.

Description

A 17-year-old Swedish female athlete named S.J. recently joined the athletic center where you work as a dietitian. Her swimming coach recommended she do extra physical training at the gym three times a week in addition to the daily early morning swimming practices to increase her strength and endurance. He also said it would be good for her to talk to a dietitian. S.J. actively trains as an elite competitive swimmer all year round. The styles she excels at are breast-stroke and butterfly, for which she won two medals at national junior competitions last year. She is the rising star of the regional competitive swimming club in her age group and has been chosen as captain of the girls' junior group for the coming year.

During the summer, S.J. works as a lifeguard and swimming instructor at a children and youth sports camp a few hours away from home. She loves children and enjoys showing them how to water play. She also likes giving swimming lessons to older children. During school, she teaches at a local pool on Saturdays.

S.J. is finishing high school in a health science concentration this year and needs high grades to enter college. This is not easy because of her heavy training schedule, but S.J. is quite a perfectionist and determined adolescent. She also has high aspirations. Two years ago, her parents took her on a trip to the Olympics and she had the time of her life. She hopes that she will be accepted to a university sports medicine program next year and plans to join the university swimming team. She dreams about qualifying for the next Olympic games in 2 years.

Therefore, S.J. is usually on the go, except on Sundays, which are reserved for time at home with her parents and two younger sisters. On Sundays, S.J. does grocery shopping, laundry, and cooking with her mother. She sometimes takes her sisters to the nearby fast food restaurant in the afternoon.

Last time S.J. came to the athletic center, she asked for an appointment with you to have more information about healthy eating. You are delighted and are now preparing for that meeting.

1. What are the key nutritional needs of adolescents?

2. What are some challenges for today's adolescents in order to meet their nutritional needs?

3. What are the special nutritional needs of female versus male adolescents?

4. What are some challenges for today's female adolescents to meet their nutritional needs?

5. What are the key nutritional needs of athletes, including swimmers like S.J.?

6. Which nutrient should be the main source of energy in the diet of athletes in order to favor optimal performance, especially during prolonged exercise and for endurance sports? Explain.

7. Do athletes need to adopt a high-protein diet or take protein/amino acid supplements to meet their protein needs? Explain.

8. What are the special nutritional needs of female versus male athletes?

9. What are the key nutritional needs of female teenage athletes like S.J.?

10. What is the "Female Athlete Triad"?

11. What are the consequences of the "Female Athlete Triad"?

12. What do you perceive are some challenges for S.J. to meet her nutritional needs?

13. Fill in each blank space with an appropriate word.

   a) _____ is involved in muscle contraction. Low blood levels of this mineral are associated

   with skeletal muscle b) _____.

Case Follow-up

You finally meet with S.J. Together, you talk about healthy eating and she has many questions for you. She wants to know what fluids she should be drinking while training, and if you recommend that she consume sports foods and supplements to increase her performance. She says that many of her teammates are consuming some sports foods and also some types of nutritive or nonnutritive supplements.

14. What should athletes drink when they exercise intensely or for a long period of time? (Water? Fruit juice or beverage? Soda pop? Sports drinks?)

15. Is thirst a good gauge of the need to drink fluids? Explain.

16. How much fluid should athletes drink when exercising? How often should they drink?

17. What are sports foods? Give some examples.

18. Do you recommend that S.J. consume sports foods? Explain.

19. What are sports supplements? Give some examples.

20. List some of the sport supplements or dietary supplements most commonly used by athletes.

21. Do you recommend S.J. take sports and dietary supplements? Explain.

3.5 Nutrition in Adulthood

REVIEW THE INFORMATION

1. Fill in each blank space with the most appropriate choice provided in parentheses.

   Adulthood represents a period of about a) _____ (55, 60, 65, or 70) years. Early or young

   adults are of age b) _____ (16–25, 18–40, 19–30, or 21–35) years old. Although most young

   adults have attained their maximum stature, they reach their peak bone density around c) _____ (25, 30, 35, or 40) years old. Their muscle mass will also continue to increase if they continue to be physically active. Most individuals have an active lifestyle and achieve their peak physical capacity during early adulthood.

   In our busy societies, adults tend to eat more often at d) _____ (home, work, restaurants,

   or *relatives'*) and to buy more e) _____ (pre-prepared, convenience, ready-to-eat, or *all three answers*) foods than their parents did. Some individuals are so busy that they forget to pay attention to their lifestyle and food habits.

   Middle-age adults are between f) _____ (26 and 54, 31 and 64, 36 and 59, or 41 and 69) years of age. Midlife is marked by hormonal changes, which have an impact on nutritional status, including

g) _____ (menarche, menopause, or climacteric) in men and h) _____ (menarche, menopause, or climacteric) in women. Many middle-aged adults become less active and tend to gain weight during this period, which makes them more at risk for developing chronic diseases, such as

i) _____ (type 2 diabetes mellitus, hyperlipidemia, cardiovascular disease, or all three answers). The pleasure of preparing and sharing everyday food or special occasion meals with family members, relatives, friends, and community members at home or in various settings is an important part of the social life of adults and contributes to their quality of life and enjoyment of living. Food security, however, is

an issue for some adults, who have limited access to j)_____ (affordable, nutritious, culturally acceptable, safe, or all four answers) foods.

For adults of all ages, having sound eating and nutritional habits will positively influence their

k) _____ (physical, mental, future, or all three answers) health and well-being. Late adults or the elderly are of age l) _____ (55, 60, 65, or 70) years old and over.

2. What activities are common to young adults?

_____

_____

_____

_____

_____

_____

3. What activities are common to middle adults?

_____

_____

_____

_____

_____

4. Explain what *health* means.

_____

_____

5. Explain the statement "good health is a lifelong journey."

_____

_____

_____

6. What factors influence the eating behaviors of adults?

_____

_____

_____

_____

_____

_____

7. What BMI range is associated with the lowest risk of developing health problems in adult men and women?

_____

8. What BMI ranges are associated with an increased or high risk of developing health problems in adult men and women?

_____

_____

_____

_____

_____

9. What are the positive effects of healthy eating and physical activity in young and middle adults?

_____

_____

_____

_____

10. What is a *chronic disease*?

_____

_____

11. What are *risk factors* for chronic diseases?

_____

_____

12. A poor diet can promote the development of which chronic diseases?

_____

_____

13. What is a *dietary supplement*?

_____

_____

_____

_____

14. Which of the following foods are rich in vitamin E? Circle them.

Grapefruit juice	Pistachios	Sunflower seeds	Hazelnuts	Brazil nuts	Oatmeal
Safflower oil	Cauliflower	Sherbet	Wheat germ	Mayonnaise	Mango
Corn oil	Yellow beans	Cod liver	Molasses	Canola oil	Avocado
Milk	Pears	Pita bread	Coconut	Almonds	
Onions	Mushrooms	Yogurt	Salmon	Peanuts	

15. What are nutrient-dense foods?

_____

16. Give some examples of nutrient-dense foods.

_____

_____

17. What is an empty-calorie food?

_____

18. Give some examples of empty-calorie foods.

_____

_____

19. Explain the statement "there is no good or bad food."

_____

_____

_____

_____

_____

_____

_____

UNDERSTAND THE CONCEPTS

1. During what period of the life cycle are bones remodeled to become more dense and thicker?

_____

2. Why are women at risk of iron deficiency in early adulthood?

_____

_____

3. Why is the Estimated Energy Requirement (EER) of young adult women different from that of young adult men?

_____

_____

4. Why does the basal energy expenditure of middle adults decline compared to that of young adults?

_____

_____

5. What is menopause?

_____

_____

6. What is climacteric?

_____

_____

7. Women who experience menopause are on average between the ages of

   a) 40 and 45   d) 55 and 60
   b) 45 and 50   e) 60 and 65
   c) 45 and 55

8. What is a *determinant of health*?

   _____

   _____

9. What are the main determinants of health? Explain what each of them entails.

   _____

   _____

   _____

   _____

   _____

   _____

   _____

   _____

10. What are the N.H.A.N.E.S.?

   _____

   _____

   _____

   _____

   _____

   _____

11. What have we learned about the health status of U.S. adults from N.H.A.N.E.S.?

   _____

   _____

   _____

   _____

   _____

12. What is "Healthy People 2010"?

   _____

   _____

   _____

   _____

   _____

13. What are the two ultimate goals of "Healthy People 2010"?

   1) _____

   2) _____

14. Indicate if the following nutritional practices are HEALTHY and helpful practices or potentially UNHEALTHY practices.

    a) _____: Ordering the large or super-sized meals to get more for your money and making an effort to eat it all.

    b) _____: Serving and eating a small or medium portion of food at a time

    c) _____: Drinking coffee or caffeine-containing beverages instead of breakfast

    d) _____: Eating slowly and taking the time to chew well

    e) _____: Smoking cigarettes or using drugs to curb your appetite

    f) _____: Taking a moment to ask yourself if you are still hungry before taking second helpings

    g) _____: Replacing meals by eating many snacks throughout the day

    h) _____: Making dinner the main meal of the day, then lying on the couch or going to bed

    i) _____: Skipping breakfast or lunch to stay lean

    j) _____: Sharing your large or super-sized food servings with family members or friends

    k) _____: Learning to enjoy the way food tastes naturally, without extra salt, fat, sugar, and condiments

    l) _____: Drinking soda pop throughout the day

    m) _____: Not eating breakfast or lunch because you do not have time in your hectic daily schedule

    n) _____: Drinking diet soda pop as the main fluid source throughout the day

    o) _____: Asking for the regular instead of large or super-sized at a restaurant

    p) _____: Drinking water as the main fluid source throughout the day

    q) _____: Consuming meal replacement shakes or bars instead of having regular meals

    r) _____: Planning meals and a list (mentally or in writing) before going to shop for groceries

    s) _____: Enjoy eating and treating yourself, without excess

    t) _____: Resisting the temptation to eat when you are not hungry

    u) _____: Making a conscious effort not to eat when hungry to stay lean

    v) _____: Going for a walk after lunch or dinner

    w) _____: Eating at sporadic and irregular times every day

    aa) _____: Stopping eating when you feel full, even if more food is offered to you

    bb) _____: Eating meals while doing something else (e.g., working, driving, watching television)

    cc) _____: Trying a bite of the food to see if you like it before adding extra salt, sugar, condiments, and fat, in case it does not need any

    dd) _____: Regularly going to all-you-can-eat buffet restaurants

    ee) _____: Making breakfast the main meal of the day

    ff) _____: Gulping down food in a rush without chewing or realizing how much you just ate

    gg) _____: Eating high-fat and high-energy foods at fast food restaurants every day

    hh) _____: Weighing yourself on a weekly or monthly basis to check if your body weight is stable or increasing/decreasing and readjusting your lifestyle pattern if necessary

    ii) _____: Taking your health for granted and not paying attention to what you eat and how much you eat jj) _____: Restricting your intake to a very limited variety of foods, possibly excluding some food group(s)

kk) _____: Eating regular meals, and possibly snacks, every day

15. How does physical activity help with weight management?

_____

_____

_____

16. Which dietary component has a high energy density and is frequently implicated in the development of obesity and other chronic diseases? _____

17. What is cholesterol?

_____

_____

18. In what foods is dietary cholesterol found?

_____

_____

_____

19. Why is cholesterol not an essential nutrient?

_____

_____

20. How are dietary fat and cholesterol transported in the blood?

_____

_____

_____

21. Where is cholesterol stored in the body?

_____

22. How does the body use cholesterol?

_____

_____

_____

23. What are LDLs?

_____

24. What happens when the diet is high in fat, saturated fat, and cholesterol?

_____

_____

_____

25. What are the long-term consequences of diets high in fat, saturated fat, and cholesterol?

_____

_____

_____

26. What are antioxidants?

   _____

   _____

27. Which micronutrient prevents fats from being oxidized? _____

28. What are hyperlipidemias?

   _____

   _____

   _____

29. What is type 2 diabetes mellitus?

   _____

   _____

   _____

30. What is heart disease?

   _____

   _____

   _____

31. What is cardiovascular disease?

   _____

   _____

   _____

32. Which of the following statements are true about the way adults learn?

   a) They usually wait for others to provide them with information.
   b) They all learn the same way.
   c) They have the same overall background of previous knowledge.
   d) They can be at different motivational stages.
   e) They always have to be pushed to learn and change.
   f) They can have a different background of education.
   g) They prefer that others (e.g., health care professionals) decide what is best for them.
   h) They have different perceived needs.
   i) They like to be involved in their learning.
   j) They want to understand and know why.
   k) They have varied life experiences.
   l) They have very similar needs and concerns.
   m) They prefer personalized information.
   n) They can be at different developmental stages.
   o) They are independent and often seek information and answers to their questions on their own.

33. Adults may or may not be ready to modify and improve their lifestyle habits, depending on the stage of change they are at.

   1- What are the stages of change?
   2- Explain each of them in terms of lifestyle habits.

   _____

   _____

   _____

_____

_____

_____

_____

_____

_____

_____

_____

_____

34. What are some of the community nutrition programs for adults in your area? Explain what they are.

_____

_____

_____

_____

_____

_____

_____

_____

35. What is the enrichment of food?

_____

_____

36. What is the fortification of food?

_____

37. Give some examples of fortified foods.

_____

38. What is the difference between a *natural food* and a *natural product*?

_____

39. What is an organic food?

_____

40. What is a genetically modified organism (GMO) or genetically modified food?

_____

_____

41. Give some examples of GMO foods found in some markets.

_____

_____

_____

_____

42. What are prebiotics?

_____

_____

43. What are probiotics?

_____

_____

44. Indicate whether the following statements are TRUE or FALSE, and justify your answers.

a) _____ : Many adults take dietary supplements.

Justification: _____

_____

b) _____ : Taking dietary supplements and natural products is necessary for good health.

Justification: _____

_____

c) _____ : Taking dietary supplements guarantees good health and prevents disease.

Justification: _____

_____

d) _____ : Taking a dietary supplement compensates for not eating healthy.

Justification: _____

_____

e) _____ : Too many vitamins and minerals is better than not enough.

Justification: _____

_____

_____

f) _____ : Food does not provide the same nutrient quality as it is used to provide; therefore, adults must take dietary supplements to meet their daily needs.

Justification: _____

_____

_____

g) _____ : It is better to take a dietary supplement of one nutrient than a multivitamin and mineral supplement.

Justification: _____

_____

h) _____: The safety and efficacy of numerous natural products or compounds has not been determined.

Justification: _____

_____

i) _____: Adults often take dietary supplements or herbal/natural products in an attempt to lose weight.

Justification: _____

_____

45. According to the Dietary Reference Intake guidelines, what are the Recommended Dietary Allowances for **iron** and the Adequate Intakes for **calcium** for women between 19 and 50 years of age (nonpregnant and nonlactating women)?

a) 15 mg/day for iron and 1200 mg/day for calcium
b) 18 mg/day for iron and 1000 mg/day for calcium
c) 12 mg/day for iron and 1300 mg/day for calcium
d) 27 mg/day for iron and 1300 mg/day for calcium
e) 13 mg/day for iron and 800 mg/day for calcium

46. Why is the calcium AI higher for middle adults than for young adults?

_____

47. The intake of four micronutrients tends to be especially low in people not eating any animal food sources. Which micronutrients are they?

_____

48. The two nutrients most lacking in the average adult diet, especially that of women, are

a)_____ and b) _____.

49. In general, a diet containing less than _____ kcal/day (_____ kJ/day) is nutritionally inadequate for an adult and is likely to be deficient in some nutrients.

INTEGRATE YOUR LEARNING

1. What health problems are associated with being overweight or obese?

_____

_____

2. Of what is waist circumference measurement an indicator?

_____

_____

3. What waist circumference cut-off values are associated with an increased risk of developing health problems?

_____

_____

4. What health problems are associated with being underweight?

_____

_____

5. Indicate whether the following statements are TRUE or FALSE, and justify your answer.

a) _____: Lifestyle changes are difficult, but possible.

Justification: _____

_____

_____

b) _____: There is no quick, effortless, and magical solution to obesity prevention and treatment.

Justification: _____

_____

_____

c) _____: There is no substitute for nutritionally adequate and sound dietary habits to keep the body healthy.

Justification: _____

_____

_____

d) _____: Very few overweight or obese people are able to lose weight.

Justification: _____

_____

_____

e) _____: Slim and active people do not have to pay attention to what they eat.

Justification: _____

_____

_____

f) _____: Physically active individuals can eat what they want and do not have to worry about chronic diseases.

Justification: _____

_____

_____

g) _____: "Learning" is different from "being informed."

Justification: _____

_____

_____

h) _____: "Knowing" is different from "doing."

Justification: _____

_____

_____

6. According to the guidelines for body weight classification in adults, the BMI range associated with a healthy body weight for most individuals and the least risk of developing health problems is

   _____ kg/m^2.

7. According to the guidelines for body weight classification in adults, obesity can be defined as excess body

   fat accumulation with a body mass index of _____ kg/m^2.

8. According to the present BMI interpretation guidelines, individuals with a BMI of *a)* _____

   are classified as obese class 1, those with a BMI of *b)* _____ as obese class 2, and those

   with a BMI of *c)* _____ as obese class 3 (or extremely obese).

9. You and a work colleague decide to eat lunch at the cafeteria. Your colleague is sedentary and obese. The menu offered is the following:

   ### Appetizers
   Cream of broccoli soup
   Chicken noodle soup
   Garden salad with balsamic vinaigrette
   Fried spicy cheese sticks
   Nachos plate (corn chips, sour cream, tomato salsa, and cheese)

   ### Entrees
   Hamburger and homemade French fries
   Large club sandwich (white bread, mayonnaise, bacon, sliced tomatoes, chicken)
   Fish and chips (fried fish, homemade chips, coleslaw)
   Individual 9" meat lover's pizza (pepperoni, cheese, bacon, ham, ground beef)
   Submarine sandwich (whole wheat 7" bun, mozzarella cheese,
   shaved lean chicken and ham, lettuce, mustard)

   ### Desserts
   Apple pie served hot with vanilla ice cream and caramel
   Assorted glazed danishes
   Fresh fruit salad
   Low-fat fruit yogurt
   Carrot cake
   Brownies with chocolate ice cream and hot fudge

   ### Beverages
   (available in regular or large size)

Cola pop	Diet cola pop
Orange pop	Ginger ale
Bottled water	Vegetable juice
Milk 1% fat	Pure orange juice
Coffee	Tea

Specialty coffee: Hazelnut and cream

If you had to recommend a healthy lunch for your middle-aged colleague and yourself from this cafeteria menu, what would you recommend? Justify your choices.

Appetizer: _____

Entree: _____

Dessert: _____

Beverage: _____

Justification: _____

_____

10. What are the main "Healthy People 2010" objectives related to the nutrition and the body weight of adults?

_____

_____

_____

_____

11. What types of diets contribute to an increased risk of developing these chronic diseases?

   a) Type 2 diabetes mellitus: _____

   _____

   b) Hypertension: _____

   _____

   c) Cardiovascular disease/atherosclerosis: _____

   _____

   d) Cancer: _____

   _____

12. Which food contains cholesterol?
   a) Butter   d) Nuts
   b) Margarine   e) Seeds
   c) Legumes

13. Give 10 tips for adults to select healthy foods at the grocery store.

   1) _____

   _____

   2) _____

   _____

   3) _____

   _____

   4) _____

   _____

   5) _____

   _____

   6) _____

   _____

   7) _____

   _____

8) _____

_____

_____

9) _____

_____

10)_____

_____

14. Indicate what the DRI recommendations are for the following nutrients during early and middle adulthood. *(DRI recommendation tables can be found in the appendix section at the end of this book.)*

KEY DRI RECOMMENDATIONS FOR EARLY AND MIDDLE-AGE ADULTS							
Nutrients	DRIs	Females*			Males		
		19–30 years	31–50 years	51–64 years	19–30 years	31–50 years	51–64 years
Protein	RDA (g/kg/day) and [g/day]						
Protein	AMDR (% of energy)						
Carbohydrate	RDA (g/day)						
Carbohydrate	AMDR (% of energy)						
Fat	AMDR (% of energy)						
Total fiber	AI (g/day)						
Total water	AI (L/day)						
Calcium	AI (mg/day)						
Vitamin D	AI (µg/day)						
Vitamin C	RDA (mg/day)						
Iron	RDA (mg/day)						
Vitamin A	RDA (µg/day)						
Vitamin E	RDA (mg/day)						
Folate	RDA (µg/day)						
Vitamin B_{12}	RDA (µg/day)						

* Nonpregnant and nonlactating females. For pregnant and lactating women, refer to appropriate DRI recommendations specific to pregnancy and lactation.

15. Answer the following questions using the summary table of key DRI recommendations for adults you completed in question 14.

a) What is the principal source of energy for adults, according to the AMDRs?

_____

b) Are protein RDAs the same for adults of all ages? Explain.

_____

_____

c) Which micronutrients have the same RDAs for females and males aged 19–64 years?

_____

d) Which micronutrients have the same AI recommendations for both female and male adults?

_____

e) Which micronutrients have the same RDAs for both early and middle adults?

_____

f) Which micronutrients have higher AI recommendations for adults aged 51–64 years than younger adults?

_____

g) Which micronutrients have higher RDAs for male than female adults?

_____

h) Which micronutrient has a higher RDA for female than male adults aged 19 to about 50 years?

_____

CHALLENGE YOUR LEARNING

CASE STUDY

Objectives

One objective of this case is to understand how complex individual health can be, as well as how multiple factors in someone's life can promote the development of disease. While change can be difficult, it is possible to help reduce the risk factors and help prevent the development of chronic diseases and their complications.

Another objective of this case is to highlight the importance of health care professionals constantly updating themselves on new information available, as well as being critical about information, such as that found on the Internet.

Description

B.D. is a 50-year-old archeologist. He started to work in the field when he was only 15 years old, helping his father, who ran a successful archeological consulting business. "Those were the good old days!" he tells you, when he would follow work crews all around the country looking for arrowheads, running from site to site. He would sleep content at night, tired from working hard physically, digging in the fields almost every workday, looking for discoveries. "I did that for 30 years!" he tells you with a proud smile on his face. "I was slim and strong like a young tree!" he continues. "There was no need to go to the gym back then, and I could eat everything I wanted! Mom would give us pancakes and fried eggs every morning for breakfast, and she would make sure to have meat pie and freshly made cake ready by dinner time when we came back."

In his 20s, B.D. used to party hard with his friends on the weekends. Some of his friends had a band, and that is how he met his wife. He was drinking alcohol and smoking cigarettes regularly every day then, but he reduced these behaviors at 34 years old when they had twins. From then on, B.D.'s life changed, with a lot of added stress. He had to work more hours to support his new family responsibilities and make ends meet while his wife was raising the twins at home and taking care of her mother at the same time.

Ten years later, his father passed away unexpectedly from a stroke at the age of 63. B.D. was left with the archeological business and his mother to take care of. Although B.D. had been working for his father all these years and truly enjoyed doing archeology in the field, he found it extremely challenging to become a businessman as well. He realized how hard his father must have been working to keep the business rolling with all of the employees to support and supervise. B.D. did not want to disappoint his mother and wife and took over the lead of the business, as his father had asked. He was spending countless sleepless nights worrying about the possibility of having to let lifelong employees go, as the business's profit margin was getting slimmer.

His new lifestyle as a small business owner was one that was sedentary and frustrating; he would spend hours sitting at his father's desk doing budgetary plans and things he did not like. Although he managed to do all right with the company's finances, he was extremely stressed. One way he could relieve part of his stress was to eat the traditional family homemade foods his wife and mother were ever so lovingly preparing for him. His mother would tell him, "Your father would be so proud of you, son!" as she would serve him his favorite foods, just like when he was working in the field. By the time he reached 55 years old, B.D. was an obese man and was diagnosed with hypertension, hyperlipidemia, and type 2 diabetes mellitus by his family physician. The same year, his mother had a cerebrovascular accident. She told B.D. that her own father (B.D.'s maternal grandfather) was obese and had diabetes mellitus.

1. What chronic disease(s) is B.D. suffering from?

2. For each chronic disease listed in question 1, identify what the risk factors were that favored their development in B.D.

3. What determinants or factors are influencing B.D.'s health? Explain.

4. For what other chronic disease(s) is B.D. at risk?

5. What is atherosclerosis?

6. What is the *metabolic syndrome* or *syndrome X*? Explain.

7. What possible lifestyle changes could B.D. make to improve his health?

8. At what stage of change is B.D.? Explain your answer.

9. What is ephedra?

10. Should B.D. be taking ephedra? Explain why.

11. What is a nutraceutical?

12. What are functional foods?

13. What are some examples of functional foods?

   1- For each functional food, indicate what is/are the key component(s).
   2- For each key component, indicate what are the associated potential health benefits.

14. What are phytochemicals?

15. What is leptin?

16. How can you find out if certain health information obtained from the Internet is credible and trustworthy?

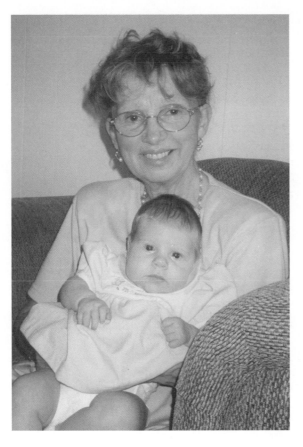

Photo provided by Isabelle Giroux, 2006.

3.6 Nutrition in Aging

REVIEW THE INFORMATION

1. Elderly individuals are _____ years old and older.

   a) 55   b) 65   c) 75   d) 85   e) 95

2. The **young old** are elderly individuals

   a) between 55 and 64 years old
   b) between 65 and 74 years old
   c) between 75 and 84 years old

   d) 85 years old and older
   e) 95 years old and older

3. The **aged** are elderly individuals

   a) between 55 and 64 years old
   b) between 65 and 74 years old
   c) between 75 and 84 years old

   d) 85 years old and older
   e) 95 years old and older

4. The **oldest old** are elderly individuals

   a) between 55 and 64 years old
   b) between 65 and 74 years old
   c) between 75 and 84 years old

   d) 85 years old and older
   e) 95 years old and older

5. Elderly individuals represent almost _____% of the overall population in Canada and the United States.

   a) 10   c) 30   e) 50
   b) 20   d) 40

6. What age category is increasing most quickly in the United States and Canada?

   _____

7. What is the current life expectancy in the United States and Canada?

   a) Just over 71 years old   d) About 85 years old
   b) About 75 years old   e) Almost 90 years old
   c) Just over 79 years old

8. Life expectancy is

   a) the same for both men and women   d) decreasing
   b) longer for women   e) staying the same
   c) longer for men

9. What is the life span of humans?

   a) About 100 years   c) About 110 years   e) About 120 years
   b) About 105 years   d) About 115 years

10. What is the principal cause of illness and death in Canada and the United States?

    a) Diabetes mellitus   d) Chronic obstructive lung disease
    b) Cancer   e) Ischemic heart disease
    c) Pneumonia and influenza

11. Explain what quality of life means.

    _____

    _____

    _____

    _____

12. What factors impact quality of life?

    _____

    _____

    _____

13. What elements can <u>reduce</u> the quality of life of aging individuals? Provide at least six elements and give an example to illustrate and explain how each element impairs quality of life.

    1- Element: _____

       Example: _____

    _____

    _____

    _____

    _____

    _____

    _____

2- Element: _____

Example: _____

_____

_____

_____

_____

_____

_____

_____

3- Element: _____

Example: _____

_____

_____

_____

_____

_____

_____

_____

4- Element: _____

Example: _____

_____

_____

_____

_____

_____

_____

_____

5- Element: _____

Example: _____

_____

_____

_____

_____

_____

6- Element: _____

Example: _____

_____

_____

_____

_____

_____

14. What elements can <u>increase</u> the quality of life of elderly individuals? Provide at least six elements. Give an example to illustrate and explain how each element contributes to quality of life.

1- Element: _____

Example: _____

_____

_____

_____

_____

_____

2- Element: _____

Example: _____

_____

_____

_____

_____

_____

3- Element: _____

Example: _____

_____

_____

_____

_____

_____

4- Element: _____

Example: _____

_____

_____

_____

_____

_____

5- Element:_____

   Example:_____

   _____

   _____

   _____

   _____

   _____

   _____

6- Element:_____

   Example:_____

   _____

   _____

   _____

   _____

   _____

   _____

15. Which of these foods is rich in insoluble fiber?

   a) Casserole with green peas   d) Oatmeal cereal
   b) Lentil salad   e) Wheat bran muffin
   c) Barley soup

16. Which nutrient is required for the metabolism of folate?

   a) Thiamin (vitamin B_1)   d) Pyridoxine (vitamin B_6)
   b) Riboflavin (vitamin B_2)   e) Cobalamin (vitamin B_{12})
   c) Niacin (vitamin B_3)

17. These foods are a source of vitamin B_{12}, <u>except</u>

   a) apple   d) milk
   b) beef steak   e) egg
   c) liver

18. These foods are a source of folate, <u>except</u>

   a) asparagus   d) orange
   b) oil   e) corn
   c) egg

19. Pumpkin, mango, sweet potatoes, and apricots are foods rich in

   a) ascorbic acid   d) phylloquinone (vitamin K)
   b) β-carotene   e) riboflavin
   c) tocopherol

20. These foods are a source of vitamin B_6, <u>except</u>

   a) oatmeal   d) potato
   b) banana   e) butter
   c) tomato

21. Kiwi fruit, strawberries, broccoli, sweet peppers, and tangerines are a source of

    a) ascorbic acid   d) thiamin
    b) β-carotene   e) riboflavin
    c) niacin

22. These foods are a source of zinc, <u>except</u>

    a) meat   d) nuts
    b) grains   e) milk products
    c) vegetable shortening

UNDERSTAND THE CONCEPTS

1. What factors influence the aging process?

   _____

   _____

   _____

   _____

   _____

2. What modifications in body composition occur in the elderly years?

   _____

   _____

3. What causes these modifications in body composition to occur in the elderly years?

   _____

   _____

   _____

   _____

   _____

   _____

4. Why do many elderly people die from infectious diseases and their complications?

   _____

   _____

   _____

   _____

   _____

5. What alimentary tract problems are associated with the elderly years? Give some examples of problems found in each of the following parts of the alimentary tract.

   1- Oral cavity: _____

   2- Stomach: _____

   3- Intestines: _____

6. When is the fastest bone loss happening in females?

    _____

7. What is osteoporosis?

    _____

    _____

    _____

8. What are the two main types of osteoporosis and their characteristics?

    1- Type: _____

    Characteristics: _____

    _____

    _____

    _____

    2- Type: _____

    Characteristics: _____

    _____

    _____

    _____

9. What is the term for a condition associated with aging that is characterized by chronic inflammation of the stomach accompanied by a diminished size and functioning of the gastric mucosa and glands?

    _____

10. Explain why there is a reduction in energy requirements in the elderly years.

    _____

    _____

    _____

11. Why do elderly individuals often suffer from constipation?

    _____

    _____

    _____

12. Adequate intake of vitamin E, ascorbic acid, and carotenoids is associated with a reduced incidence of _____ in aging adults.

    a) osteoporosis   d) arthritis
    b) dysphagia   e) senile dementia
    c) cataracts

13. Indicate the DRI recommendations for elderly individuals in this table. *(You can refer to the DRI recommendation tables in the appendix section at the end of this book.)*

KEY DRI RECOMMENDATIONS FOR ELDERLY MALES AND FEMALES

Energy and Nutrients	DRIs	51–70 year old Females	51–70 year old Males	≥71 year old Females	≥71 year old Males
Water	AI (L/day)				
Total fiber	AI (g/day)				
Iron	RDA (mg/day)				
Vitamin D	AI (µg/day)§				
Vitamin C	RDA (mg/day)				
Zinc	RDA (mg/day)				
Vitamin A	RDA (µg/day)§				
Vitamin E	RDA (mg/day)				
Vitamin B6	RDA (mg/day)				
Folate	RDA (µg/day)§				
Vitamin B12	RDA (µg/day)§				

§ Micrograms (mcg) per day.

14. What is osteoarthritis?

_____

_____

15. What can help to alleviate osteoarthritic pain in overweight or obese individuals?

_____

_____

16. What dysfunctions are associated with inadequacies in folate and vitamins B_1, B_3, B_6, and/or B_{12}?

_____

17. Why is it recommended that elderly individuals meet their vitamin B_{12} needs mainly by consuming foods fortified with the vitamin or with a supplement?

_____

_____

18. Which easily available foods are fortified with vitamin B_{12}?

_____

19. What are reasons why many elderly people have a suboptimal folate status?

_____

_____

20. Elevated serum homocysteine concentrations, an independent risk factor for coronary artery disease, can result from _____ deficiencies.

    a) ascorbic acid and/or tocopherol
    b) selenium and/or magnesium
    c) thiamin, niacin, and/or riboflavin
    d) retinol and/or β-carotene
    e) folate, pyridoxine, and/or cobalamin

21. There is a reduced capacity of the body to synthesize and activate _____ with aging, which often contributes to inadequacy in that micronutrient in older adults, especially if they are homebound and have a low milk intake.

    a) calcium
    b) phosphorus
    c) vitamin D
    d) riboflavin
    e) vitamin E

22. What BMI range, according to present guidelines, is associated with the lowest risk of mortality from chronic diseases in elderly individuals?

    _____

23. Which micronutrient is better absorbed and stored by older adults than by younger adults?

    _____

24. In otherwise healthy older adults, low iron status can result from decreased iron absorption due to
    _____ .

25. Deficiency in which nutrient resembles symptoms associated with aging, such as dermatitis, reduced taste acuity, and appetite?

    _____

26. What term refers to "taking many medications concurrently," which is frequent in the elderly?

    _____

27. What are the 10 leading causes of death in the United States and Canada?

    _____

    _____

    _____

28. Which of these leading causes of death are related to nutrition and diet?

    _____

29. Which of these leading causes of death are possibly related to alcohol?

    _____

30. Many diseases are multifactorial in etiology. Indicate what risk factors can contribute to the development of the following diseases.

    1- **Obesity**

    a) Diet-related risk factors: _____

    _____

    _____

    _____

    b) Other risk factors: _____

    _____

    _____

    _____

2- **Cancer**

a) Diet-related risk factors: _____

_____

_____

_____

b) Other risk factors: _____

_____

_____

_____

3- **Type 2 diabetes mellitus**

a) Diet-related risk factors: _____

_____

_____

_____

b) Other risk factors: _____

_____

_____

_____

4- **Hypertension**

a) Diet-related risk factors: _____

_____

_____

_____

b) Other risk factors: _____

_____

_____

_____

5- **Osteoporosis**

a) Diet-related risk factors: _____

_____

_____

_____

b) Other risk factors: _____

_____

_____

_____

6- **Cardiovascular and heart disease**

a) Diet-related risk factors: _____

_____

_____

_____

b) Other risk factors: _____

_____

_____

_____

7- **Dental and oral disease**

c) Diet-related risk factors: _____

_____

_____

_____

d) Other risk factors: _____

_____

_____

_____

31. Indicate whether the following statements are TRUE or FALSE, and justify your answer.

1- _____: Elderly people do not need to drink milk since their bones are not growing anymore.

Justification: _____

_____

_____

_____

2- _____: Consumption of milk and milk products causes mucus formation.

Justification: _____

_____

_____

_____

3- _____: Elderly individuals who have problems chewing often have a low intake of vitamin B_{12} and folate.

Justification: _____

_____

_____

_____

4- _____: Diuretics and anti-inflammatory medications are commonly taken by elderly individuals to treat illness and can result in a poor folate status.

Justification: _____

_____

_____

_____

5- _____: Long-term oral intake of corticosteroids for the treatment of inflammation increases the need for calcium and vitamin D.

Justification: _____

_____

_____

_____

6- _____: Antacids reduce the absorption of folate, thiamin, and vitamin A.

Justification: _____

_____

_____

_____

32. What nutrition programs are available to promote the health of seniors in your community?

_____

_____

_____

_____

_____

_____

INTEGRATE YOUR LEARNING

1. What are the consequences of gum disease, loss of teeth, and poorly fitted dentures?

_____

_____

_____

2. What is dysphagia?

_____

3. What sensory losses associated with aging can impair food intake?

_____

4. What are the consequences of atrophic gastritis?

_____

_____

_____

_____

_____

_____

5. What is the impact of atrophic gastritis on vitamin B_{12} metabolism and status? Explain.

_____

_____

_____

_____

_____

_____

6. What are the consequences of intestinal bacterial overgrowth?

_____

_____

_____

_____

_____

_____

7. Why are antibiotics less effective against bacterial infection in malnourished individuals?

_____

_____

_____

_____

_____

_____

8. Why does improper iron supplementation in malnourished individuals actually increase the risk of developing infection or worsen an infectious condition?

_____

_____

_____

_____

_____

_____

9. Which elderly individuals are more at risk for malnutrition?

_____

_____

_____

_____

_____

_____

10. Why are the iron needs of elderly women less than those of women in their early adulthood?

_____

_____

11. Which elderly individuals are more at risk of iron deficiency anemia?

_____

_____

_____

_____

_____

_____

_____

12. Why are the calcium needs of elderly individuals higher than those of young and middle adults?

_____

_____

13. Why are the vitamin D needs of elderly individuals higher than those of young and middle adults?

_____

_____

_____

_____

_____

14. Why are the vitamin B_6 needs of elderly individuals higher than those of young and middle adults?

_____

_____

15. Why is dehydration a risk in older adults?

_____

_____

_____

_____

_____

_____

16. What are complications of dehydration in older adults?

_____

_____

17. Why is estimating dietary recommendation standards for elderly individuals such a difficult task?

_____

_____

18. Explain why many aging individuals gain weight and become overweight or obese.

_____

_____

_____

19. What is hyperhomocysteinemia?

_____

_____

_____

CHALLENGE YOUR LEARNING

CASE STUDY

Objectives

This case study will help you better understand the life changes associated with aging and the very difficult situations in which elderly individuals often find themselves as they grow older.

It will also help you realize why many elderly individuals are at risk of malnutrition and what can be done to help them have a better quality of life and prevent the complications of their disease states.

Description

C.B. is a 78-year-old woman who lives in the country. Her two beloved sons are raised and long gone. They have their own families with young children and are busy professionals in another city, more than 8 hours away by car from their mother. Even though they keep in touch by phone and send her photos in the mail, she only sees them a few times a year. C.B.'s husband passed away 10 years ago from a myocardial infarction. She has been feeling lonely, sad, and depressed since then. She used to play the piano magnificently, but she stopped, as her religion required, when her husband died. She soon forgot the notes and her hands became too stiff to play due to arthritic pain. C.B.'s arthritis problems make it her hard for her to walk freely and her handwriting is not readable anymore. She is constantly afraid of losing her balance and falling, but she refuses to use her cane. She also has osteoporosis, cataracts, and Alzheimer disease.

C.B. lives with her 82-year-old sister, who has uncontrolled type 2 diabetes mellitus and short-term memory loss. They both still live in the old house where they grew up with six other siblings and where C.B. raised her sons with her husband. They spend most of their day listening to music on the radio, caring for their pet bird, and reliving the past as they rock in their chairs in the living room. They sometimes go onto the porch, where they have another set of comfortable rocking chairs for when the weather is warm, but they otherwise stay in the house all day. They do not talk much to one another as they suffer from mild hearing loss, but they enjoy one another's peaceful company and they do many things together. They usually have a long nap every afternoon.

C.B. and her sister usually have three meals a day: oatmeal made with water and a banana for breakfast; chicken noodle soup with soda crackers and white bread with butter for lunch with fruit gelatin for dessert; and usually oatmeal made with water and a couple of commercial mini-caramel cakes for dinner. Each meal is accompanied by black tea with ginger cookies to dip into the tea. A couple of times per week, they have a ham sandwich or grilled cheese on white bread with commercially prepared coleslaw for lunch. Otherwise, their diet is almost always the same every day. C.B. does not like the taste of milk and milk products, but her sister sometimes eats ice cream. They are both constipated and are taking mineral oil to help relieve that problem.

A kind teenage boy living across the street cuts the grass for them weekly in the summer months and gets groceries for them once a week from the corner store where he works. Otherwise, the sisters have very little social interaction, as they are afraid to walk outside the house for fear of falling.

1. Why is C.B. at risk of malnutrition?

2. Why is C.B.'s sister at risk of malnutrition?

3. What can be done to decrease their risk of malnutrition? Give four suggestions.

   1- _____

   2- _____

   3- _____

   4- _____

4. Why are C.B. and her sister constipated?

5. What can be done to help relieve constipation? Give 10 recommendations.

   1- _____

   2- _____

   3- _____

   4- _____

   5- _____

   6- _____

   7- _____

   8- _____

   9- _____

   10- _____

6. Why is it not recommended to take mineral oil as a laxative?

7. What physiologic changes happen in the brain as a result of aging?

8. What nutrient deficiencies are associated with reduced brain function?

9. What is Alzheimer disease?

10. C.B. and her sister would have benefited from nutrition screening and intervention. What tools are used in your community to perform nutrition screening of elderly individuals?

Case Follow-up

C.B.'s sister did not monitor her blood glucose levels and her diabetes mellitus became out of control. She often forgot to take her medications. One night, she felt weak in the dark on the stairs and fell unconscious at the bottom of the stairs. She was brought to the hospital emergency room in an ambulance, but she passed away from diabetic coma and trauma from her bad fall.

C.B. firmly insisted that she wanted to continue living in the old house even though her sons wanted her to move into a nursing home. C.B. could not afford the monthly cost of the nursing home and did not want her sons to have to pay for her. She was also frightened by the idea of moving out of the house where she had lived all of her life. However, C.B. was very lonely and visibly depressed by the absence of her best friend and sister.

In the following months, C.B. was losing weight and her dentures did not fit anymore. She got sick eating food that had gone bad without her realizing it, because of her poor eyesight. She had acute diarrhea and became dehydrated, frail, and confused. One morning she filled a bath and forgot about it, so it overflowed. She then noticed water on the floor, but as she remembered about the bath, she slipped on the wet floor and broke her hip. She was brought to the hospital emergency room and was admitted to the palliative care unit of the hospital. Since her admission in palliative care, she has been crying regularly, not eating, refusing nutrition support, and not recognizing her sons when they come to visit her.

11. Why did C.B. become malnourished?

12. What is palliative care?

Nutrition in Diverse Cultures and Communities

INTRODUCTION

Part 4 focuses on the fact that sociocultural, ethnic, and religious practices and beliefs have a strong influence on people's food choices and eating patterns. Individuals from different cultures and communities often have typical eating patterns that can be quite different from mainstream North American society. In this chapter we will take a closer look at some cultural eating patterns, including those adopted by vegetarian, Jewish, Hispanic, and Aboriginal (Indian, Inuit, and Métis) communities. We will also discuss some factors influencing the food choices of individuals from diverse cultural groups and communities, and how these factors impact the nutritional status of the individuals.

The individuals in a cultural group may follow the dietary patterns typical of their culture or community with more or less emphasis, according to their personal choice at a given period in their life. In addition, the prominent cultural group in a society usually influences the smaller cultural groups, while the reverse can also be true. Furthermore, some people come from a multicultural family where the parents are each from a different culture or community background.

Dietitians must be culturally aware. They have to take into consideration the culture and community background of individuals, as well as their beliefs and resources, when assessing nutritional needs and making nutritional recommendations to help their clients. To be useful, a dietitian's dietary recommendations have to be realistic and include practical examples individualized to the client's daily life. To accomplish this, dietitians have to understand the chosen dietary beliefs/rules/laws and habits of their clients, and know which foods they select and which meals they usually prepare.

As part of their work, dietitians assist individuals from various backgrounds, including those with limited resources, to attain the healthiest dietary habits possible. They often use teaching tools to favor clear communications with their clients, especially those with low literacy levels or those speaking a language different from their own.

4.1 Vegetarian Nutrition

REVIEW THE INFORMATION

1. Define who *vegetarians* are.

   _____

   _____

2. Define who *semi-vegetarians* are.

   _____

   _____

3. Define who *vegans* are.

   _____

   _____

4. What are *vegetarian diets*?

   _____

   _____

5. What are the main reasons why people choose to be vegetarian?

   _____

   _____

   _____

   _____

   _____

6. Is vegetarianism a new trend? Explain your answer.

   _____

   _____

7. Which one(s) of the following cultural groups promote(s) vegetarianism?

   a) Hindu   b) Buddhist   c) Greek   d) Jain   e) All of the above

8. What are some of the vegetarian options often offered by restaurants, including fast food restaurants?

   _____

   _____

9. Identify some vegetarian restaurants/caterers in your area or restaurants offering a selection of vegetarian options.

   _____

   _____

10. Identify some vegetarian foods available at the grocery stores in your area. *(Note: If you are not aware of them, take a look at the meat alternative and dairy substitute sections of your supermarket and you will discover many products.)*

    _____

    _____

11. Identify some vegetarian food companies and brand-name products available in your area.

_____

_____

UNDERSTAND THE CONCEPTS

1. What proportion of adults follows vegetarian diets in the United States and Canada?

   a) 2.5% and 4.0%, respectively
   b) 4.5% and 6.0%, respectively
   c) 6.5% and 8.0%, respectively
   d) 8.5% and 10.0%, respectively
   e) 10.5% and 12.0%, respectively

2. How many adult people follow vegetarian diets in the United States and Canada?

   a) 0.8 million and 500,000, respectively
   b) 1.8 million and 600,000, respectively
   c) 2.8 million and 700,000, respectively
   d) 3.8 million and 800,000, respectively
   e) 4.8 million and 900,000, respectively

3. Indicate whether the following statements are TRUE or FALSE.

   a) _____: Vegetarians are more often males than females.

   b) _____: Vegetarians are more likely to live in small cities than large cities.

   c) _____: Vegetarians are more likely to live on the west or east coast.

4. For each vegetarian diet, indicate which foods are usually included (✓) and which ones are omitted (**X**).

COMPOSITION OF THE MAIN VEGETARIAN DIETS								
Foods	Lacto-ovo-vegetarian	Lacto-vegetarian	Ovo-vegetarian	Vegan	Macrobiotic	Fruitarians	Pesco-vegetarian	Polo-vegetarian
Fruits								
Vegetables								
Legumes								
Nuts and seeds								
Grains								
Milk and milk products								
Fortified soy products								
Eggs								
Meat								
Poultry								
Fish and seafood								
Comments								

5. How are vegetarian diets different from the typical North American diet? Explain.

_____

_____

_____

_____

_____

_____

_____

_____

_____

6. Why is the interest in vegetarianism increasing?

_____

_____

_____

_____

_____

_____

_____

_____

_____

_____

7. Which nutrient needs are at risk of not being met by some vegans?

_____

_____

8. Which fortified foods can help vegetarians, and especially vegans, to meet all of their micronutrient needs?

_____

_____

9. What is the Protein Digestibility Corrected Amino Acid Score?

_____

_____

_____

10. Which of these proteins has the highest Protein Digestibility Corrected Amino Acid Score?

a) Soy protein concentrate   c) Wheat gluten   e) Black bean protein

b) Beef protein   d) Egg white protein

11. The main inhibitor of iron and zinc absorption in vegetarian diets is

    a) soluble fiber   c) caffeine   e) calcium
    b) phytate   d) insoluble fiber

INTEGRATE YOUR LEARNING

1. Explain the following statement: *The dietary habits of vegetarians can vary quite considerably. An individual assessment is therefore needed to determine the nutritional quality of the diet of a person who says he or she is vegetarian.*

2. What is the position of dietitians on vegetarian diets?

3. How can dietetic professionals help vegetarians?

4. Vegetarian diets are associated with lower risk of which diseases?

5. Why is energy adequacy important for vegetarians to meet their protein needs?

6. Why is variety important for vegetarians to meet their protein needs?

_____

_____

_____

_____

_____

_____

CHALLENGE YOUR LEARNING

CASE STUDY

Objectives

You will see with this case that the diet of vegetarians has to be well planned to adequately meet the needs of the individual through the different parts of the life cycle, especially in the periods of increased requirements, such as pregnancy and lactation.

In addition, even though vegetarians are often more health aware than many individuals in our society and strive to be the healthiest they can be, they sometimes lack the understanding of what their nutritional requirements are (i.e., what nutrients they need, how much, and why) and what the food sources of these nutrients are. Since dietitians are experts in this field, they can help vegetarians and teach them how to have a well-balanced diet that meets all of their nutritional needs.

Description

Mrs. J.L. is a slim, active 28-year-old elementary school music teacher. She has a successful career and a loving husband. Recently, she and her husband were very excited to find out that she is pregnant, as they both adore children. They just bought a house in town and the timing is perfect for them to have a baby.

Her family physician is referring J.L. to you because she is in the second trimester (4 months pregnant) and has only gained 0.7 lb (0.3 kg) so far. Her pre-pregnancy weight was 114 lb (52 kg) and her height is 5'7". She had nausea a few times during the first trimester, but not anymore. Other than that, J.L. has not been diagnosed with any illness that would explain her lack of pregnancy weight gain.

Mrs. J.L. say, "I have always been slim and health conscious, even as a child. I saw my father suffering through such a long and terrible fight with cancer. I was in my first year of university when he passed away and we decided, my twin sister and I, to become vegan."

Mrs. J.L. admits that she is worried for her baby and she is hoping that you will help her gain weight and build her strength. She indicates that she has continued to eat three regular meals a day when she became pregnant and started to take a daily prenatal multivitamin and mineral supplement. She has been making an effort to drink more fluids in the last 5 months, at least 4 liters (4.2 quarts or about 17 cups) of water throughout the day. She does not have the appetite to eat more. She does not restrict her energy intake. She is willing to modify some of her dietary choices during pregnancy if you can convince her that it will be beneficial for her baby.

This is what she states realistically represents her actual daily food intake.

Breakfast:

1 cup (237 mL)	**Oatmeal**	regular, cooked, made with water
½ cup (118 mL, 75 g)	**Banana**	½ medium, raw, sliced
½ cup (4 fluid oz, 118 mL)	**Pineapple juice**	unsweetened, canned

Lunch:

½ cup (4 fluid oz, 118 mL)	**Soy beverage**	fortified
1⅓ cup (316 mL)	**"Four bean salad":**	
3 Tbsp (45 mL, 31 g)	Chickpeas	cooked
3 Tbsp (45 mL, 38 g)	Lentils	cooked
3 Tbsp (45 mL, 34 g)	Soybeans	cooked
3 Tbsp (45 mL, 34 g)	Red kidney beans	cooked
¼ cup (59 mL, 25 g)	Cauliflower	fresh, raw, chopped
¼ cup (59 mL, 22 g)	Broccoli	fresh, raw, chopped
1 Tbsp (15 mL)	Canola oil	
1 tsp (5 mL)	Mustard	prepared, yellow
1 medium (98 g)	**Peach**	fresh, raw

Dinner:

½ cup (4 fluid oz, 118 mL)	**Tomato juice**	canned
2 cups (474 mL)	**Stir-fry:**	
1 cup (237 mL)	Brown rice	cooked
3½ oz (100 mL)	Snow peas	fresh, cooked
½ cup (118 mL)	Tomato	medium, fresh, chopped, and cooked
3½ oz (100 mL)	Yellow beans	fresh, cooked
2 tsp (10 mL)	Canola oil	
2 Tbsp (30 mL)	Soy sauce	
½ cup (118 mL)	**Orange sherbet**	

1. What was Mrs. J.L.'s pre-pregnancy BMI?

2. What is your interpretation of her pre-pregnancy body weight?

3. What is the pregnancy weight gain recommendation for Mrs. J.L., based on her pre-pregnancy body weight?

4. How much weight should Mrs. J.L. have gained by now? Explain.

5. Which nutrients are especially at risk of not being met in *pregnant vegans*?

6. What is her daily energy intake based on her present food intake?

7. What is her energy need?

8. Is her energy intake adequate to meet her needs? Explain.

9. What is her daily protein intake based on her present food intake?

10. What is her protein need?

11. Is her protein intake adequate to meet her needs? Explain.

12. What is her intake of micronutrients based on her present food intake?

13. What are her micronutrient needs?

14. Is she meeting her micronutrient needs? Explain.

15. What are the fluid needs during pregnancy?

16. Is Mrs. J.L. meeting her fluid needs? Explain.

17. Give three practical and realistic recommendations to help Mrs. J.L. meet her energy needs.

18. Give three practical and realistic recommendations to help Mrs. J.L. meet her protein needs.

19. Give three practical and realistic recommendations to help Mrs. J.L. meet her calcium needs.

20. Give three practical and realistic recommendations to help Mrs. J.L. meet her iron needs.

21. Give three practical and realistic recommendations to help Mrs. J.L. meet her vitamin B_{12} needs.

22. Give three practical and realistic recommendations to help Mrs. J.L. meet her folate needs.

23. Give three practical and realistic recommendations to help Mrs. J.L. meet her zinc needs.

24. Give three practical and realistic recommendations to help Mrs. J.L. meet her linolenic acid needs.

4.2 Kosher Nutrition

REVIEW THE INFORMATION

1. Sharing food is part of many community special events, sociocultural traditions, and religious rituals throughout the year.
   1- Describe 10 special events that take place in your social environment.
   2- Indicate what particular foods are shared at each event.
   3- Are some of these special events Jewish celebrations? If so, indicate which ones.

   a) Special event: _____

   Food shared: _____

   b) Special event: _____

   Food shared: _____

   c) Special event: _____

   Food shared: _____

   d) Special event: _____

   Food shared: _____

   e) Special event: _____

   Food shared: _____

   f) Special event: _____

   Food shared: _____

   g) Special event: _____

   Food shared: _____

   h) Special event: _____

   Food shared: _____

   i) Special event: _____

   Food shared: _____

   j) Special event: _____

   Food shared: _____

2. What are the main Jewish holiday celebrations?

_____

_____

_____

_____

3. There are over _____ million Jews in the United States, which is about _____ % of the population.

   a) 2; 0.3   b) 4; 1.3   c) 6; 2.3   d) 8; 3.3   e) 10; 4.3

4. There are over _____ Jewish people in Canada, with the majority residing in Toronto and Montreal.

   a) 50,000   b) 150,000   c) 250,000   d) 350,000   e) 450,000

UNDERSTAND THE CONCEPTS

1. The largest group of Jews in North America is the group of Ashkenazic Jews, who are mainly from

   _____ descent.

   a) German   c) Polish   e) all of the above
   b) Russian   d) Romanian

2. The Sephardic Jews are descended from Jews originating from _____ and who migrated to North America in the early 1600s.

   a) Spain   c) North Africa   e) all of the above
   b) Portugal   d) around the Mediterranean

3. Ashkenazic Jews enjoy _____, which are foods typically consumed in eastern and central Europe.

   a) rye breads   c) knishes   e) a, b, and c
   b) borschts   d) hummus

4. Meat stews with legumes, vegetables, and fruits enjoyed by Sephardic Jews originated from

   a) Spain   c) Portugal   e) a, b, and c
   b) North Africa   d) Romania

5. What are the three main religious denominations within Judaism?

   _____

6. Associate each of the Jewish terms and foods listed below with their description.

Kosher	Cholent	Treif (or Trefe or Traif)	Kashrut
Torah	Sabbath (or Shabbat)	Rosh Hashanah	Hanukkah
Challah (or Hallah)	Pareve	Latkes	Fleischig
Passover (or Pesach)	Borscht	Bar (or Bat) Mitzvah	Milchig
Yom Kippur	Matzoh		

   1- _____ Word meaning proper or fit to consume, in reference to religious law

   2- _____ This Day of Atonement or repentance is the holiest day of the Jewish year. This holy day of complete fast (no food or water) is observed in autumn (8 days following Rosh Hashanah) to ask God to forgive the sins committed during the previous year. The fast starts at sundown prior to the holy day and continues until sundown the next day.

   3- _____ The Jewish dietary laws

   4- _____ Word to characterize milk and milk products and foods or meals containing milk or milk products

5- _____ A crispy, flat unleavened bread made with flour and water. It is eaten during Passover and symbolizes the bread that the Jewish people ate when they fled from Egypt.

6- _____ The first five books of the Bible, written by Moses, from which the Jewish dietary laws are derived

7- _____ Word meaning food nonproper or ritually unfit to consume. It is a synonym for nonkosher.

8- _____ A type of soup prepared with beets, cabbage, spinach, or sorrel. Beef or, alternatively, dairy (sour cream or yogurt) is added in the preparation.

9- _____ Word meaning rest and referring to the day of rest that the Jewish people observe from sundown on Friday to sundown on Saturday, and which is considered to be the most important day of the week.

10- _____ A type of stew, which is often prepared on Friday before the Sabbath, left in the oven on low heat overnight, and eaten on Saturday. This recipe originated from Europe and there are many varieties. This meal-in-a-pot usually contains beef, beans, and potatoes.

11- _____ Potato pancakes served on Hanukkah. They are prepared with grated potatoes and chopped onions, then fried in oil.

12- _____ Term indicating that a food is neutral or does not contain meat or milk products. A neutral food can be eaten with a food or meal containing meat or milk products.

13- _____ A type of bread considered to be the Sabbath bread and served at the Friday evening meal in preparation for the Sabbath. In addition to being served during the Sabbath, this bread is also shared on other holidays. It is yeast bread made with eggs, which is often braided.

14- _____ A holy day celebrating the start of the Jewish New Year

15- _____ It means "festival of lights" and refers to a festive holiday celebrated in December.

16- _____ A very important holiday that takes place over 8 days and is celebrated in the spring. It memorializes the exodus of Jewish people from Egypt and their liberation from bondage. A different set of dishes is used during this holiday.

17- _____ Word indicating the presence of meat or meat byproduct in a food or meal

18- _____ Means "commandment age" and refers to the ceremony during which a young Jew takes on the religious responsibilities of adulthood

7. Explain the main Jewish dietary laws.

_____

_____

_____

_____

_____

_____

_____

_____

_____

_____

_____

_____

_____
_____
_____
_____
_____
_____
_____
_____
_____
_____
_____

8. How are kosher foods identified in the food industry?

_____
_____
_____
_____
_____

9. Categorize the following foods as **milchig**, **fleischig**, **pareve**, or **treif**.

a) Egg: _____

b) Pasta: _____

c) Coffee with milk: _____

d) Baked products containing lard: _____

e) Tea: _____

f) Fresh fruits: _____

g) Cheeseburger: _____

h) Meatless lasagna: _____

i) Duck: _____

j) Meat with blood: _____

k) Rice with butter: _____

l) Fish with fins and scales (e.g., halibut, salmon, haddock, tuna): _____

m) Vegetables: _____

n) Crustaceans (e.g., clams, oysters): _____

o) Animals that die a natural death: _____

p) Shellfish (e.g., lobster, clams, shrimp, crabs): _____

q) Fish-like mammals (e.g., turbot, catfish, shark, whale): _____

r) Salad with creamy dressing and bacon pieces: _____

s) Beans: _____

t) Cattle, deer, sheep, and goat: _____

u) Chicken, pheasant, turkey, and duck: _____

v) Vegetable oil: _____

INTEGRATE YOUR LEARNING

1. Jewish dietary laws and customs are followed more closely by _____ Jews and less closely by

   _____ Jews.

   a) reform; conservative   c) orthodox; conservative   e) reform; orthodox

   b) conservative; orthodox   d) orthodox; reform

2. What factors influence the dietary habits of Jews? Explain.

   _____

   _____

   _____

   _____

3. What should dietitians take into consideration when helping Jewish clients? Explain.

   _____

   _____

   _____

   _____

4. Identify the main kosher certification symbols and kosher-certifying agencies in your area.

   _____

   _____

   _____

   _____

   _____

5. What would **KD** found on the food label of the box of your favorite cereal bar mean?

   _____

   _____

   _____

6. Why are kosher-certified foods usually more expensive than nonkosher foods?

   _____

   _____

   _____

   _____

7. Does "kosher style" on a food label indicate that the food is kosher certified? Explain.

   _____

   _____

   _____

   _____

8. According to the strict Jewish dietary laws, the following foods are neutral <u>except</u>

   a) coffee with sugar   c) fruit salad   e) vegetable juice with lemon
   b) baked beans   d) vegetables with butter

9. According to the strict Jewish dietary laws, which one of the following foods is allowed?

   a) Catfish   c) Eggnog   e) Baked products containing lard
   b) Shellfish   d) Peanut butter

10. According to the strict Jewish dietary laws, which one of the following foods is allowed?

   a) Gelatin   c) Shark   e) Ham
   b) Shrimp   d) Haddock

CHALLENGE YOUR LEARNING

CASE STUDY

Objectives
This case is intended to help you test your understanding of the needs of observant Jewish individuals, to see if you can help them follow the kosher dietary laws with respect to their individual choices, and to test your resourcefulness.

Description
Mrs. J.M. has been admitted this morning to the long-term care institution where you work as a dietitian. This is what she receives for lunch after her arrival: chicken and broccoli cream soup, ham and cheese sandwich on whole wheat bread, apple pie, and a glass of milk. She tells you that she does not mean to be difficult, but that she cannot accept this meal because she is keeping kosher. She is 79 years old. She looks frail and underweight and the nursing staff is worried about her not eating.

1. Explain the reasons why Mrs. J.M. cannot eat the meal offered to her if she is keeping kosher.

2. Explain what you would say to Mrs. J.M.

3. What could be quickly offered to her in substitution for that lunch that would be appropriate to meet her needs?

Case Follow-up
Mrs. J.M. explains that she is a Hasidic Jew. She says that she usually eats a dairy meal for lunch such as lokshen kugel, salad, and tea with milk. She tells you: "There is no rush for you to bring me food tomorrow, as it is Yom Kippur. My daughter will likely bring me some leckach tonight."

4. What is a Hasidic Jew?

5. What is a lokshen kugel?

6. What is leckach?

7. What does Mrs. J.M. mean by "There is no rush for you to bring me food tomorrow, as it is Yom Kippur"?

Case Follow-up
You inform the physician that Mrs. J.M. is underweight and has signs of muscle wasting, but that she intends to celebrate Yom Kippur tomorrow. The physician replies that Mrs. J.M. has hypertension and diabetes mellitus, and that she should be eating on a regular basis because of her medical condition and the medications she is taking.

8. Is Mrs. J.M. obligated to respect the restrictions of Yom Kippur? Explain.

9. Who should be consulted to provide answers to questions about kashrut or waiver for medical reasons?

10. Do the Jewish dietary laws allow oral nutritional supplements? Explain.

11. Mrs. J.M. needs to be on a sodium-restricted diet because of her hypertension. Will there be a problem because Mrs. J.M is keeping kosher? Explain.

4.3 Hispanic Nutrition

REVIEW THE INFORMATION

1. Hispanic people represent the _____ largest and most quickly expanding cultural group in the United States.

   a) first   b) second   c) third   d) forth   e) fifth

2. What group constitutes the largest subgroup of Hispanic people?

   _____

3. Mexican Americans live mainly in New Mexico and _____. Many also live in large urban areas.

   a) California   b) Texas   c) Colorado   d) Arizona   e) all of the above

4. Which foods are popular Mexican favorites served in restaurants all over North America?

   _____

   _____

UNDERSTAND THE CONCEPTS

1. Which cultures have influenced the traditional diet of Mexican people?

   _____

2. Which staples are used for the basis of Mexican cuisine?

   _____

   _____

3. Describe the following traditional Mexican foods.

   a) Guacamole: _____

   _____

   b) Albondigas: _____

   _____

   c) Atole: _____

   _____

   d) Bolillo: _____

   _____

   e) Burrito: _____

   _____

    f) Chorizo: _____

_____

    g) Quesadilla: _____

_____

    h) Taco: _____

_____

4. What foods are believed to be "cold" foods?

_____

_____

5. What foods are believed to be "hot" foods?

_____

_____

6. What is the significance of "cold" and "hot" foods?

_____

_____

_____

_____

_____

_____

7. Mexican American communities represent the fastest growing group of American

    a) children   b) teenagers   c) young adults   d) middle adults   e) older adults

INTEGRATE YOUR LEARNING

1. Briefly describe the diet of Mexican Americans today.

_____

_____

_____

2. What are the nutritional advantages of the traditional Mexican diet?

_____

_____

_____

3. What are the limitations of the traditional Mexican diet?

_____

_____

_____

4. Which mainstream American foods are now being consumed more often by Mexican Americans?

_____

_____

5. What factors affect the contemporary Mexican American diet?

_____

_____

_____

_____

6. What is the prevalence of type 2 diabetes mellitus among Mexican Americans, compared with that of Anglo-Americans?

_____

_____

_____

_____

CHALLENGE YOUR LEARNING

CASE STUDY

Objectives

This case study will help you understand the contemporary Mexican American culture and eating patterns, as well as the influence of socioeconomic factors on daily food choices.

Description

Mr. J.A. is a hard-working, middle-aged Mexican American. He is 43 years old and has a healthy body weight. J.A. lives in Chicago with his wife and their young children. He works long days as a waiter in a popular downtown Mexican restaurant, while his wife takes care of their two preschool children. He often ends up working on weekends as well to ensure that they are able to meet their financial needs. His lunch and dinner are provided for him at the restaurant. Although the timing of his lunch and dinner vary every day depending on the restaurant's clientele, he is allowed to choose what he wants to eat. Mr. J.A. is not a picky eater, but he does not tolerate milk products and prefers to exclude them from his diet. Because he works in a restaurant, he sometimes does not feel like eating, as he sees food all day long.

He typically eats the following:

Breakfast: 1 cup (237 mL) beans refried in lard
½ cup (118 mL) chorizo pieces
2 corn tortillas (6 inches, 15 cm, or 26 g each tortilla)
1 cup (8 fluid oz, 237 mL) coffee

Lunch: 1 cup (237 mL) beans refried in lard
2 corn tortillas (6 inches, 15 cm, or 26 g each tortilla)
1 cup (237 mL) Mexican rice fried in 1 Tbsp oil
1 can (1½ cups, 12 fluid oz, 355 mL) soft drink

Dinner: 1 cup (237 mL) ground beef fried in 1 Tbsp oil
1 cup (237 mL) beans refried in lard
2 corn tortillas (6 inches, 15 cm, or 26 g each tortilla)
2 Tbsp (30 mL) chili sauce
1 cup (8 fluid oz, 237 mL) lemonade drink

1. Does Mr. J.A. have a healthy diet? Explain why.

2. What is the energy and nutrient content of Mr. J.A.'s diet? Is he meeting his needs?

3. What changes can Mr. J.A. make to his diet to better meet his dietary needs? Take into consideration his cultural traditions.

4. What could help improve Mr. J.A.'s appetite? Give four practical suggestions.

5. Prepare an example of a healthy menu that Mr. J.A. could follow to help him meet his dietary needs. Take into consideration his cultural traditions and the fact that he has financial limitations.

4.4 Nutrition and Aboriginal People

REVIEW THE INFORMATION

1. What are synonyms for *Aboriginal people*?

   _____

2. What are the main groups of Aboriginal people in North America?

   _____

3. Give examples of traditional Aboriginal animal foods.

   _____

   _____

   _____

   _____

   _____

   _____

   _____

   _____

4. Give examples of traditional Aboriginal plant foods.

   _____

   _____

   _____

   _____

   _____

   _____

   _____

   _____

5. Give examples of traditional Aboriginal beverages.

_____

_____

_____

6. In the United States, the population of American Indians and Alaskan Natives includes more than _____ federally recognized tribes.

   a) 220   b) 330   c) 440   d) 550   e) 660

7. There are over _____ million people of Aboriginal descent in Canada and about _____% live on a reserve, while the rest live off of a reserve.

   a) 0.2; 18   b) 0.4; 28   c) 0.6; 38   d) 0.8; 48   e) 1.0; 58

UNDERSTAND THE CONCEPTS

1. Identify some of the distinct North American Aboriginal tribes.

_____

_____

_____

_____

_____

_____

_____

_____

_____

_____

_____

_____

_____

_____

2. Define who Metis people are.

_____

_____

_____

_____

_____

_____

_____

_____

3. The traditional diet of Northern Indians and Inuit is based on what foods?

_____

_____

_____

_____

_____

_____

_____

_____

_____

_____

_____

4. Define the following traditional Aboriginal foods.

a) Indian succotash: _____

_____

_____

b) Taniga: _____

_____

_____

c) Pemmican: _____

_____

_____

d) Indian ice cream: _____

_____

_____

e) Bannock: _____

_____

_____

f) Fry bread: _____

_____

_____

g) Light bread: _____

_____

_____

h) Alkaad or Navajo cake: _____

_____

_____

5. What are some of the traditional Aboriginal food-related activities?

_____

_____

_____

_____

6. What is the impact of geographic location on the traditional diet of Indian and Inuit nations?

_____

_____

_____

_____

7. Which foods were introduced in the diet of Aboriginal people after the arrival of Europeans in North America?

_____

_____

8. What are Aboriginal people eating today? Explain.

_____

_____

_____

_____

_____

_____

_____

_____

9. What are the benefits of including traditional Aboriginal foods in the diet? Explain.

_____

_____

_____

_____

_____

_____

10. What are the risks associated with the consumption of traditional Aboriginal foods nowadays? Explain.

_____

_____

_____

_____

_____

_____

_____

11. Which traditional Aboriginal meats are low in fat?

_____

_____

_____

12. Which traditional Aboriginal foods are excellent sources of iron?

_____

_____

_____

13. Which traditional Aboriginal foods are excellent sources of zinc?

_____

_____

_____

14. Which traditional Aboriginal foods are excellent sources of vitamin A?

_____

_____

_____

15. Which traditional Aboriginal foods are excellent sources of calcium?

_____

_____

_____

INTEGRATE YOUR LEARNING

1. What is the nutritional value of traditional Aboriginal foods? Explain.

_____

_____

_____

_____

_____

_____

_____

2. Which of the following traditional meat source(s) is/are low in fat, being only 1%–5% fat?

   a) Clams and oysters
   b) Walrus and seal
   c) Ptarmigan and white fish
   d) Moose and caribou
   e) All of the above

3. Which of these traditional iron sources has the highest source of iron, providing 40–70 mg/100-g (3½-oz) serving?

   a) Dry meat from beluga and narwhal
   b) Meat from walrus and seal
   c) Liver from caribou and moose
   d) Meat from caribou, moose, and rabbit
   e) Flesh from fish and clams

4. Which of these sources of calcium has(have) the highest source of calcium, containing 250–500 mg/per 100-g (3½-oz) serving?

   a) Clams and mussels
   b) Bannock
   c) Fireweed
   d) Fish head and skin
   e) Willow leaves and kelp (seaweed)

5. These traditional Aboriginal foods are a very high source of vitamin A, except

   a) caribou liver
   b) moose liver
   c) seaweed
   d) seal liver
   e) beluga liver

6. These traditional Aboriginal foods are a good source of ascorbic acid, except

   a) bakeapple and strawberries
   b) wild rice
   c) red and white currants
   d) fireweed dandelion greens

7. Which of these traditional Aboriginal foods is/are a very good source(s) of zinc, providing 6–9 mg/100-g (3½-oz) serving?

   a) Polar bear meat
   b) Moose meat
   c) Beluga meat
   d) Narwhal meat
   e) All of the above

8. Indicate whether the following statements are TRUE or FALSE, and justify your answers.

   a) _____: In the past, many Aboriginal communities believed that overeating was an offense, and therefore, being overweight was uncommon for Aboriginal individuals.

   Justification: _____

   _____

   _____

   b) _____: Young Aboriginal people tend to prefer store-bought foods, which are replacing a lot of the traditional foods preferred by their elders.

   Justification: _____

   _____

   _____

   c) _____: The incidence of overweight and obesity in most Aboriginal populations is presently about the same as that of the rest of the North American population.

   Justification: _____

   _____

   _____

   d) _____: The health status of most Aboriginal individuals has become significantly poorer compared with the average health of North American people.

   Justification: _____

   _____

   _____

e) _____: The life expectancy of people in most Aboriginal tribes has improved but is still less than that of non-Aboriginal people in North America.

Justification: _____

_____

_____

f) _____: The incidence of pregnant women developing diabetes mellitus is the same for Aboriginal and non-Aboriginal populations.

Justification: _____

_____

_____

g) _____: Alcohol abuse is one of the most serious health and social problems faced by many Aboriginal communities.

Justification: _____

_____

_____

CHALLENGE YOUR LEARNING

CASE STUDY

Objectives

This case will help you understand how the lifestyle and eating patterns of young contemporary Aboriginal people has changed and the challenges associated with these changes, such as the challenges faced by individuals living off of a reserve.

Description

F.B. is a pleasant, sociable, and mature young woman. She is the receptionist at the Aboriginal Community Access Center where you work as a nutritionist. F.B. is an Oneida. She has been living downtown for 2 years, but always visits her mother on the weekend. Her mother lives on a reserve with F.B.'s younger sisters and brothers. The reserve is only a 1-hour drive away. F.B. enjoys her independence and the busy city life, but looks forward to a more traditional family life on the weekend. She gives generous support to her mother and grandparents, who are raising her siblings. F.B. also helps her family by giving part of her salary to her mother so that she can make ends meet.

F.B. is 26 years old, sedentary, and significantly overweight. F.B. is 5′5″ tall and currently weighs 175 lb. She says that her weight has increased since she has been living in town. F.B. lives alone in a small apartment she rents near the Aboriginal Community Access Center. She is currently taking a computer programming class in the evening at a nearby community college and has made some good friends. F.B. and her friends go out after class two to three times a week. They have a couple of favorite pubs downtown where they like to have a drink.

This morning, F.B. looks tired but excited. She tells you in a flash that she met this very nice man in town last night and that she will see him again tonight. Later on in the morning, F.B. comes by your office and asks if you would be willing to help her lose weight, because "you know best about these things," she says with a smile. You reply that you will be delighted to meet with her at lunchtime to discuss her lifestyle habits.

This is what she remembers eating yesterday, which was a Tuesday:

Breakfast:	3 pieces/slices of bacon (about 24 g cooked)
	1 large egg fried in bacon grease (46 g)
	1 cup (237 mL) diced potatoes fried in bacon grease
	2 slices of toasted white bread (30 g each)
	2 tsp (10 mL) butter per toast
	1 cup (8 fluid oz, 237 mL) coffee
	2 tsp (10 mL) sugar
Early morning snack:	1 glazed doughnut (47 g)
	1 cup (8 fluid oz, 237 mL) coffee
	2 tsp (10 mL) sugar
Late morning snack:	1 cup (8 fluid oz, 237 mL) coffee
	2 tsp (10 mL) sugar
	1 chocolate candy bar (2 oz, 57 g)
Lunch:	2 slices white bread (30 g each)
	2 slices beef lunchmeat bologna (1 oz, 28 g each)
	1 Tbsp (15 mL) mayonnaise
	1 frosted cupcake (30 g)
	1 can (1½ cups, 12 fluid oz, 355 mL) cola soda pop
Afternoon snack:	4 sandwich-type cookies (10 g each)
	1 can (1½ cups, 12 fluid oz, 355 mL) orange drink
Supper:	6 oz (168 g) fried beefsteak
	1 cup (237 mL) mashed potatoes
	1 cup (237 mL) canned corn kernels,
	with 1 Tbsp (15 mL) butter
	1 cup (8 fluid oz, 237 mL) tea
	2 tsp (10 mL) sugar
Evening snack:	1 serving of French fries (about 20 fries, 100 g)
	2 beers (12 fluid oz, 1½ cups, or 356 mL each)
	throughout the evening

1. Who are Oneida people?

2. What is F.B.'s body mass index?

3. What is your qualitative analysis of F.B.'s diet from what she ate yesterday? Explain.

4. What is your quantitative analysis of F.B.'s diet from what she ate yesterday?
   Use a *table of nutrient contents of foods* or *food composition and diet analysis software* to quantify the content of F.B.'s diet in terms of energy, macronutrients, and micronutrients.

5. List six questions you would ask F.B. in order to better understand her overall dietary pattern.

6. What practical feedback would you give F.B. on her dietary intake? Prepare four recommendations to help her improve her diet and list them in order of priority.

7. What advice will you give F.B. when she asks you how to lose weight? Explain.

8. Do you have any hypothesis as to why F.B. is not including milk and milk products in her diet? Explain.

9. What are your suggestions to help F.B. meet her calcium needs?

Case Follow-up

F.B. has now been dating that man for a year. This has been a great motivation for her to have a healthier lifestyle. F.B. has progressively lost her excess body weight by eating healthier and walking with her partner every night. They are now planning a family and F.B. asks you the following questions.

10. Is it true that some traditional Aboriginal foods are not good to eat anymore because of environmental contamination? Which foods are now at risk of being contaminated and why?

11. Why should I not consume liver from moose, caribou, seal, or beluga if my partner and I are trying to conceive?

Nutrition Care Process

INTRODUCTION

Since clinical nutrition is a medical intervention to help individuals with their health, the first goal of this section is to introduce you to medical care and the medical terminology and documentation systems used in health care institutions (Part 5.1). The second goal of this section is to make you familiar with the different elements of the nutrition care process (Parts 5.2 to 5.7), while keeping in mind ethics, jurisprudence, and quality of care (Part 5.8).

5.1 Medical Care and Records

REVIEW THE INFORMATION

1. Who are health care providers?

   _____

   _____

2. Who are the *clients* of a dietitian working in a health care setting?

   _____

   _____

   _____

3. What is the multidisciplinary health care team?

   _____

   _____

   _____

4. What is a medical record?

   _____

   _____

   _____

5. What are the primary purposes of medical records?

_____

_____

_____

UNDERSTAND THE CONCEPTS

1. What types of personal and health information are found in medical records?

_____

_____

_____

_____

_____

2. What are the four main components of the medical record and what information does each component contain?

a) Component: _____

Content: _____

_____

_____

_____

_____

_____

b) Component: _____

Content: _____

_____

_____

_____

_____

_____

c) Component: _____

Content: _____

_____

_____

_____

_____

_____

d) Component: _____

Content: _____

_____

_____

_____

_____

_____

3. Is there a specific order for each component in a medical record? Explain your answer.

_____

_____

_____

_____

_____

_____

_____

4. What does charting mean?

_____

_____

5. Who completes the charting?

_____

6. When is the charting done?

_____

_____

7. What is the meaning of the following medical abbreviations and symbols frequently used in charting?

Important notes: *Even though these medical abbreviations and symbols are utilized by numerous English-speaking health care professionals and health care institutions around the world, you should always verify which medical abbreviations are approved for use in your specific institution and understood by its multidisciplinary health care team members. This list is not a complete list.*

@ _____

A_{1C} _____

AA _____

Asmt _____

Abd _____

a.c. _____

ad lib _____

AIDS _____

Alb _____

Amts _____

ASAP _____

BEE _____

BG _____

BGC _____

bgm _____

b.i.d. _____

BMR _____

BMI _____

BP _____

BSA _____

BUN _____

BW _____

Bx _____

c̄ _____

Ca _____

CABG _____

CAD _____

cath _____

CBC _____

CBW _____

cc _____

CC _____

CDE _____

CF _____

CHD _____

CHF _____

CHO _____

Chol or chol _____

Cl _____

cm _____

CNS _____

CNSD _____

c/o _____

COPD _____

Cr _____

CRF _____

CVA _____

CVD _____

d _____

DAT _____

def. _____

Diet Rx _____

DM _____

D_5NS _____

DOB _____

DRI _____

D_5W _____

Dx _____

Ⓔ _____

EAA _____

ECG _____

EFA _____

e.g. _____

elec. or lytes _____

EN _____

esp. _____

ESRD _____

ETOH _____

f _____

FBS _____

Fe _____

FH _____

fl _____

fn _____

FTT _____

Fx _____

g _____

GDM _____

GERD _____

GI _____

gluc _____

GRF _____

GTT _____

GYN _____

h _____

Hb or Hgb _____

HBP _____

Hct _____

HDL _____

Hg _____

HIV _____

HN _____

H/O _____

h.s. or H.S. _____

HTN _____

ht _____

Hx _____

IBD _____

ibid _____

IBW _____

i.c. _____

ICU _____

ID _____

IDDM _____

idem _____

i.e. _____

i.m. or I.M. _____

in or " _____

i.v. or I.V. _____

K _____

Kcal or kcal _____

Kg or kg _____

KJ or kJ _____

L _____

Ⓛ _____

lb _____

lbs _____

LBM _____

LBW _____

LDL _____

LDL-c _____

LES _____

liq. _____

LLQ _____

LUQ _____

Lytes _____

μL _____

MAMC _____

max. _____

mcg _____

MCT _____

MD _____

meds. _____

mEq _____

Mg _____

MI _____

min. _____

mmol _____

MODY _____

mos. _____

mOsm _____

MVI _____

N _____

Ⓝ _____

Na _____

NA _____

Nb _____

NCP _____

neg _____

NG _____

NICU _____

NPO _____

N/V or N&V _____

O_2 _____

OB _____

OGTT _____

OR _____

OT _____

oz _____

P _____

p.c. _____

PG-SGA _____

PEG _____

PEM _____

PHx _____

PKU _____

PN _____

p.o. or po _____

P.O. _____

prn _____

Pro _____

Pt _____

Pt Ed _____

PUFA _____

q.AM _____

q.d _____

q.2d _____

q.h _____

q.4h _____

q.i.d _____

q.o.d _____

Qty _____

® _____

RBC _____

RD _____

RD/N _____

RDA _____

REE _____

rep. _____

RLQ _____

RN _____

RNP _____

R/O _____

RPh _____

RUQ _____

Rx _____

sec _____

Ser alb _____

Sgx _____

SOB _____

S/P _____

S&S _____

Sx _____

t _____

Δt _____

°T _____

tbsp _____

tsp _____

TB _____

TEE _____

TEN _____

TG _____

t.i.d. _____

t.i.d.a.c. _____

TLC _____

TPN _____

Tx _____

UBW _____

UL _____

UUN _____

Vit. _____

VLDL _____

vs _____

v/v _____

WBC _____

wk _____

WNL _____

w/o _____

wt _____

WW _____

x3 _____

y.o. or yo   _____

yrs   _____

Zn   _____

μ   _____

_____

↓   _____

↑   _____

∅   _____

~   _____

3x   _____

♀   _____

♂   _____

≥   _____

≤   _____

%   _____

Δ   _____

8. What is the nutrition care process?

_____

_____

9. What are the steps of the nutrition care process? Describe each step.

_____

_____

_____

_____

_____

_____

_____

_____

_____

10. What is the nutrition care plan?

_____

_____

_____

11. What is the HIPAA law in the United States <u>or</u> the PIPEDA law in Canada?

_____

_____

_____

INTEGRATE YOUR LEARNING

1. Explain why the medical record of a client has to be kept confidential.

   _____

   _____

   _____

2. What do multidisciplinary health care team members do?

   _____

   _____

3. What are standards of care?

   _____

   _____

   _____

4. What is a clinical pathway?

   _____

   _____

   _____

5. What do clinical pathways contain?

   _____

   _____

   _____

6. What charting style is appropriate for medical records?

   _____

   _____

   _____

   _____

   _____

7. How should an error be corrected in the medical record?

   _____

   _____

8. What is the difference between the initial care plan and the progress notes?

   _____

   _____

   _____

   _____

   _____

   _____

9. What can happen if the charting of care provided for a client is not appropriately done due to the following problems? Give some examples.

a) Incomplete charting:

_____

_____

_____

Example: _____

_____

b) Charting not performed in a timely fashion:

_____

_____

_____

Example: _____

_____

c) Charting not clear, legible, and using the correct medical abbreviations:

_____

_____

_____

Example: _____

_____

d) Charting not kept confidential:

_____

_____

_____

Example: _____

_____

e) Charting not individualized and patient centered:

_____

_____

_____

Example: _____

_____

CHALLENGE YOUR LEARNING

CASE STUDY

Objectives

You are now ready to use what you have learned about documenting clients' health information in their medical records, using appropriate medical terminology and abbreviations.

Description

You are a clinical nutrition assistant working with the dietitian in cardiology at St. Mary's Hospital. She is asking you to assist her with the nutrition assessment of a client this afternoon. You go right away to read the initial nutrition care plan she recently charted in the client's medical record (shown below) to understand the client's nutritional problem and see what has to be done.

EXAMPLE OF INITIAL NUTRITION CARE PLAN

Nutrition Services   Name of client
St. Mary's Hospital   Address
                                                                          Physician

<u>**Initial Nutrition Care Plan**</u>

Sept. 13, 2007, 10:00 AM

M.P. is a 75 y.o. African American ♂ Pt admitted for Ⓛ femoral arterial graft after arterial occlusion due to atherosclerosis. PHx of vascular problems: HBP × 5 yrs, CVA '03, infarction c̄ hospitalization in spring. ∅ ETOH & smoking × 2 yrs
ht = 5'8″

CBW = 117 lb BMI = 17.8 kg/m² ↓   UBW = 160 lb Ⓝ
Diet/calorie count: 1080 kcal (4540 kJ), 42 g pro., ↓ fat + salt, ↑ fiber intake
Labs N/A yet
P.O. meds. known to cause anorexia: haloperidol decanoate

↓ 43 lb in last 6 mos. (27% BW) due to P.O. anorexia and ↓ appetite since infarction. Pt at ↑ PEM risk. Diet/ calorie count shows insufficient Ⓔ & pro. intake. Pt willing to take oral suppl. @ hospital.

***Overall goal**: To help M.P. ↑ Ⓔ & pro. intake to prevent wt ↓, favor gradual wt ↑, and improve his nutritional status during hospitalization.*

***Specific objectives**:*

1. *Pt. Ed. + support to aid M.P. gradually ↑ Ⓔ & pro. intake.*
2. *To offer M.P. oral suppl. t.i.d.i.c. to help recover wt lost.*
3. *To assess + monitor M.P.'s nutritional status q.d. until improved.*

***Plan of action**:*

- *High Ⓔ, high pro. diet c̄ oral suppl. AM, PM, at bedtime started today.*
- *Asmt of M.P.'s nutr. status this PM: Scored PG-SGA, skinfolds, Ser.alb., N balance.*
- *Dietary counseling started this AM: M.P. shown how to ↑ Ⓔ & pro. intake.*
- *No restricting diet Rx, encourage M.P. to continue limiting dietary fat + salt.*

_____ *Laura Ann Philp, RD*

1. Translate the initial nutrition care plan. Make sure your handwriting is legible and that you use the correct meaning of the medical abbreviations and symbols.

2. Explain the advantages and disadvantages of using medical abbreviations and symbols in charting.

3. What is a femoral arterial graft?

4. What is haloperidol decanoate and why was it given to the client?

5. What is an oral nutritional supplement?

6. Why is an oral nutritional supplement given to this client?

7. Give some examples of complete oral nutritional supplements.

8. Many health care institutions are now using electronic charting or have at least part of their patient health information accessible through an electronic database. What are the <u>advantages</u> and <u>disadvantages</u> of electronic charting and medical records?

5.2 Nutrition Care Plan

REVIEW THE INFORMATION

1. What is clinical nutrition?

2. What are synonyms for clinical nutrition?

3. Where can dietitians work in clinical practice?

4. Who are clinical dietetic technicians?

5. What is defined as the course of action for meeting the client's nutritional needs based on the assessment of data collected?

6. Which term better defines "an ongoing collection of information that documents a client's individualized health care"?

   a) Health database   c) Progress notes   e) Health problem list
   b) Narrative notes   d) Medical record

7. What is the last step of the nutrition care process?

UNDERSTAND THE CONCEPTS

1. What main types of responsibilities do dietitians working in clinical practice have? Provide an example for each type of responsibility.
   Here is an example:
   > Type of responsibilities: *Supervisory responsibilities*
   > Example: *Dietitians give functional supervision and guidance to assigned technical and support personnel (e.g., clinical nutrition assistants).*

   a) Type of responsibilities: _____

   Example: _____

   _____

   _____

   b) Type of responsibilities: _____

   Example: _____

   _____

   _____

   c) Type of responsibilities: _____

   Example: _____

   _____

   _____

   d) Type of responsibilities: _____

   Example: _____

   _____

   _____

2. List the six main *clinical* responsibilities of dietitians in health care settings. An example is provided to help you.

   1- *Assessing the nutritional status of clients*

   2- _____

   3- _____

   4- _____

   5- _____

   6- _____

3. What are some of the responsibilities of clinical nutrition assistants?

   _____

   _____

   _____

   _____

   _____

   _____

   _____

4. Give some examples of standard problem-oriented formats used for charting care plans, including nutrition care plans.

_____

_____

_____

_____

_____

_____

_____

_____

_____

5. Explain what a *SOAP note* is.

_____

_____

_____

6. What are the three nutrition diagnosis components?

_____

_____

_____

INTEGRATE YOUR LEARNING

1. Indicate whether the following duties dietitians perform are related to their clinical responsibility of assessment, nutrition diagnosis, planning, implementation, monitoring and evaluation, discharge planning, or documentation of records.

   a) To refer and liaise with community nutrition services to ease the transfer of a client _____

   b) To ensure that a nutrition screening of all hospital clients is performed shortly after their admission

   _____

   c) To review on an ongoing basis the care provided to a client and progress made toward meeting the

   goals of care _____

   d) To evaluate the nutritional status of clients found at nutritional risk and of those referred by physicians

   _____

   e) To recommend a nutrition care plan to meet a client's dietary requirements _____

   f) To accomplish a nutrition care plan through nutrition counseling and education _____

   g) To determine the nutritional needs of a client based on data collected _____

   h) To chart the initial nutrition care plan for a client in his or her medical record _____

   i) To liaise with the patient foodservice technician to ensure that an appropriate modified diet is

   provided _____

j) To provide nutrition education to a client before he or she leaves the hospital so that he or she can manage his or her disease at home _____

k) To review the current hospital standards of nutritional care _____

l) To identify and state the nutrition problem a client has in his or her medical record, along with the signs and symptoms of that problem _____

m) To ask a client to share and explain his or her food choices and eating patterns based on his or her ethnic and religious beliefs _____

n) To ask a patient care support aid to provide feeding assistance to a client at mealtime _____

o) To communicate the food likes and dislikes of a client to the patient foodservice technician _____

2. In which section of the SOAP note would you chart the information below: subjective data (**S**), objective data (**O**), assessment of data (**A**), or plan of care (**P**)?

a) _____ Result of a laboratory test performed at the hospital

b) _____ Patient-centered and measurable overall treatment goal

c) _____ Age, gender, and chief complaint of the client

d) _____ List of medications prescribed by the treating physician

e) _____ Specific objectives including patient education

f) _____ Usual body weight and dietary intake information given by the client

g) _____ Factual information observed by a health care professional

h) _____ Dietitian's evaluation of the nutritional status

i) _____ Present or previous lifestyle habits or socioeconomic factors indicated by the client during an interview

j) _____ Recommendations by the dietitian for the physician's approval

k) _____ Family's perception of the problem with the health of the client

l) _____ Detailed plan of action, including work completed, in progress, and planned

m) _____ Physical examination data from the physician

n) _____ Dietitian's analysis and interpretation of data

o) _____ Calculated energy intake from observed food intake by the client at the hospital

p) _____ Dietitian's judgment of the problem based on the data collected

q) _____ Steps, activities, and interventions to implement, monitor, and evaluate the nutritional care provided to the client

r) _____ Measured height and weight at the hospital

s) _____ Evaluation of the acceptance of the diet prescribed and of the need for patient education

3. What are *measurable* goals?

_____

_____

_____

CHALLENGE YOUR LEARNING

CASE STUDY

Objectives

This case is asking you to chart a nutrition care plan using a standard charting format, just like the dietitian would do after a nutrition interview and education session with the client. To accomplish this, you will need to organize and synthesize the relevant information provided.

Description

Mrs. H. Brown asked her family physician to refer her to a registered dietitian to help her lose some weight. The physician encouraged her and gave her the contact information of your private dietetic practice.

While interviewing Mrs. Brown on the afternoon of September 14, she says, "I have been heavy since I started as a businesswoman in the 1980s. My weight has been increasing since then. I have a lot of stress in my life. I am always on the go and I usually meet my clients at the restaurant in the afternoon. I do not eat breakfast, but I stay up late at night and I tend to snack while driving or watching television.

The fact is that my young brother recently had a cerebrovascular accident and he is now paralyzed and in a wheelchair. He even needs some help to eat, like a baby! It breaks my heart to see him. Last week, he told me that this could also happen to me if I do not take care of my health, so I went to see my doctor. Dr. D. Bower prescribed me some Xenical (orlistat) and he said you could help me lose some weight and feel better. I do not want to end up like my brother! Do you think you can help me lose some weight? Give me a diet and I will follow it."

After hearing this, you feel that Mrs. Brown is ready to make significant improvements to her lifestyle and will most likely make efforts to follow your recommendations to help her adopt healthier eating patterns, which should translate into a healthier body weight in the long run. You encourage her in her desire to adopt a healthier lifestyle. You tell her that you will help her, but that she will be the leader, the one who will be making the necessary efforts and changes.

You ask Mrs. Brown to tell you about her usual daily dietary intake. Based on this information, you find that her daily diet provides her with about 3210 kcal (13,400 kJ) and that 45% of this energy comes from fat. Mrs. Brown is 55 years of age and sedentary, and smokes three to five cigarettes a day. She consumes the equivalent of four meals a day, including a late evening meal. She says that she does not like citrus fruits.

Mrs. Brown currently weighs 215 lb. Her height is 5'9". You determine that her total energy expenditure is about 1990 kcal (8300 kJ)/day, and you judge that her energy intake should be gradually reduced to 2150 kcal (9000 kJ)/day to help her lose weight.

The overall goal for Mrs. Brown is education for a gradual weight loss to help her reach a healthier body weight and prevent the complications of obesity.

One of your specific objectives is to support Mrs. Brown in adopting a healthy lifestyle and eating patterns, including having regular meals and exercising every day. Another specific objective is patient education to favor self-monitoring of her food intake, management of her stress, and a weight loss of 1 to 2 lb/week. Your last specific objective is to monitor Mrs. Brown's progress monthly.

You advise Mrs. Brown to consume three regular meals daily, including a breakfast. You ask her to complete a 7-day food record to show you at the next meeting in a month. At that visit, you will look at the 7-day food intake record and discuss healthy food options with her as well as what initial changes she is ready to make to begin to improve her diet.

In the following visits, you plan to set weight management goals and strategies with Mrs. Brown. You also plan to use MyPyramid (or Canada's Food Guide to Healthy Eating) as a teaching tool, as well as to counsel her to help her reduce her snacking and make healthy low-fat choices at the restaurant. Finally, Mrs. Brown agrees to come back on a monthly basis for follow-up and nutrition counseling.

1. Write a **SOAP note** based on the case information described. Use correct medical abbreviations and symbols. Make sure your handwriting is easy to read.

2. Use **focus charting** (DAR format) this time to chart the nutrition care plan based on the information provided.

3. Write a **DAP note** based on the same information.

5.3 Nutrition Interview

REVIEW THE INFORMATION

1. What is an interview?

2. What is a nutrition interview?

3. What skills are necessary for dietitians to perform a good nutrition interview?

UNDERSTAND THE CONCEPTS

6. What are the purposes of the nutrition interview?

7. What are the parts of the nutrition interview, and what are the purposes of each part?

_____

_____

_____

_____

_____

_____

8. How can confidentiality and privacy be respected during a nutrition interview?

_____

_____

_____

_____

_____

_____

9. Different types of questions can be asked to gather information during a nutrition interview.

a) What is the difference between *primary* and *secondary* questions?

_____

_____

_____

b) What is the difference between *open-ended* and *closed* questions?

_____

_____

_____

c) What is the difference between *neutral* and *leading* questions?

_____

_____

_____

10. Which of the following words or phrases tend to be found at the beginning of *productive* questions? Explain your reasoning.

What   Where   How   Do you   Tell me about   Why

_____

_____

11. Which of the following words or phrases tend to be found at the beginning of *nonproductive* questions? Explain your reasoning.

What   Where   How   Do you   Tell me about   Why

_____

_____

_____

12. There are different ways of responding to clients' statements during an interview, including using probing responses. What are some types of probing responses?

_____

_____

_____

_____

_____

_____

13. What are understanding responses?

_____

_____

14. A client recently diagnosed with breast cancer tells you the following during a nutrition interview: "*My mother died from cancer. It is so unfair that I had to get it too. All my life, I have always been watching what I am eating to be healthy. I cannot just leave my husband and the kids right now. They need me. I am too young. Isn't there a vitamin supplement I could take to fight it off? Tell me everything you know. Please tell me what to do and I will do it.*"

    Give an example of what an understanding response could be.

_____

_____

_____

_____

15. Give examples of ineffective responses to clients' statements.

_____

_____

_____

_____

_____

16. What is *patient-centered* care?

_____

_____

_____

_____

17. The hospital where you work is the regional cancer center of a large, multiethnic area of the city. Your clients are of various regional and cultural backgrounds. Many of your clients do not read English and some have difficulty understanding it. The clients' socioeconomic level ranges from low to high, and so does their level of education.

    a) What barriers to communication are you likely to face with your clients?

_____

_____

_____
_____
_____
_____
_____
_____
_____
_____

b) What can you do as a dietetic professional to reduce these barriers to communication with your clients?

_____
_____
_____
_____
_____
_____
_____
_____
_____
_____
_____

INTEGRATE YOUR LEARNING

1. What can be done (verbally and nonverbally) to help establish the first contact during the opening of the nutrition interview?

_____
_____
_____
_____
_____
_____
_____
_____
_____

2. What can be said to break the ice during the opening of the nutrition interview?

_____
_____

_____

_____

_____

_____

_____

_____

_____

_____

3. Determine if the following questions are primary (**P**) or secondary (**S**) questions.

a) _____ What are your eating habits during the week?

b) _____ What do you eat at the cafeteria at work for lunch with your colleagues?

c) _____ What type of pizza do you usually eat at the cafeteria for lunch?

d) _____ Where do you usually eat?

e) _____ Tell me about what you eat on the weekends.

f) _____ How often do you eat at a restaurant during the weekend?

g) _____ Which restaurants do you usually go to with your family every weekend?

h) _____ What is your favorite meal at the restaurant you go to on the weekend?

i) _____ How often do you consume snack foods?

j) _____ When you eat snack foods in the evening, what snack foods do you eat?

k) _____ How many crackers do you eat when you eat crackers in the evening?

l) _____ What types of crackers do you like to eat in the evening?

m) _____ Please tell me about your cultural food practices and beliefs.

n) _____ How much soy beverage do you think you consume on average daily?

o) _____ You told me you are vegetarian. What types of foods do you include in your diet?

p) _____ Which Kosher dietary laws do you usually observe?

q) _____ Please describe what you like and dislike to drink.

4. Determine if the following questions are open ended (**O**) or closed (**C**).

a) _____ What do you usually drink during the day?

b) _____ Do you drink water during the day?

c) _____ How many cups of coffee do you drink in a typical day?

d) _____ What type of milk do you put in your coffee?

e) _____ What do you like to eat in the morning?

f) _____ Do you have lunch?

g) _____ Is there any food you avoid?

h) _____ Tell me about the foods you consume when you are on the go.

i) _____ Do you snack as a way of coping with stress?

j) _____ What are your favorite foods?

k) _____ Are you hungry at mealtime?

l) _____ How do you think you could reduce the amount of fat in your diet?

m) _____ What do you think are possible reasons why you have been losing weight?

n) _____ What factors have influenced your choice to become vegan during adolescence?

o) _____ At what time do you usually have dinner?

p) _____ Do you observe particular religious holidays?

q) _____ What is your favorite fruit?

r) _____ Would you be willing to incorporate more whole grain products in your diet?

s) _____ How do you feel in the afternoon when you do not take time to eat lunch?

t) _____ What happens when you consume milk products?

5. Determine if the following questions are neutral (**N**) or leading (**L**).

a) _____ Who is involved in the preparation of meals in your household?

b) _____ Does your wife always prepare every single meal for you?

c) _____ How many meals and snacks do you usually have every day?

d) _____ You eat breakfast, don't you?

e) _____ Are you telling me that you are one of those people who does not eat breakfast?

f) _____ Did you skip breakfast again?

g) _____ You are still not eating breakfast, are you?

h) _____ What do you have for breakfast in the morning, cereal or toast?

i) _____ What do you usually eat in the evenings?

j) _____ What types of restaurants do you go to?

k) _____ Do you really enjoy these greasy foods?

l) _____ What beverages do you enjoy on a regular basis?

m) _____ Why do you keep on eating fried foods when you know your blood cholesterol is high?

n) _____ Don't you know you should be making an effort to avoid alcohol?

o) _____ Where on earth did you learn that milk is bad for adults?

p) _____ Don't tell me you like fast food?

q) _____ What is your excuse for not eating vegetables this time?

r) _____ What are your feelings toward including iron-rich foods in your diet, including meat?

s) _____ What are your favorite meals?

t) _____ Are there foods you dislike or avoid?

u) _____ Do you have any food allergies or intolerance?

6. Paraphrase the following statements from clients.

a) "You told me that I should reduce my salt intake because of my high blood pressure, but I do not know how I can do it when I eat fast food on the go all the time."

_____

_____

b) "I feel bad coming to see you because I know we discussed that it would be good for my health to re- duce my salt intake, but I have not been able to do it. I am sorry. I do not want to waste your time."

_____

_____

c) "I gave up on eating the fattening fast foods I used to enjoy so much every day, sometimes twice a day, and I lost 10 lb already."

_____

_____

d) "It is hard for me to reduce my sugar intake as my husband and children really like it when I bake and prepare our favorite cupcakes and pies."

_____

_____

CHALLENGE YOUR LEARNING

CASE STUDY

Objectives
This case is an opportunity to help you learn the best interview technique possible when interviewing a client. Expertise in interviewing clients comes with practice, so you are encouraged to actually role-play the case to help you visualize what you would do and say. You can practice in front of a mirror to see yourself and also practice with a peer. You can even arrange to videotape the interview and view it afterwards to evaluate your skills.

Description
B.R. is a 49-year-old Polish man recently diagnosed with hypercholesterolemia, due to high blood low-density lipoprotein cholesterol (LDL-chol) concentration. Mr. B.R. is an astronomy faculty member at a nearby university and is a very active man who walks to work almost every day. Dr. M. Bower has referred him to you, as you are one of the dietitians of the hospital's outpatient lipid clinic. Mr. B.R. has an appointment with you at 2:00 p.m. this afternoon for a nutrition assessment and education on how to have a healthy diet that is low in fat, especially saturated fat and cholesterol. The only information you have from the physician is that he is slim and that his father has had hypercholesterolemia for quite a number of years.

1. How would you get ready for the appointment with Mr. B.R.?

2. It is 2:00 p.m. and Mr. B.R. knocks on the door of your office. How would you greet him? Describe in detail your verbal and nonverbal communication with Mr. B.R. as you open the interview.

Case Follow-up
The opening of the interview with Mr. B.R. is going well. Mr. B.R. is talkative and has acknowledged that he is interested in getting your expertise on what would help him with his hypercholesterolemia problem. You are now getting to the body of the interview and starting the nutrition assessment.

3. What can you say to Mr. B.R. to switch the focus of the conversation toward the assessment of his usual dietary habits?

Case Follow-up

As you continue the interview, Mr. B.R. honestly tells you that he did not think he would ever suffer from hypercholesterolemia like his overweight father, as he is slim and regularly exercises by walking to work almost every day. He admits that he thought only overweight and obese people could develop hypercholesterolemia. He said that he did not pay attention to his diet in the past and ate high-fat fast foods on a regular basis, but that he is now willing to make an effort to reduce the amount of fat, saturated fat, trans fatty acids, and cholesterol in his diet.

4. Paraphrase this information for the client.

5. Time has passed and you now need to close the interview with Mr. B.R. How do you proceed? Describe your verbal and nonverbal communication with Mr. B.R. as you close the interview.

5.4 Nutrition Screening

REVIEW THE INFORMATION

1. What is a screening process?

_____

_____

2. What is a nutrition assessment?

_____

_____

3. Define malnutrition.

_____

_____

_____

4. Give some examples of malnourished individuals you might see in hospitals.

_____

_____

_____

_____

_____

_____

5. Who performs the nutrition screening of clients in hospitals?

_____

_____

_____

UNDERSTAND THE CONCEPTS

1. Explain the following statement: "Nutritional imbalances and malnutrition can go unnoticed unless a nutrition assessment is performed."

_____

_____

_____

2. What are the different methods of nutrition assessment?

_____

_____

3. What is nutrition screening?

_____

_____

4. What is the purpose of nutrition screening?

_____

_____

5. What characteristics or factors are associated with an increased risk of malnutrition in clients, and can be used as part of a nutrition screening?

_____

_____

_____

_____

_____

_____

6. Identify some nutrition screening tools.

_____

_____

_____

_____

_____

_____

7. Which of these nutrition screening tools have specifically been developed for elderly individuals?

_____

_____

_____

_____

8. What are the following types of malnutrition?

a) Marasmus: _____

_____

b) Kwashiorkor: _____

_____

c) Marasmic-kwashiorkor: _____

_____

9. Estimation of the fluid status

1- Define the following terms:

a) Dehydration: _____

_____

b) Euvolemia: _____

_____

c) Overhydration: _____

_____

d) Edema: _____

_____

e) Ascites: _____

_____

2- What are signs and symptoms of dehydration?

_____

_____

3- What are signs and symptoms of overhydration?

_____

_____

10. Who provides nutritional care to clients found at <u>low</u>, <u>moderate</u>, and <u>high</u> nutritional risk during nutrition screening?

_____

_____

11. Clients at high nutritional risk have to be screened within _____ of hospital admission.

a) 12 hours   b) 24 hours   c) 36 hours   d) 2 days   e) 3 days

12. Miss J.S. is a 43-year-old woman coming to the St. Mark's Regional Diabetes Center to meet with you for an initial nutrition interview. Miss J.S.'s height is 5′4″. She tells you that her weight has always been stable (around 160 lb), but that a year ago she started to become very ill. At the interview, you measure her weight to be 140 lb. You find in her medical record that she was diagnosed with breast cancer 12 months ago.

a) What is her usual BMI?

_____

_____

b) What is your interpretation of her usual BMI?

_____

_____

c) What is her percent weight change?

_____

_____

d) What is your interpretation of her percent weight change?

_____

_____

e) Calculate her current percent UBW.

_____

_____

f) What is your interpretation of her current percent UBW?

_____

_____

INTEGRATE YOUR LEARNING

1. What is important to keep in mind when selecting a nutrition screening tool?

_____

_____

_____

_____

_____

2. The "Determine Your Nutritional Health checklist" of the Nutrition Screening Initiative is based on warnings signs of nutritional risk forming the acronym DETERMINE. Which warning signs are they?

D: _____

E: _____

T: _____

E: _____

R: _____

M: _____

I: _____

N: _____

E: _____

3. What is the basis of the Scored Patient-Generated Subjective Global Assessment?

_____

_____

_____

_____

4. What are the advantages of the Scored Patient-Generated Subjective Global Assessment?

_____

_____

5. What signs of reduced muscle mass are often evident during the physical examination of a malnourished client?

_____

_____

6. What signs of reduced fat stores are often evident during the physical examination of a malnourished client?

_____

_____

7. What is the Mini Nutritional Assessment (MNA)? Explain what it involves.

_____

_____

_____

_____

_____

8. What is the process of identifying individuals who have risk factors that place them at potential risk for nutritional problems?

a) Dietary assessment   c) Laboratory testing   e) Clinical assessment
b) Nutrition screening   d) Medical diagnosis

9. Which of the following is designed for the detection of subclinical nutritional deficiencies?

a) Physical examination   c) Anthropometric assessment   e) Biochemical data
b) Diet history   d) Medical history

10. Mr. Lopez is a 48-year-old patient coming to your outpatient clinic for a nutrition interview and assessment. Mr. Lopez is 5'10" tall and thinks he currently weighs about 130 lb. You measure him on the clinic's weigh scale, however, and record a weight of 124 lb. On the previous progress notes in his medical chart, you find out that his weight 3 months ago was 150 lb with no prior loss or gain.

a) What is his present BMI?

_____

_____

b) What is your interpretation of his present BMI?

_____

_____

c) What is his IBW calculated from a BMI of 22.0 kg/m^2?

_____

_____

d) What is his weight change?

_____

_____

e) What is his percent weight change (from UBW)?

_____

_____

f) What is your interpretation of his percent weight change?

_____

_____

g) At what percentage of his UBW is he presently?

_____

_____

h) What is your interpretation of his percent UBW?

_____

_____

CHALLENGE YOUR LEARNING

CASE STUDY

Objectives

You are aware of the usefulness and importance of screening hospital clients for nutritional imbalances. This case study will now ask you to integrate the concepts you have learned and to practice doing the nutrition screening of a hospital client.

Description

M.V. is a 26-year-old client hospitalized early this morning in preparation for surgery, as part of the treatment for his duodenal cancer. The physician in charge ordered intravenous fluids and NPO until surgery tomorrow. The plan is to install a PEG-J tube during the surgery, so that M.V. can receive enteral nutrition below the cancer site after surgery.

You start a nutrition assessment right away to see if he is at nutritional risk. You find in the medical chart's database that his UBW is 161 lb, but that he has been suffering from diarrhea, abdominal cramps, and anorexia in the last 9 months. In the last 2 weeks, he was unable to put on his shoes because his feet were swollen. He has also been having steatorrhea.

At your request, M.V. reports on the Scored Patient-Generated SGA form that he currently weighs 111 lb and is 5'4" tall. Six months ago, he weighed 154 lb. One month ago he weighed 106 lb.

This is what you see when you look at M.V.: M.V. appears frail. He does not have the stamina to stand. His shoulders are squared and his acromions protrude. His scapula bones are very prominent. There is a deep indentation in the area between his thumb and forefinger when these fingers touch. His feet and ankles are visibly swollen.

1. What is his current BMI?

2. What is your interpretation of his current BMI?

3. What was his usual BMI?

4. What is your interpretation of his usual BMI?

5. What is his body weight change in the last month?

6. What is your interpretation of his body weight change in the last month?

7. What is his percent body weight change in the last 6 months?

8. What is your interpretation of his percent body weight change in the last 6 months?

9. At what percentage of his UBW is he presently?

10. What is your interpretation of the percent UBW?

11. What is your interpretation of this clinical sign: "His shoulders are squared and his acromions protrude"?

12. What is your interpretation of this clinical sign: "His scapula bones are very prominent"?

13. What is your interpretation of this clinical sign: "There is a deep indentation in the area between his thumb and forefinger when these fingers touch"?

14. Why are M.V.'s feet and ankles swollen?

15. What is your interpretation of M.V.'s nutritional status based on the Scored Patient-Generated SGA?

16. What is a PEG-J feeding tube?

5.5 Complete Nutrition Assessment

REVIEW THE INFORMATION

1. What is defined as the evaluation of the nutritional status of individuals?

   _____

   _____

2. What are other terms for *complete* nutrition assessment (as opposed to partial nutrition assessment or nutrition screening)?

   _____

   _____

3. Which types of clients need a complete nutrition assessment?

   _____

   _____

4. Fill in each space with the appropriate choice from the lists provided in parentheses.

   Nutrition assessment is the a) _____ (*first, second, third, or fourth*) step of the nutrition care process.

   Nutrition b) _____ (*problem, diagnosis, monitoring, or screening*) is based on the nutrition assessment and allows the dietitian to identify the nutrition-related c) _____ (*etiologies, problems, signs and symptoms, outcomes*) the client has, as well as their

   d) _____ (*etiology, problem, signs and symptoms, or outcomes*) or cause, and their

   e) _____ (*etiology, problem, signs and symptoms, or outcomes*) or defining characteristics.

UNDERSTAND THE CONCEPTS

1. What are the five components of the complete nutrition assessment?

   1- _____

   2- _____

   3- _____

   4- _____

   5- _____

2. What are known as the *ABCD findings*?

   _____

   _____

   _____

   _____

   _____

3. What is included in the medical history data?

   _____

   _____

   _____

   _____

4. What are anthropometric and body composition data?

   _____

   _____

   _____

   _____

5. What are anthropometric indexes? Give some examples.

   _____

   _____

   _____

   _____

6. How are anthropometric data from clients evaluated?

   _____

   _____

   _____

   _____

   _____

7. What are biochemical data?

   _____

   _____

8. Why are biochemical data useful?

_____

_____

9. What are the limitations of biochemical data?

_____

_____

10. What are some of the main biochemical measures of visceral (nonskeletal) protein status?

_____

_____

11. What hematologic biochemical measurements are used to measure iron status and determine if there is presence of anemia?

_____

_____

_____

_____

_____

_____

12. What are the main biochemical measures of blood lipid status and cardiovascular health?

_____

_____

_____

_____

_____

13. What are clinical data? Give an example.

_____

_____

14. What are the limitations of clinical data?

_____

_____

15. What are dietary assessment data?

_____

_____

INTEGRATE YOUR LEARNING

1. How can the ideal or healthy body weight of an adult be determined?

_____

_____

2. Visceral protein measurements are an indicator of protein status.

    1- What is the half-life of the following visceral proteins?

        a) Albumin: _____

        b) Transferrin: _____

        c) Thyroxine-binding prealbumin: _____

        d) Retinol-binding protein: _____

    2- Which of these visceral proteins has the fastest turnover?

        _____

    3- Therefore, which of these visceral proteins is more sensitive to acute nutritional changes?

        _____

    4- Which organ secretes many plasma proteins, including albumin, transferrin, and prealbumin?

        _____

    5- What happens to the blood concentration of visceral proteins when clients are dehydrated or overhydrated?

        _____

        _____

        _____

3. Aside from the measurement of visceral protein concentrations, what are other biochemical methods of estimating the protein status of clients?

    _____

    _____

    _____

4. Complete this table by identifying which nutrient deficiencies may cause these clinical signs of malnutrition in clients.

CLINICAL SIGNS OF MALNUTRITION RESULTING FROM NUTRIENT DEFICIENCIES	
Clinical Signs of Malnutrition	**Possible Nutrient Deficiencies**
a) Alopecia (baldness)	
b) Pellagra	
c) Rickets, osteoporosis	
d) Anemia	
e) Tooth decay	
f) Goiter, cretinism	
g) Scurvy	
h) Cheilitis	

(continued)

CLINICAL SIGNS OF MALNUTRITION RESULTING FROM NUTRIENT DEFICIENCIES
(continued)

Clinical Signs of Malnutrition	Possible Nutrient Deficiencies
i) Angular stomatitis	
j) Atrophic lingual papillae and glossitis	
k) Scaly, erythematous rash about the mouth and chin and on nasolabial folds and the palm of hands	
l) Impaired night vision, blindness	
m) Neural tube defects (e.g., spina bifida)	
n) Beriberi	

CHALLENGE YOUR LEARNING

CASE STUDY

Objectives
This case is asking you to perform a complete nutrition assessment for a client. You will need to consider all of the medical history data and ABCD findings in order to form an overall picture of the nutritional status of the client.

Description
Mr. T.P. is 68 years old and of French descent. He spends quiet time with his dog in his little old house near the city. His wife passed away 10 years ago in a car accident. Fortunately, he has enough money to live well and stay in their house. Mr. T.P.'s two sons had to move out of town a year ago for work, but faithfully call him once a week. Mr. T.P. often feels lonely and isolated. For the last week his sons had not been able to reach him, even though they left numerous messages on his answering machine. They started to become worried after not talking to him for many days. They decided to come visit him and found him in bed. Mr. T.P. said he had been too tired to come out of bed for the last 5 days, so they took him to the nearest hospital, where he was admitted for an assessment.

At first, you find the following information in his medical record: ht = 5'7"; CBW = 105 lb.

		HEMATOLOGIC TEST VALUES OF MR. T.P.*			
Blood Tests	Results in Conventional Units	Reference Ranges in Conventional Units$^\psi$	Results in International Units	Reference Ranges in SI Units$^\psi$	Interpretation of Results (Normal, High, or Low)
Serum Albumin	2.3	3.2–4.6 g/dL	23	32–46 g/L	
Serum Ferritin	15	20–150 ng/mL	15	20–150 µg/L	
CBC					
Total WBC count	3.9×10^3	$4.8–10.8 \times 10^3/\mu L$	3.9×10^6	$4.8–10.8 \times 10^6/L$	
Total RBC count	4.5×10^6	$4.7–6.1 \times 10^6/\mu L$	4.5×10^{12}	$4.7–6.1 \times 10^{12}/L$	
Hct	39	42%–52%	0.39	0.42–0.52	
Hb	11	14–18 g/dL	1.71	2.17–2.79 mmol/L	
MCV (of RBC)	72	80–94 μ^3	72	80–94 fL	
MCH (of RBC)	22	27–31 pg	0.34	0.42–0.48 fmol	

*CBC, complete blood count; RBC, red blood cells; Hct, hematocrit; Hb, hemoglobin; WBC, white blood cells; MCV, mean corpuscular volume; MCH, mean corpuscular hemoglobin; μ = mc (micro).
$^\psi$ Reference range values from Stegman JK, publisher. Stedman's Medical Dictionary for the Health Professions and Nursing. Illustrated 5th Ed. Baltimore: Lippincott Williams & Wilkins, 2005:177–191.

Afterwards, you gain additional information while doing the complete nutrition assessment:

Mid-upper-arm circumference: 8.7 inches (22.0 cm)
Mid-upper-arm muscle area: 19.5 inches^2 (31 cm^2)
Triceps skinfold thickness: 0.16 inch (4.0 mm)
Elbow breadth: 3.36 inches (74 mm)

Finally, you obtain the following information during an interview with Mr. T.P.:

He used to weigh about 145 lb, but he fell on an ice patch and broke his right leg last winter. Since then, he has had very little appetite, feels weak, and has lost weight progressively during the last 6 months. He stays around the house and calls the grocery store for home delivery once a week.

Mr. T.P. said that he had always been healthy before breaking his leg. He never took any medications. He does not keep alcohol at home and he smokes a pipe of tobacco after dinner.

While talking to Mr. T.P., you observe some hollowing near his temples, as well as protrusion of his clavicles and shoulder bones. He is telling you that his hair is now dry and dull, and that he is losing it easily.

Mr. T.P. said that since he broke his leg, his usual daily intake has included the following:

Breakfast:
1 medium banana, fresh (118 g)
1 slice of white enriched bread (25 g)
1 tsp (5 mL) butter
1 Tbsp (15 mL) black cane molasses
1 cup (237 mL) tea, brewed

Lunch:
1½ cup (355 mL) tomato soup made from:
- 1 cup (237 mL) tomato juice, canned
- ½ cup (118 mL) spaghettini noodles, wheat, cooked
5–7 crackers (15–21 g)
½ cup (118 mL) apple juice, canned, unsweetened

Dinner:
1 cup (237 mL) Special K cereal
1 cup (237 mL) homogenized milk
½ cup (118 mL) peach gelatin dessert mix prepared with water
1 cup (237 mL) herbal tea

1. What do you know about his medical history?

2. What do you know about his social history?

3. What do you know about his dietary history?

4. What is your interpretation of his bone frame size based on his elbow breadth?

5. What is his current body mass index? Give your interpretation.

6. What is his ideal body weight? (Calculate using BMI formula.)

7. What is his ideal body weight, using the Hamwi method?

> *Reminder:*
>
> *IBW for Men = 106 lb for 5 feet + 6 lb/inch over 5 feet (or −6 lb/inch under 5 feet)*
>   *Add 10% for large bone frame or remove 10% for small bone frame*
> *or*
>
> *IBW for Men = 48.18 kg for 150 cm + 1.1 kg/cm over 150 cm (or −1.1 kg/cm under 150 cm)*
>   *Add 10% for large bone frame or remove 10% for small bone frame*

8. What is his weight change?

9. What is his percent weight change? Give your interpretation.

10. What is his percent usual body weight? Give your interpretation.

11. What is his percent ideal body weight? Use the IBW you calculated in question 6 and give your interpretation.

12. What is your interpretation of his triceps skinfold thickness?

13. What is your interpretation of his mid-upper-arm circumference and mid-upper-arm muscle area?

14. What does the serum albumin and total WBC count help you to evaluate?

15. What is your interpretation of his serum albumin concentration?

16. What do the serum hematocrit and hemoglobin levels tell you?

17. What do the serum ferritin concentration, mean corpuscular volume, and mean corpuscular hemoglobin tell you?

18. List the clinical signs and their interpretation.

19. What other clinical signs would you look for?

20. Use nutrition analysis software to estimate his usual daily energy and protein intake.

21. Is his energy intake adequate? Justify.

22. What is his protein requirement?

23. Is his protein intake adequate? Justify.

24. What is his fluid intake?

25. Is his fluid intake adequate? Justify.

26. What is his iron intake?

27. Is his iron intake adequate? Justify.

28. What is your overall assessment of Mr. T.P.'s nutritional status based on the medical history data and ABCD findings? Explain.

5.6 Dietary Assessment

REVIEW THE INFORMATION

1. What is a dietary assessment?

   _____

   _____

2. What is the effect of diet on health?

   _____

   _____

3. What factors influence the diet of people (e.g., their eating habits, food choices, etc.)?

   _____

   _____

   _____

   _____

   _____

4. What <u>additional</u> factors have an impact on the dietary intake of <u>hospital clients</u>? Provide seven different factors and explain how they impact dietary intake.

   1- _____

   _____

   _____

   2- _____

   _____

   _____

   3- _____

   _____

   _____

4- _____

_____

_____

5- _____

_____

_____

6- _____

_____

_____

7- _____

_____

_____

5. How can diet be used to help clients?

_____

_____

_____

_____

_____

_____

6. What factors affect the dietary <u>needs</u> of individuals?

_____

_____

_____

_____

UNDERSTAND THE CONCEPTS

1. What are the steps of the dietary assessment?

_____

_____

_____

2. What information about the dietary intake of clients is important to collect during the dietary assessment?

_____

_____

_____

_____

_____

3. How can information about the dietary intake of clients be collected?

_____

_____

_____

_____

_____

4. How can the energy and nutrient intake of a client be quantified?

_____

_____

_____

_____

_____

_____

5. What are exchange lists?

_____

_____

6. How can the diet of clients be evaluated for its adequacy?

_____

_____

_____

_____

_____

_____

_____

7. What methods can be used to estimate the daily energy requirements of healthy adults?

_____

_____

_____

_____

_____

8. What methods can be used to estimate the daily energy requirements of adults under clinical stress conditions?

_____

_____

_____

_____

9. What is the most accurate method used to estimate daily energy requirements in health care settings, and what are the limitations of that method?

_____

_____

_____

_____

_____

_____

10. What are the modified Harris-Benedict equations?

_____

_____

_____

_____

_____

_____

_____

_____

_____

_____

11. What are the daily estimated protein requirements of healthy adults and of adults under clinical stress conditions?

_____

_____

_____

_____

_____

12. How are fluid requirements estimated?

_____

_____

_____

_____

_____

_____

INTEGRATE YOUR LEARNING

1. What is a diet history?

   _____

   _____

   _____

   _____

   _____

2. What are the advantages and disadvantages of these different dietary assessment methods?

ADVANTAGES AND DISADVANTAGES OF USING DIFFERENT DIETARY ASSESSMENT METHODS		
Dietary Assessment Methods	Advantages	Disadvantages
a) 24-hour dietary recall		
b) Self-administered food frequency questionnaire		
c) 3-day food record including a weekend day		
d) Diet history		
e) Direct observation		

3. Quantify the energy and macronutrient intake provided by the following usual daily intake using the Diet Count Form (also called Calorie Count Form) provided.

   Breakfast: 1 cup (8 fluid oz, 237 mL) orange juice
   2 pieces whole wheat bread, toasted (25 g each)
   4 tsp (20 mL) margarine
   4 tsp (20 mL) honey

   Morning snack: 1 cup (8 fluid oz, 237 mL) coffee with 1 tsp (5 mL) sugar

Lunch: 1 cup (237 mL) cooked rice
2 tsp (10 mL) margarine
½ cup (118 mL) cooked green peas
1½ oz (44 g) cooked lean ground beef patty
1⅓ cup (10⅔ fluid oz, 316 mL) regular cola pop

Afternoon snack: 1 small apple, fresh (106 g, 2½ inches or 6 cm diameter)
1 cup (8 fluid oz, 237 mL) water

Dinner: 1½ cup (35 mL) cooked pasta
½ cup (118 mL) tomato sauce
1 medium carrot, raw (72 g)
1 cup (8 fluid oz, 237 mL) milk, 2% fat

DIET COUNT FORM					
Food	Portion	Number of Portions	Carbohydrate (g)	Protein (g)	Fat (g)
Starch/bread	½ cup, 118 mL or 1 slice		15	3	
Fruit	½ cup, 118 mL or 1 small		15		
Vegetable	½ cup or 118 mL		7	2	
Milk:	½ cup or 118 mL				
- Nonfat			6	4	0
- 1% fat			6	4	1
- 2% fat			6	4	2
- Whole			6	4	4
Meat:	1 oz or 28 g				
- Very lean				7	0–1
- Lean				7	3
- Medium fat				7	5
- High fat				7	8
Fat	1 tsp or 5 mL				5
Sugar	1 tsp or 5 mL		5		
Others:					
Iced cake	1 small slice		65	4	4
Pie	⅙ of 9 inches (23 cm)		50	4	16
Soft drink	1 cup, 8 fluid oz or 237 mL		22		
Fruit gelatin	½ cup or 118 mL		18	2	
Total (g)					
			× 4 kcal/g or 17 kJ/g	*× 4 kcal/g or 17 kJ/g*	*× 9 kcal/g or 37 kJ/g*
Total					
TOTAL ENERGY	= _____				
% of Energy					

4. Use the Harris-Benedict equation below to calculate the daily energy need of this client based on his estimated total energy expenditure (TEE). The client is a 33-year-old Chinese man weighing 178 lb, measuring 5'11" tall, and who performs standing work (activity factor of 1.8).

   Reminder:

   BEE for men (kcal/day) = 66.47 + 13.75 W (kg) + 5.003 H (cm) − 6.775 A (years)

   or

   BEE for men (kcal/day) = 65 + 6.2 W (lb) + 12.7 H (inches) − 6.8 A (years)

   or

   BEE for men (kJ/day) = 278 + 58 W (kg) + 21 H (cm) − 28.5 A (years)

   _____

   _____

   _____

   _____

5. Mr. B.B. is an elderly man who has just been admitted to the Long Point Long-Term Care Institution, where you are the registered dietitian, because he could not live on his own anymore. Mr. B.B. is not eating much and seems depressed, and you are concerned about the adequacy of his energy and protein intake. He is 72 years old, presently weighs 175 lb, and measures 6'3". He tells you that his usual body weight was more like 210 lb when his wife was still alive, 5 years ago, to cook him his favorite foods. Mr. B.B. tells you that he still takes care of himself and walks to church (5-minute slow walk each way) every morning rain or shine.

   a) What is his basal energy expenditure, using the Harris-Benedict equation?

   _____

   _____

   _____

   _____

   b) What is his total energy need?

   _____

   _____

   _____

   c) What is his protein requirement per pound (or kilogram) of body weight?

   _____

6. During a nutrition interview, you ask Mrs. L.B., a patient with dyslipidemia type IIa, to tell you everything she ate or drank yesterday. She says that she has a pretty good memory for these things and that yesterday was a typical food intake day for her. You quickly analyze her food intake and realize that her daily protein intake is about 85 g, her daily fat intake is 96 g, and her daily carbohydrate intake is 120 g.

   a) What is the amount of energy coming from dietary proteins?

   _____

   b) What is the amount of energy coming from dietary fats?

   _____

   c) What is the percentage of energy coming from dietary fats?

   _____

   _____

7. Miss A. is a 32-year-old ambulatory patient with COPD. Her PO recovery is prolonged and you are concerned that her energy intake might not be adequate to meet her needs. As part of the nutrition assessment, you perform a diet count (or calorie count) and find that her Pro intake is about 50 g/day, her CHO intake is about 150 g/day, and her fat intake is about 40 g/day. You calculate her total energy expenditure to be 2240 kcal/day.

a) How much energy is coming from dietary protein?

_____

b) How much energy is coming from dietary carbohydrate?

_____

c) How much energy is coming from dietary fat?

_____

d) What is her total daily energy intake?

_____

e) What is the percent energy coming from dietary protein?

_____

f) If her energy intake is not adequate to meet her needs, by how many kilocalories (or kilojoules) per day should it be decreased or increased?

_____

_____

8. M.H. is a 53 y.o. ♀ who has recently received a Dx of mild colon cancer (benign tumor without metastases). M.H. has been admitted to the hospital c̄ CC of abd pain @ LLQ and is on a DAT. M.H. is presently confined to bed or chair. M.H.'s actual BW and ht are 120 lbs and 5′3″, respectively. M.H. does not have signs of muscle wasting. The Ser alb concentration of M.H. is presently Ⓝ.

a) What is M.H.'s basal energy expenditure in kJ/day, based on the Harris-Benedict equation?

Reminder:

BEE for women (kcal/day) = 655.10 + 9.563 W (kg) + 1.85 H (cm) − 4.676 A (years)

or

BEE for women (kcal/day) = 655 + 4.3 W (lb) + 4.3 H (inches) − 4.7 A (years)

or

BEE for women (kJ/day) = 2743 + 40 W (kg) + 7.7 H (cm) − 19.7 A (years)

_____

_____

_____

b) What is M.H.'s total daily energy need?

_____

_____

_____

c) What is M.H.'s dietary protein requirement in g/day, according to the adult Recommended Dietary Allowance for protein and her current body weight?

_____

_____

d) What is M.H's fluid requirement, in fluid oz/lb (or mL/kg) body weight, based on her age?

CHALLENGE YOUR LEARNING

CASE STUDY

Objectives

The dietary assessment is a key part of the comprehensive assessment of the nutritional status of clients. This case will be good practice for you to quickly assess the dietary intake of a client using a Diet Count Form (or Calorie Count Form) and to estimate his main dietary needs. The case will also be an opportunity to review anthropometric data.

Description

Mr. J.G. is a 32-year-old patient who broke several long bones in a car accident a week ago. Luckily, he did not suffer from multiple trauma, burns, or head injury. He is normally very active, but presently has to stay in bed most of the time to recover from the accident. His height is 6′2″ and his usual weight is 172 lb. His current weight is 167 lb and he is presently in a mild catabolic state. He has a large bone frame. Mr. J.G. is vegetarian and seems a little depressed. You are wondering if his energy and protein intake are meeting his requirements for recovery.

The dietetic technician provides you with a list of his food intake from the previous day at the hospital:

Breakfast:	½ cup (4 fluid oz, 118 mL) orange juice, pure
	1 cup (237 mL, 47 g) bran flakes
	1 cup (8 fluid oz, 237 mL) skimmed milk
	½ cup (118 mL) applesauce, unsweetened, canned
	1 cup (8 fluid oz, 237 mL) coffee, with 2 tsp (10 mL) granulated sugar
Lunch:	¾ cup (6 fluid oz, 180 mL) tomato juice, canned
	1½ cup (355 mL) cooked pilaf rice, plain
	½ cup (118 mL) green beans, boiled
	1 slice whole wheat bread (25 g)
	1 Tbsp (15 mL) soft margarine
	½ cup (4 fluid oz, 118 mL) apple juice, pure
	1 pear, small, raw (139 g)
Dinner:	1 cup (8 fluid oz, 237 mL) skimmed milk
	1 cup (237 mL) cooked elbow noodles, plain
	1 tsp (5 mL) soft margarine
	½ cup (118 mL) baby carrots, boiled
	1 slice pumpernickel bread (25 g)
	1 tsp (5 mL) soft margarine
	½ cup (118 mL) peaches, canned in juice
	1 cup (8 fluid oz, 237 mL) tea, with 2 tsp (10 mL) granulated sugar

1. What is Mr. J.G.'s current BMI? Give your interpretation of this information.

2. What is his IBW, according to the Hamwi method?

Reminder:
> IBW for Men = 106 lb for 5 feet + 6 lb/inch over 5 feet (or −6 lb/inch under 5 feet)
> Add 10% for large bone frame or remove 10% for small bone frame

or

> IBW for Men = 48.18 kg for 150 cm + 1.1 kg/cm over 150 cm (or −1.1 kg/cm under 150 cm)
> Add 10% for large bone frame or remove 10% for small bone frame

3. What is his weight change?

4. What is his percent weight change? Give your interpretation.

5. What is his percent UBW? Give your interpretation.

6. What is the percent IBW? (Use the IBW found using the Hamwi method.) Give your interpretation.

7. Perform a diet count (or calorie count) to estimate the energy and protein intake of Mr. J.G., based on his food intake of yesterday.

8. What is his energy intake in kcal/day or kJ/day?

9. What is his protein intake in g/day?

10. How much energy comes from dietary protein?

11. What is the percent of energy coming from dietary protein?

12. What is the percent of energy coming from dietary carbohydrate?

13. What is the percent of energy coming from dietary fat?

14. What is the basal energy expenditure, using his CBW?

Reminder: Modified Harris-Benedict Equations Method

For men: BEE (kcal/day) = 66.47 + 13.75 W (kg) + 5.003 H (cm) − 6.775 A (years)

or

BEE (kcal/day) = 65 + 6.2 W (lb) + 12.7 H (in) − 6.8 A (years)

or

BEE (kJ/day) = 278 + 58 W (kg) + 21 H (cm) − 28.5 A (years)

Activity Factors:
- Bed rest/chair-bound   1.05–1.2
- Work sitting with limited movements   1.4–1.5
- Work sitting with movement   1.6–1.7
- Work/activity standing   1.8–1.9
- High activity level/vigorous work   2.0–2.4

Clinical Stress Factors:
- After Sgx w/o complication   1.0–1.1
- Peritoneal infection   1.05–1.25
- Cancer   1.1–1.45
- Multiple and/or long bone Fx   1.1–1.3
- Sepsis   1.2–1.4
- Severe/acute infection   1.2–1.6
- Fever*   1.2 per degree Celsius over 37
- Closed head wound/injury   1.3
- HIV infection   1.3
- Infection + trauma   1.3–1.55
- Multiple trauma   1.4
- Burn injury   1.5–2.1

* degrees Celsius (°C) = [degrees Fahrenheit (°F) − 32] × 5/9

DIET COUNT FORM FOR J.G.

Food	Portion	Number of Portions	Carbohydrate (g)	Protein (g)	Fat (g)
Starch/bread	½ cup, 118 mL or 1 slice		15	3	
Fruit	½ cup, 118 mL or 1 small		15		
Vegetable	½ cup or 118 mL		7	2	
Milk:	½ cup or 118 mL				
- Nonfat			6	4	0
- 1% fat			6	4	1
- 2% fat			6	4	2
- Whole			6	4	4
Meat:	1 oz or 28 g				
- Very lean				7	0–1
- Lean				7	3
- Medium fat				7	5
- High fat				7	8
Fat	1 tsp or 5 mL				5
Sugar	1 tsp or 5 mL		5		
Others:					
Iced cake	1 small slice		65	4	4
Pie	⅙ of 9 inches (23 cm)		50	4	16
Soft drink	1 cup, 8 fluid oz or 237 mL		22		
Fruit gelatin	½ cup or 118 mL		18	2	
Total (g)					
			× 4 kcal/g or 17 kJ/g	× 4 kcal/g or 17 kJ/g	× 9 kcal/g or 37 kJ/g
Total					
TOTAL ENERGY	= _____				
% of Energy					

15. What is the energy need, using the total energy expenditure formula?

16. What stress factor did you use to calculate the total energy expenditure? Explain.

17. What activity factor did you use to calculate the total energy expenditure? Explain.

18. What is Mr. J.G.'s protein need in g/day, based on his CBW and on daily protein requirements of clients under clinical stress conditions?

Reminder:

Daily Protein Requirements for Clients in Clinical Stress Conditions

- For maintenance:	1.0 g	per kg (2.2 lb)
- For repletion:	1.3–2.0 g	per kg (2.2 lb)
- In catabolic states:	1.2–2.0 g	per kg (2.2 lb)
- After an operation:	1.0–1.5 g	per kg (2.2 lb)
- In sepsis:	1.2–1.5 g	per kg (2.2 lb)
- For refeeding syndrome:	1.2–1.5 g	per kg (2.2 lb)
- For multiple trauma:	1.3–1.7 g	per kg (2.2 lb)
- For burn injury:	1.8–2.5 g	per kg (2.2 lb)

19. Estimate Mr. J.G.'s fluid intake from what he drank at mealtime yesterday.

20. Compare Mr. J.G.'s fluid intake to the adequate intake of total water.

21. Compare Mr. J.G.'s food intake from the previous day to the recommendations of MyPyramid (or Canada's Food Guide).

22. What is your overall assessment of Mr. J.G.'s current diet? Explain.

23. Provide three practical and realistic suggestions to help Mr. J.G. meet his current energy, protein, and fluid needs.

    1) _____

    2) _____

    3) _____

5.7 Nutrition Counseling and Education

REVIEW THE INFORMATION

1. Explain the following statement: "Providing nutrition information is not enough to cause changes in eating behaviors."

    _____

    _____

2. What are three important components of the communication process?

    1) _____

    2) _____

    3) _____

3. What is the type of care given in clinical settings that is based on a helping relationship and partnership in solving the client's problem?

    _____

4. Give eight characteristics of effective nutrition teaching tools.

    1) _____

    2) _____

    3) _____

    4) _____

    5) _____

6) _____

7) _____

8) _____

UNDERSTAND THE CONCEPTS

1. What is nutrition counseling?

_____

_____

_____

2. What is the basis for nutrition counseling?

_____

3. What skills are necessary to perform nutrition counseling?

_____

_____

_____

_____

4. Why is it important for the dietitian to determine the client's readiness and motivation to change and to tailor the counseling approach accordingly?

_____

_____

_____

5. What are the stages of behavior change? Explain each stage.

_____

_____

_____

_____

_____

_____

_____

_____

_____

_____

_____

6. What is the basis of patient-centered care?

_____

_____

_____

7. What is the ultimate goal of nutrition counseling?

_____

8. What is the appropriate versus inappropriate body language and setting for a nutrition interview and/or counseling session?

APPROPRIATE VERSUS INAPPROPRIATE BODY LANGUAGE AND SETTING FOR COUNSELING	
Appropriate Body Language and Setting	Inappropriate Body Language and Setting

9. What is active listening?

_____

_____

10. What can be done in order to prepare for a nutrition counseling session?

_____

_____

_____

_____

_____

_____

11. What should be done during a nutrition counseling session?

_____

_____

_____

_____

_____

_____

_____

_____

12. What should be done after a nutrition counseling session?

_____

_____

_____

_____

_____

INTEGRATE YOUR LEARNING

1. Explain the following statement: "The client becomes the expert; the dietitian is the expert-maker."

_____

_____

_____

2. What is the basis of the helping relationship through which the dietitian helps the client?

_____

_____

_____

_____

3. How should the intervention of the dietitian be tailored in the following situations?

   a) The client has no willingness or motivation to change his or her current eating behaviors.

   _____

   _____

   b) The client is uncertain about making a change, mainly because he or she does not believe in his or her ability to change.

   _____

   _____

c) The client wants to improve his or her lifestyle and dietary habits, but does not know where to start.

_____

_____

4. Why are eating habit changes difficult to make and sustain?

_____

_____

_____

_____

5. Why is promoting compliance of clients to dietary recommendations not easy to do?

_____

_____

_____

_____

_____

6. You have a counseling session scheduled with Mrs. S.V. this morning to help her with her constipation problem, at the request of her physician.
   Mrs. S.V. is an 83-year-old Greek woman who lives with her daughter. Her understanding of the English language is limited. She comes from a large family of farmers. She never attended school and does not know how to read. She is poor and dependent on her daughter for resources necessary for daily living.
   What should you keep in mind during the counseling session to communicate effectively with Mrs. S.V.?

_____

_____

_____

_____

_____

_____

_____

CHALLENGE YOUR LEARNING

CASE STUDY

Objectives
This is an opportunity for you to test your understanding of client counseling concepts and see how you could help a client who is in need of behavioral change. Keep in mind to always respect the client, who is the leader in the decision-making process.

Description
Ms. R.G.M. is an obese, single, sedentary, 33-year-old Caucasian woman. She works long hours in a corner store open 24 hours a day and lives in an apartment build-

ing next to the store. She has barely enough money to pay the monthly rent, and the rest of her income goes to taking care of her elderly mother, since they do not have enough money for her to be in a senior retirement facility. Ms. R.G.M. is a hard worker and rarely complains about her situation. She loves her mother and promised to take good care of her. She always stays nearby in case her mother needs help, so she can come quickly.

Ms. R.G.M. has been feeling sick for the last few months. She feels more and more tired and weak all the time. She barely has the energy to take care of her mother anymore. The physician diagnosed her with type 2 diabetes mellitus and had her start medication and insulin treatments. He asked her to meet with the dietitian to improve her diet and lose weight.

Ms. R.G.M. is now feeling a little better and is meeting with you today for a nutrition assessment. When you ask her what she usually eats during the day, she tells you that she does not eat on a regular basis, but rather has snacks throughout the day. "I start working at 3:00 a.m., so I do not have time to have breakfast before I leave the apartment. I usually sip soda pop during the day and I have a chocolate bar, vanilla cup cake, or granola bar when there are no clients around at the store. I often have a frozen pizza with mom for dinner. I do not know why the doctor wanted me to meet with you, as I do not eat that much for it to be a problem. I have always been at this weight and that is not about to change. I do not have money to go to the fancy restaurants and order nice pieces of meat, you know."

1. What is your interpretation of what Ms. R.G.M. is telling you?

2. In what stage of behavioral change is Ms. R.G.M. presently? Explain why.

3. Is Ms. R.G.M. motivated to change? Explain your answer.

4. What actions can be taken to help Ms. R.G.M.?

5. What are some barriers that make it harder for Ms. R.G.M. to make behavioral changes?

5.8 Ethics, Jurisprudence, and Quality of Care

REVIEW THE INFORMATION

1. What are some of the overall responsibilities of dietitians working in clinical practice?

_____

_____

_____

_____

_____

_____

2. How are professional standards of practice for dietitians established?

_____

_____

3. What is a quality assurance or quality control program?

_____

_____

_____

_____

4. Which federal law protects patient rights by ensuring protection of personal information, including health information?

_____

_____

UNDERSTAND THE CONCEPTS

1. What are the standards of professional performance (United States) or professional standards of practice (Canada) of dietitians?

_____

_____

_____

_____

_____

_____

2. Why is the registration of dietitians necessary?

_____

_____

3. How can dietitians be professional?

_____

_____

_____

_____

4. How can dietitians ensure their competence?

_____

_____

_____

_____

5. What is a code of ethics?

_____

_____

6. What is a professional misconduct regulation?

_____

_____

7. What are some of the legal duties of dietitians?

_____

_____

_____

_____

8. What are the confidentiality obligations?

_____

_____

_____

_____

9. Indicate whether the following statements about the privacy of personal information are TRUE or FALSE.

   a) _____ Clients have the legal right to have access to their medical chart.

   b) _____ A dietitian who makes a mistake when charting in the medical record of a client has the duty to correct the erroneous information.

   c) _____ Medical charts have to be kept for 5 years after the last visit of the client.

10. When do dietitians need to obtain informed consent from their clients? Give examples.

_____

_____

_____

_____

_____

_____

_____

11. How should dietitians gain informed consent from their clients for treatment?

_____

_____

_____

_____

_____

_____

_____

12. What are record-keeping guidelines?

_____

_____

_____

13. According to the law, when is it mandatory for dietitians to report inappropriate patient care or information related to a client?

_____

_____

_____

_____

14. What is a controlled act?

_____

_____

15. Can dietitians perform the following controlled acts?

a) _____ To communicate a diagnosis to a client or his or her family

b) _____ To prescribe a drug or vitamin supplement

c) _____ To put an instrument beyond the larynx

d) _____ To give an injection in a tissue below the dermis

e) _____ To dispense or sell drugs or vitamin supplements

f) _____ To give an order for medical treatment or diagnosis procedure

16. What does *quality health care* refer to?

_____

_____

_____

17. What are the main obligations of dietitians under the HIPAA (in the United States) and PIPEDA (in Canada) laws and their related regulations?

_____

_____

_____

_____

_____

_____

_____

_____

18. What is evidence-based practice, and why is it desirable?

_____

_____

_____

_____

_____

INTEGRATE YOUR LEARNING

1. You have been working for 2 years as a registered dietitian in the United States. You and your husband are moving to Canada for a sabbatical year. Can you start working as a dietitian in Canada? Explain why.

_____

_____

_____

_____

2. Here are 10 rules to guide the patient–clinician relationship and help to increase the quality of health care. Please explain what each rule means and how it should be applied in practice.

1- "Safety should be a system property."

_____

_____

_____

2- "Transparency to the client is necessary."

_____

_____

_____

3- "Client needs should be anticipated."

_____

_____

_____

4- "Waste should be continuously reduced."

_____

_____

_____

5- "Cooperation among health care professionals should be a priority."

_____

_____

_____

6- "Care should be based on a continuous helping relationship."

_____

_____

_____

7- "Care should be customized to clients' needs and values."

_____

_____

_____

8- "The client should be the source of control."

_____

_____

_____

9- "Knowledge should be shared and information should flow freely."

_____

_____

_____

10- "Decision making should be evidence-based."

_____

_____

_____

3. Explain what systems and requirements are in place to protect health care clients.

_____

_____

_____

_____

_____

_____

_____

_____

_____

_____

_____

_____

_____

_____

_____

_____

CHALLENGE YOUR LEARNING

CASE STUDY

Objectives

The objective of this case is to integrate your knowledge of ethics, jurisprudence, and quality of care and use it to guide the decisions you are making as part of concrete day-to-day work situations. The case will also ask you to apply your knowledge of the nutrition care process, and you will need to use your judgment to determine what is in the best interest of the client.

Description

You started to work as a contract dietitian in a large 50-bed long-term care institution last month. Since they did not have a dietitian for a while, you initially performed a nutrition screening of all of the residents. You are now overwhelmed with the number of residents requiring your intervention due to nutritional risk and the very small amount of time (15 minutes) you have to help each resident every month. In order to help more residents every day, you decide to perform as many nutritional assessments and interventions as possible during the day. You then take part of the medical records home with you at night, chart your nutrition care plans in the evening, and insert everything (the information you took plus your charted notes) in the clients' medical record early the following morning.

1. Is this the appropriate way to deal with the amount of work? Explain your position.

2. What negative consequences are associated with the way the problem of work overload was dealt with?

3. What should be done if the charting in the medical record is delayed?

4. What would have been a correct way to deal with the situation?

Case Follow-up

You notice that a resident, Mrs. B.W., is moderately malnourished due to poor dietary intake resulting from ill-fitting dentures. The client lost weight due to pneumonia a few months ago and her dentures are not fitting properly, so she does not wear them. You perform resident meal rounds at lunchtime and you observe that Mrs. B.W. is having a hard time chewing on her gums and is often choking on meat and bread. You switch Mrs. B.W. to a pureed diet to reduce the need for chewing. The next day, a nurse tells you that Mrs. B.W., who is 80 years old, is quite upset, has not touched her last two meals, and has told the nurse, "I do not want to eat that baby food at my age! Give me real food!"

5. Was it the proper way to try to help Mrs. B.W.? Explain your position.

6. List some negative consequences that may result from the intervention you described in question 5.

7. What would have been a correct way to deal with the situation?

8. What could be done now?

Regular and Modified Diets

INTRODUCTION

Dietitians working in health care facilities have the responsibility of ensuring that all clients receive appropriate nutrition to meet their nutritional needs consistent with their health condition and individual requirements. While many clients require a regular diet (Part 6.1) during their hospital stay, some clients benefit from a diet modified in consistency (Part 6.2) or in nutrient composition (Part 6.3) in order to help in the prevention or treatment of their disease. Moreover, certain clients need nutrition support in addition to, or instead of, an oral diet to help them meet their nutritional needs. Nutrition support can be provided as oral supplements or through specialized nutrition routes, such as enteral nutrition or parenteral nutrition, which we will discuss in Part 7.

6.1 Regular Diet in Health Care Institutions

REVIEW THE INFORMATION

1. Give six meal-planning principles known to promote good health.

   _____

   _____

2. What do you perceive are the seven main challenges in trying to meet the nutritional needs of all the clients in a hospital at any given time while operating within health care resource constraints? Briefly explain each challenge.

   1) _____

   _____

   _____

   2) _____

   _____

   _____

3) _____
_____
_____

4) _____
_____
_____

5) _____
_____
_____

6) _____
_____
_____

7) _____
_____
_____

3. What are outsourced food products? Why do many hospitals include outsourced products in their menu?

_____
_____
_____
_____
_____
_____

UNDERSTAND THE CONCEPTS

1. What is a *regular diet*, in reference to food offered to patients in hospitals?

_____
_____
_____
_____

2. What are other names given to the hospital's *regular diet*?

_____
_____

3. What are some of the characteristics of the typical regular diet in hospitals?

_____
_____
_____
_____

4. What is a selective menu?

_____

_____

_____

_____

5. What is a cyclical menu?

_____

_____

_____

_____

6. Give some examples of computerized foodservice software systems used by hospitals.

_____

_____

_____

_____

7. What information is inputted into computerized foodservice software systems?

_____

_____

_____

_____

8. What is a menu template?

_____

_____

_____

_____

INTEGRATE YOUR LEARNING

1. Describe in detail the process that takes place from the diet order to the meal being served to a hospital client. Indicate who is involved in the different steps of the process (dietitian, physician, dietetic technician/nutrition assistant, patient support workers, etc.).

_____

_____

_____

_____

_____

_____

_____

_____
_____
_____
_____
_____
_____
_____
_____
_____
_____
_____
_____

2. If you had just been admitted to the hospital, what type of meal would you receive?

_____
_____
_____
_____

3. What are 10 reasons why a hospitalized client may not eat?

1) _____
_____

2) _____
_____

3) _____
_____

4) _____
_____

5) _____
_____

6) _____
_____

7) _____
_____

8) _____
_____

9) _____
_____

10) _____
_____

CHALLENGE YOUR LEARNING

CASE STUDY

Objective

Planning a healthy menu may seem easy. Planning a menu for a large number of people can be difficult. Planning a menu for numerous hospital clients with diverse nutritional needs while simultaneously trying to work within a limited budget is even more challenging!

Therefore, the objective of this case is to realize the importance of standardization and careful planning in the implementation of a new hospital menu or in making changes to an existing menu. Standardization and careful planning are two key components to successfully implement and deliver nutritious and enjoyable meals, which will concurrently meet the patients' nutritional needs.

The first step is to plan the regular or general diet. Keep in mind that the foods in the regular diet should be fairly easy to modify to later plan the modified diets necessary to meet the needs of the clients requiring specialized diets modified in consistency and/or composition.

Description

You have been promoted to assistant foodservice supervisor of a 300-bed acute care hospital facility. The foodservice of the hospital is centralized in a food production center, where food is prepared and meals are cold-plated. Trays are then distributed to three hospital wings, where meals are reheated before being delivered to the clients in the various clinical departments. The average length of patient stay is 4 days. After getting poor results on consecutive patient satisfaction surveys performed over the last 2 years, your supervisor is asking for your help to change the menu. Up until now, the hospital has had a nonselective 21-day menu. However, you have recently convinced your supervisor that a selective menu would increase patient satisfaction and that a shorter menu cycle would decrease production costs.

1. What are patient satisfaction surveys?

2. Outline a realistic menu template for a 7-day selective cyclic menu to be offered to the clients of the acute care hospital. Keep in mind the meal-planning principles that promote good health when planning the menu.

MENU TEMPLATE			
	Breakfast	**Lunch**	**Dinner**
Appetizers			
Bread and cereals			
Entrées			
Beverages			
Condiments			
Dessert			

3. Prepare a regular-diet 7-day selective cyclic menu following the standard menu template you have outlined for each day.

   Notes:

   - *Be realistic as to what could be included on the hospital menu during the summer months with a limited budget.*

   - *Include meals easily produced in large quantities that reheat well, items that most people will like, healthy foods from each food group, and enough variety to meet nutrient needs.*

   - *Include foods that can be easily modified to accommodate the diets modified in consistency or composition at a later stage of menu planning.*

REGULAR-DIET 7-DAY SELECTIVE CYCLIC MENU							
	Day 1	Day 2	Day 3	Day 4	Day 5	Day 6	Day 7
Breakfast							
Lunch							

(continued)

REGULAR-DIET 7-DAY SELECTIVE CYCLIC MENU *(continued)*							
	Day 1	**Day 2**	**Day 3**	**Day 4**	**Day 5**	**Day 6**	**Day 7**
Dinner							

6.2 Modified Consistency Diets

REVIEW THE INFORMATION

1. What types of diets are routinely offered in hospital settings?

_____

_____

_____

2. Define *consistency* of food.

_____

_____

3. What is the *texture* of food?

_____

_____

4. What are dietary fibers?

_____

_____

5. What are residues?

_____

_____

6. What is the relation between dietary fibers and residues?

_____

_____

7. What does edentulous mean?

_____

_____

8. What are reasons why patients may not wear their dentures?

_____

_____

9. What are the four physiologic phases of the normal swallow?

1) _____

2) _____

3) _____

4) _____

UNDERSTAND THE CONCEPTS

1. What are modified diets?

_____

_____

2. Give some examples of diets modified in consistency.

_____

_____

3. When does the consistency of foods served to clients need to be modified? Give some examples.

_____

_____

_____

_____

4. What is dysphagia?

_____

_____

5. What main diets for dysphagia are usually available in acute care hospitals?

_____

_____

_____

_____

_____

_____

6. What are the following modified diets and when are they indicated?

   a) **Clear liquid diet**

      Description: _____

      _____

      Indication: _____

      _____

   b) **Blenderized liquid diet**

      Description: _____

      _____

      Indication: _____

      _____

   c) **Mechanically altered diet**

      Description: _____

      _____

      Indication: _____

      _____

   d) **Diets for dysphagia**

      Description: _____

      _____

      _____

      _____

      Indication: _____

      _____

      _____

      _____

7. Which foods are included in the clear liquid diet?

   _____

   _____

   _____

8. Which foods are not included in the clear liquid diet?

   _____

   _____

   _____

9. Prepare a 1-day sample menu for a client on a clear liquid diet. Include three meals and four snacks spread throughout the day.

   _____

   _____

   _____

_____

_____

_____

_____

_____

_____

10. What is the purpose of the clear liquid diet?

_____

_____

11. What is the osmolality of liquids?

_____

_____

_____

_____

_____

12. When should the osmolarity of liquids given to clients be controlled?

_____

_____

_____

13. Which fluids are hyperosmolar? Give some examples.

_____

_____

_____

14. What is the osmolality of serum?

_____

15. Which fluids have a low osmolarity? Give some examples.

_____

_____

16. What can be done to increase the tolerance to hyperosmolar fluids?

_____

_____

_____

17. Which foods are included in the blenderized liquid diet?

_____

_____

_____

18. Which foods are not included in the blenderized liquid diet?

_____

_____

_____

19. Propose a sample 1-day menu for a young adult male client who is unable to chew after a facial surgery.

_____

_____

_____

_____

_____

_____

_____

_____

20. Which foods are recommended for clients on the mechanically altered diet?

_____

_____

_____

21. Which foods are not recommended for clients on the mechanically altered diet?

_____

_____

_____

22. Define the following medical terms related to dysphagia.

a) Achalasia: _____

_____

b) Dysarthria: _____

_____

c) Ataxia: _____

_____

d) Tremor: _____

_____

e) Dyskinesia: _____

_____

f) Xerostomia: _____

_____

g) Trismus: _____

_____

h) Aspiration: _____

_____

23. What health complications are associated with untreated dysphagia?

_____

_____

_____

24. Why is aspiration dangerous?

_____

_____

_____

25. What is the difference between overt aspiration and silent aspiration?

_____

_____

_____

26. Explain the following three types of aspiration.

    1) *Prandia* aspiration: _____

    2) *Reflux* aspiration: _____

    3) *Salivary* aspiration: _____

27. Indicate which phase of the swallow is defective when the following complications are found in dysphagia clients:

    a) Difficulty chewing (e.g., due to poor jaw movement): _____

    b) Coughing: _____

    c) Food pocketing in the jaws (e.g., due to reduced cheek tone or sensitivity): _____

    d) Bolus remaining in the esophagus (e.g., due to reduced esophageal peristalsis, narrowing of the esophagus): _____

    e) Poor bolus formation (e.g., due to poor tongue control, partial glossectomy): _____

    f) Wet "gurgly" vocal quality: _____

    g) Excessive or thick saliva: _____

    h) Drooling and food leaking out of the mouth (e.g., reduced lip tone, excessive saliva): _____

    i) Aspiration: _____

28. Give 10 examples of *neurologic* diseases or conditions that are associated with dysphagia.

    1) _____

    2) _____

    3) _____

    4) _____

    5) _____

    6) _____

    7) _____

    8) _____

    9) _____

    10) _____

29. What are the five main goals of the diets for dysphagia?

    1) _____

    2) _____

    3) _____

    4) _____

    5) _____

30. Who performs dysphagia screening and when is it performed?

    _____
    _____
    _____
    _____

31. In addition to the usual medical and nutritional assessment procedures, the evaluation of a possible swallowing disorder by the multidisciplinary health care team requires a swallowing evaluation.

    Describe the main components of the swallowing evaluation and who is involved.

    _____
    _____
    _____
    _____
    _____
    _____
    _____
    _____
    _____
    _____
    _____
    _____

INTEGRATE YOUR LEARNING

1. Is the clear liquid diet nutritionally adequate? Justify your answer.

    _____
    _____
    _____

_____
_____
_____
_____
_____

2. What are the advantages and disadvantages of giving a clear liquid diet to clients?

   1) Advantages:

   _____
   _____
   _____
   _____

   2) Disadvantages:

   _____
   _____
   _____
   _____

3. Your client on a clear liquid diet is trying to progress to a regular diet, but has gas and nausea. What are your dietary recommendations to ease his progression to a regular diet?

   _____
   _____
   _____
   _____

4. Determine the energy and macronutrient content of this sample 1-day clear liquid diet menu using the diet count form provided.

   | Breakfast: | Strawberry gelatin (½ cup, 118 mL) |
   | | Apple juice (½ cup, 4 fluid oz, 118 mL) |

   | Morning snack: | Grape juice frozen popsicle |
   | | (½ cup, 118 mL, made from pure fruit juice) |

   | Lunch: | Chicken bouillon (½ cup, 118 mL) |
   | | Strained (pulp-free) orange juice (½ cup, 4 fluid oz, 118 mL) |

   | Afternoon snack: | Ginger ale (1 cup, 8 fluid oz, 237 mL) |

   | Dinner: | Beef consommé (½ cup, 118 mL) |
   | | Peach gelatin (½ cup, 118 mL) |

   | Early evening snack: | Tea (1 cup, 8 fluid oz, 237 mL) with sugar (1 tsp, 5 mL) |

   | Late evening snack: | Lemonade (pulp-free) juice (½ cup, 4 fluid oz, 118 mL) |

5. Is the blenderized liquid diet nutritionally adequate? Justify your answer.

   _____
   _____
   _____
   _____

DIET COUNT OF CLEAR LIQUID DIET 1-DAY SAMPLE MENU

Food	Portion	Number of Portions	Carbohydrate (g)	Protein (g)	Fat (g)
Fruit	½ cup, 118 mL or 1 small		15		
Fat	1 tsp or 5 mL				5
Sugar	1 tsp or 5 mL		5		
Others:					
Soft drink	1 cup, 8 fluid oz or 237 mL		22		
Fruit gelatin	½ cup or 118 mL		18	2	
Beef/chicken bouillon/ consommé	½ cup or 118 mL		1	2	
Total (g)			*× 4 kcal/g or 17 kJ/g*	*× 4 kcal/g or 17 kJ/g*	*× 9 kcal/g or 37 kJ/g*
Total					
TOTAL ENERGY	= _____				
% of Energy					

6. Give seven practical suggestions to help clients on a liquid diet (clear liquid or blenderized liquid diet) increase their energy and nutrient intake.

1) _____

_____

2) _____

_____

3) _____

_____

4) _____

_____

5) _____

_____

6) _____

_____

7) _____

_____

7. Indicate four ways to increase the nutrient density of blenderized liquid food.

1) _____

_____

2) _____

_____

3) _____

_____

4) _____

_____

8. Explain the following statement: "Gastroesophageal reflux is premorbid in clients with dysphagia."

_____

_____

_____

_____

9. Describe the following liquid viscosities and provide some examples of each of them.

a) Thin liquid consistency

Description: _____

_____

Examples: _____

_____

b) Nectar-like liquid consistency

Description: _____

_____

Examples: _____

_____

c) Honey-like liquid consistency

Description: _____

_____

Examples: _____

_____

d) Spoon-thick liquid consistency

Description: _____

_____

Examples: _____

_____

10. Which dietary strategies would help to stimulate swallowing in clients with dysphagia?

_____

_____

_____

_____

11. What foods are less likely to be tolerated by clients with dysphagia in general?

_____

_____

_____

12. What foods are most likely to be tolerated by clients with dysphagia in general?

_____

_____

_____

_____

13. Indicate whether or not it would be recommended to offer these foods to clients on the following modified diets.

DIETS MODIFIED IN CONSISTENCY				
Foods/Modified Diets	Clear Liquid Diet	Blenderized Liquid Diet	Puréed Diet With Thick Liquids	Mechanically Altered Diet
Gelatin				
Puréed chicken				
Canned peaches				
Cooked noodles				
Mashed potatoes				
Milk pudding				
Smooth peanut butter				
Vanilla ice cream				
Applesauce				

CHALLENGE YOUR LEARNING

CASE STUDY

Objectives

An objective of this case is for you to realize that clients suffering from dysphagia often have many risk factors contributing to their problems chewing and swallowing, and that each causal factor should be addressed in an individualized nutrition care plan.

Another objective is to combine your understanding of the pathophysiology of dysphagia and your knowledge of how food consistency can be altered, to suggest ways to modify the diet of a client in order to provide him with safe, nutritious foods, which will positively influence his food intake, nutritional status, and quality of life.

Description

L.B. is a 70-year-old male with dysphagia resulting from a cerebrovascular accident. His difficulties opening his mouth, chewing solids, and swallowing thin liquids result from a permanent partial paralysis of his tongue, jaw, and cricopharyngeal muscles, especially apparent on the left side. He has been on a ground/chopped/minced diet with fluids of nectar-like viscosity for two months and his food and fluid intake is progressively declining. L.B. is also taking some antidepressants, is constipated, and is complaining of having a dry mouth. You are his dietitian at the Whitehills Long-Term Care Center, and you are trying to help him increase his food intake.

1. List and explain 10 different **risk factors** likely to be negatively affecting Mr. L.B.'s food intake.

   1) Factor #1:

      Explanation:

   2) Factor #2:

      Explanation:

   3) Factor #3:

      Explanation:

   4) Factor #4:

      Explanation:

   5) Factor #5:

      Explanation:

   6) Factor #6:

      Explanation:

   7) Factor #7:

      Explanation:

   8) Factor #8:

      Explanation:

   9) Factor #9:

      Explanation:

10)Factor #10:

Explanation:

2. For each risk factor listed, provide a realistic **suggestion** to improve Mr. L.B.'s situation in order to help him increase his food intake and nutritional status. In addition, give a practical **example** of how each suggestion can be implemented.

1) Factor #1:

Suggestion:

Example:

2) Factor #2:

Suggestion:

Example:

3) Factor #3:

Suggestion:

Example:

4) Factor #4:

Suggestion:

Example:

5) Factor #5:

Suggestion:

Example:

6) Factor #6:

Suggestion:

Example:

7) Factor #7:

Suggestion:

Example:

8) Factor #8:

Suggestion:

Example:

9) Factor #9:

Suggestion:

Example:

10)Factor #10:

Suggestion:

Example:

3. How can fluids and semisolid foods be thickened? Explain.

4. What types of drugs are known to induce dysphagia problems?

5. Plan a 1-day pureed diet menu with very thick liquids for Mr. L.B.

6.3 Therapeutic Diets and Modified Mineral Diets

REVIEW THE INFORMATION

1. What are modified or therapeutic diets?

_____

_____

_____

2. What is lactose?

_____

_____

_____

3. What is lactose intolerance?

_____

_____

_____

4. What is the difference between lactose intolerance and milk hypersensitivity?

_____

_____

_____

5. What are the risks associated with malnutrition?

_____

_____

_____

_____

6. What are the main causes of malnutrition in hospital clients?

_____

_____

_____

_____

_____

7. What are the main soluble fibers?

_____

_____

_____

8. What are the main sources of soluble fiber?

_____

_____

_____

9. What are insoluble fibers?

_____

_____

_____

10. What are the main sources of insoluble fiber?

_____

_____

_____

11. What is hypercholesterolemia?

_____

_____

_____

UNDERSTAND THE CONCEPTS

1. Give some examples of frequently used therapeutic diets.

_____

_____

_____

_____

2. Describe the following diets modified in composition. Explain when each modified diet is indicated and its purpose.

a) **Lactose-controlled diet**

Description: _____

_____

_____

_____

Indication: _____

_____

_____

_____

Purpose: _____

_____

_____

_____

b) **High-energy, high-protein diet**

Description: _____

_____

_____

_____

Indication: _____

_____

_____

_____

Purpose: _____

_____

_____

_____

c) **Sodium-restricted diets**

Description: _____

_____

_____

_____

Indication: _____

_____

_____

_____

Purpose: _____

_____

_____

_____

d) **Fat-restricted diet**

Description: _____

_____

_____

_____

Indication: _____

_____

_____

_____

Purpose: _____

_____

e) **Dietary recommendations for the management of hypercholesterolemia**

Description: _____

_____

_____

_____

Indication: _____

_____

_____

_____

Purpose: _____

_____

_____

_____

f) **Fiber-restricted diet**

Description: _____

_____

_____

_____

Indication: _____

_____

_____

_____

Purpose: _____

_____

_____

_____

g) **High-fiber diet**

Description: _____

_____

_____

_____

Indication: _____

_____

_____

_____

Purpose: _____

_____

_____

_____

h) **Gluten-free diet**

Description: _____

_____

_____

_____

Indication: _____

_____

_____

_____

Purpose: _____

_____

_____

_____

i) **Protein-restricted diet**

Description: _____

_____

_____

_____

Indication: _____

_____

_____

_____

Purpose: _____

_____

_____

j) **Iron-rich diet**

Description: _____

_____

_____

_____

Indication: _____

_____

Purpose: _____

_____

_____

_____

k) **Calcium-rich diet**

Description: _____

_____

_____

_____

Indication: _____

_____

_____

_____

Purpose: _____

_____

_____

_____

l) **Dietary recommendations for the management of diabetes mellitus**

Description: _____

_____

_____

_____

Indication: _____

_____

_____

_____

Purpose: _____

_____

_____

_____

3. What are dyslipidemias?

_____

_____

_____

_____

4. Which diets are promoted by the American Heart Association for the prevention and treatment of hyper-cholesterolemia?

_____

_____

5. Which foods are likely to contain lactose, even in small quantities?

_____

_____

_____

6. When reading food labels, which words in the list of ingredients indicate the presence of lactose?

_____

_____

7. Which sources of lactose may be better tolerated when individuals can consume small amounts of lactose?

_____

_____

_____

_____

8. Which population groups have a higher incidence of primary lactase deficiency?

_____

_____

9. What is celiac disease?

_____

_____

_____

10. What are other names for celiac disease?

_____

11. What are the signs and symptoms of untreated celiac disease?

_____

_____

_____

_____

_____

12. What is gluten?

_____

_____

_____

13. Which foods contain gluten?

_____

_____

_____

14. What is dermatitis herpetiformis?

_____

_____

INTEGRATE YOUR LEARNING

1. The intake of which nutrients may be low or inadequate if milk products are limited in the diet?

_____

_____

2. Estimate the lactose content of the following foods.

LACTOSE CONTENT OF SOME DAIRY PRODUCTS	
Dairy Products	Lactose Content (grams per cup or 237 mL)
Ice cream	
Milk (0%–2% fat)	
Cottage cheese (creamed)	
Low-fat yogurt	
Lacteeze 99% Less Lactose Milk	
Lactaid 99% Lactose-Reduced Milk	
Natrel 99.9% Lactose Free Milk	

3. Lactose-controlled diet

1) Determine the approximate lactose content of this 1-day menu using the above table of "Lactose Content of Some Dairy Products" and another reference, such as:

American Dietetic Association and Dietitians of Canada. Lactose intolerance. In: Manual of Clinical Dietetics. 6th Ed. Chicago: American Dietetic Association, 2000:211–220.

One-Day Menu

Breakfast: milk, 2% fat, 1 cup (8 fluid oz, 237 mL)
2 medium pancakes made with ½ cup (4 fluid oz, 118 mL) of 2% milk
margarine, 1 Tbsp (15 mL)
pure maple syrup, 3 Tbsp (45 mL)
coffee, 1 cup (8 fluid oz, 237 mL)
Half & Half cream, 2 Tbsp (1 fluid oz, 30 mL)

Morning snack: low-fat yogurt, 1 cup (237 mL)

Lunch: cream of mushroom soup made with ½ cup (4 fluid oz, 118 mL) of 2% milk
plain bagel, 2 oz (56 g)
butter, 2 tsp (10 mL)

cream cheese, 1 oz (28 g)
milkshake made with ½ cup (118 mL) 2% milk and ½ cup (118 mL) strawberry ice cream

Afternoon snack: ice cream cone made with ½ cup (118 mL) vanilla ice cream

Dinner: 2 slices pizza, deluxe, made with 1 oz (28 g) mozzarella cheese
orange sherbet, 1 cup (237 mL)
medium piece chocolate cake (2 oz, 56 g) with ¼ cup (4 Tbsp, 59 mL) whipped cream
milk, 2% fat, 1 cup (8 fluid oz, 237 mL)

Evening snack: tortilla chips, 3½ oz (100g) bag
sour cream, ½ cup (118 mL)
salsa, ½ cup (118 mL)

2) Revise the menu for a client with lactase nonpersistence, who can tolerate up to 20 g of lactose per day.

> ### *Revised 1-Day Menu for Client With Lactase Nonpersistence*

4. High-energy, high-protein diet

1) Determine the approximate energy and protein content of the usual daily dietary intake of a client with AIDS using the Diet Count Form provided.

One-Day Menu

Breakfast: slice of white bread (1 oz, 28 g), enriched, toasted
margarine, soft, 1 tsp (5 mL)
black coffee, 1 cup (8 fluid oz, 237 mL)

Lunch: sandwich: 2 slices of white bread (1 oz or 28 g each), enriched
regular mayonnaise, 1 Tbsp (15 mL)
1 small tomato, sliced (3 oz, 84 g)

fruit gelatin, ½ cup (118 mL)
water, 1 cup (8 fluid oz, 237 mL)

Dinner: spaghetti noodles, enriched, cooked, 1 cup (5 oz, 140 g, 237 mL)
tomato sauce, canned, ½ cup (118 mL)
applesauce, sweetened, canned, ½ cup (118 mL)
herbal tea, 1 cup (8 fluid oz, 237 mL)

DIET COUNT FORM FOR CLIENT WITH AIDS

Food	Portion	Number of Portions	Carbohydrate (g)	Protein (g)	Fat (g)
Starch/bread	½ cup, 118 mL or 1 slice (1 oz, 28g)		15	3	
Fruit	½ cup, 118 mL or 1 small		15		
Vegetable	½ cup or 118 mL		7	2	
Milk:	½ cup or 118 mL				
- Nonfat			6	4	0
- 1% fat			6	4	1
- 2% fat			6	4	2
- Whole			6	4	4
Meat:	1 oz or 28 g				
- Very lean				7	0–1
- Lean				7	3
- Medium fat				7	5
- High fat				7	8
Fat	1 tsp or 5 mL				5
Sugar	1 tsp or 5 mL		5		
Others:					
Iced cake	1 small slice		65	4	4
Soft drink	1 cup, 8 fluid oz or 237 mL		22		
Fruit gelatin	½ cup or 118 mL		18	2	
Total (g)					
			× 4 kcal/g or 17 kJ/g	*× 4 kcal/g or 17 kJ/g*	*× 9 kcal/g or 37 kJ/g*
Total					
TOTAL ENERGY	= _____				
% of Energy					

2) Revise the menu to help this client with AIDS meet his energy and protein needs, which are 2100 kcal (8780 kJ) and 100 g protein per day.

Revised 1-Day Menu for Client with AIDS

3) Verify the adequacy of your revised menu using a computerized food analysis software program (e.g., ESHA Food Processor, CBORD Diet Office, Computrition, Diet Analysis Plus, Food Smart, etc.).

Indicate here the amount of energy and protein in your revised menu.

5. Use the following table to describe the dietary recommendations of the American Heart Association for the prevention and management of hypercholesterolemia.

AMERICAN HEART ASSOCIATION DIETARY RECOMMENDATIONS FOR THE PREVENTION AND MANAGEMENT OF HYPERCHOLESTEROLEMIA		
Composition of Diet	**Dietary Guidelines for Healthy American Adults**	**Therapeutic Lifestyle Change Diet**
Total fat	Percent of energy intake	Percent of energy intake
SFA	Percent of energy intake	Percent of energy intake
PUFA, including ω-3 FA	Percent of energy intake	Percent of energy intake
MUFA	Percent of energy intake	Percent of energy intake
Cholesterol	mg/day	mg/day
Carbohydrates	Percent of energy intake	Percent of energy intake
Protein	Percent of energy intake	Percent of energy intake
Energy		

6. What are the dietary recommendations of the Canadian Working Group on Hypercholesterolemia and Other Dyslipidemias?

DIETARY RECOMMENDATIONS OF THE CANADIAN WORKING GROUP ON HYPERCHOLESTEROLEMIA AND OTHER DYSLIPIDEMIAS	
Composition of Diet	**Recommendations for the Management of Dyslipidemia and Prevention of Cardiovascular Disease**
Total fat	Percent of energy intake
SFA and *trans*-FA	Percent of energy intake
PUFA, including ω-3 FA	Percent of energy intake
MUFA	Percent of energy intake
Cholesterol	mg/day
Fiber	g/day
Carbohydrate	
Protein	
Alcohol	
Energy	

7. What nutrient deficiencies may result from severe fat maldigestion and malabsorption?

_____

_____

_____

8. What are the long-term results for an individual who is on a low-fiber diet?

_____

_____

_____

_____

9. What can result if a client usually having a low-fiber intake is suddenly given a high-fiber diet?

_____

_____

_____

_____

10. What are contraindications to a high-fiber diet?

_____

_____

_____

_____

11. What are fructooligosaccharides?

_____

_____

_____

_____

12. Why are fructooligosaccharides beneficial?

_____

_____

_____

_____

_____

13. When severe cases of celiac disease go untreated, describe what the consequences are on the digestion and absorption of the various nutrients.

_____

_____

_____

14. Reduce the sodium content of this recipe to help a client on a moderate sodium restriction of 2 g (87 mmol) sodium per day (or the equivalent of 5 g salt per day).

Pasta Salad
(Quantity: 12 portions)

5 fluid oz (150 mL)	Vegetable oil
⅓ cup (79 mL)	Lemon juice
2 Tbsp (30 mL)	Yellow mustard
2 Tbsp (30 mL)	Fresh oregano leaves
3 cups (711 mL)	Fusili pasta, cooked, drained
1½ cups (355 mL)	Canned, marinated artichokes, sliced
1½ cups (355 mL)	Crumbled feta cheese
1½ cups (355 mL)	Ham, cooked, diced
1½ cups (355 mL)	Diced raw tomatoes
1½ cups (355 mL)	Diced raw cucumber
1¼ cup (297 mL)	Sliced fresh green pepper
1 cup (237 mL)	Marinated black olives, canned
¼ cup (59 mL)	Bacon flakes, commercial
½ tsp (2.5 mL)	Salt
½ tsp (2.5 mL)	Black pepper

15. When are salt substitutes containing potassium contraindicated?

_____

_____

_____

CHALLENGE YOUR LEARNING

CASE STUDY

Objectives
This case will help you assist a client in modifying the composition of her diet in practical ways in order to help her manage her physiologic and metabolic health problems.

Description
Mrs. N.B. is a 48-year-old overweight client. She has recently been diagnosed with type 2 diabetes mellitus and hypercholesterolemia, which she is attempting to manage through progressive positive lifestyle improvements. She also complains about suffering from constipation.

Here is the 24-hour recall information that you obtained from her this morning, when she came to meet you at the Outpatient Clinic.

Breakfast:
   Rice Krispies cereal, 1 cup (237 mL, 0.9 oz, 26 g)
   honey, 1 Tbsp (15 mL)
   skim milk, ½ cup (118 mL)
   1 hard-boiled egg
   tea, ½ cup (118 mL)
   granulated sugar, 2 tsp (10 mL)

Morning snack:
   apple juice, ½ cup (118 mL)
   Mozzarella cheese, 1 oz (28 g)

Lunch:
   2 slices pumpernickel bread (1 oz or 28 g each)
   peanut butter, 1 Tbsp (15 mL)
   strawberry jelly, 1 Tbsp (15 mL)
   skim milk, ½ cup (118 mL)
   peach gelatin dessert, ½ cup (118 mL)

Afternoon snack:
   tea, ½ cup (118 mL)
   granulated sugar, 2 tsp (10 mL)
   1 small banana (2½ oz, 70 g)

Dinner:
   vegetable juice, ½ cup (4 fluid oz, 118 mL)
   iceberg lettuce, 1 cup (237 mL)
   1 medium tomato, raw, chopped (4½ oz, 126 g)
   Italian dressing, 2 Tbsp (30 mL)
   cottage cheese, 1 oz (28 g)
   chocolate ice cream, 1 cup (237 mL)
   3 chocolate chip cookies (½ oz or 14 g each)

1. Determine the fiber content of the 24-hour recall.

2. Knowing that Mrs. N.B.'s energy requirements are 1990 kcal (8320 kJ/day), what would her recommended daily fiber intake be?

3. What type(s) of fibers would you increase in her diet? Why?

4. Suggest five practical ways to help her increase her fiber intake.

PART 7

Prevention and Management of Disease

INTRODUCTION

The focus of this part is on the nutritional management of disease states as an important part of overall medical treatment available to help clients. Nutrition plays a key role in the treatment of numerous diseases, including diabetes mellitus, food allergies and intolerances, obesity, and eating disorders. Furthermore, nutrition therapy is often the initial step in the management of chronic diseases (e.g., obesity, diabetes mellitus, hypercholesterolemia, hypertension, etc.). Nutrition therapy, as part of a healthy lifestyle-changing approach to disease management, is frequently recommended to clients before medication or other more invasive, aggressive, and costly medical therapies are initiated. Even when medications are necessary, nutrition therapy is continued, as in the majority of cases nutrition and medication therapies are more effective when combined than are medication(s) alone. This is also true for nutrition therapy combined with other medical therapies, such as surgery, radiotherapy, and chemotherapy.

This part also emphasizes the importance of the prevention of disease development as opposed to simply relying on cure. This is important because diseases place a heavy burden on individuals and society, in terms of quality of life, cost, and other resources. In addition, prevention may be the only real "treatment" currently available for many diseases, including AIDS, type 2 diabetes mellitus, and cancer.

In order to appropriately use nutrition to assist clients with prevention and treatment of disease, *dietitians must continually integrate and develop their skills and knowledge in multiple areas.* Dietitians individualize their approach to benefit each unique client and use a client-centered approach for nutrition assessment and counseling (as discussed in Part 5). They keep in mind the anatomic physiology of the gastrointestinal tract (covered in Part 2) and body to understand the impact of pathology on the nutritional status of clients. They have the unique ability to help clients modify their dietary habits when needed to prevent or manage disease while ensuring that the individual's nutrient needs are being met, because they know about food and its composition (see Part 1). They combine their understanding of human behavior, life cycle (covered in Part 3), food science, and therapeutic diets (explained in Part 6) to make practical and realistic nutritional and dietary recommendations to benefit their clients in their own sociocultural (discussed in Part 4) and economic environments. Dietetics is an amazingly interesting, multidisciplinary, ever-growing, and extremely rewarding profession! As fellow dietitians say, *dietitians have the unique aptitude to turn science into food <u>and</u> to turn food into science!*

As dietitians gain experience, skills, and knowledge in some area(s) of care, they can develop specialized expertise, which is very beneficial to their clients and professional colleagues. However, dietetic interns and dietitians are responsible for developing and maintaining adequate competencies in all main areas of nutrition care.

In Part 7, we will be discussing at-risk pregnancies (Part 7.1), selected diseases in infancy and childhood (Part 7.2), adverse reactions to food (Part 7.3), obesity and eating disorders (Part 7.4), cardiovascular disease (Part 7.5), diabetes mellitus (Part 7.6), gastroesophageal reflux disease (Part 7.7), peptic ulcer disease (Part 7.8), inflammatory bowel disease (Part 7.9), diseases of the liver and pancreas (Part 7.10), gastrointestinal surgery and short bowel syndrome (Part 7.11), wasting disorders (Part 7.12), renal disease (Part 7.13), neurologic and psychiatric disorders (Part 7.14), nutrition support (Part 7.15), and food/nutrient–drug interactions (Part 7.16).

The goal here is not to discuss every single disease state, but to understand the nutritional and multidisciplinary approach to prevention and treatment of some common diseases and to integrate what you are leaning along the way.

7.1 At-Risk Pregnancies

REVIEW THE INFORMATION

1. What are the four main goals of nutrition care in pregnancy?

   a) _____

   _____

   _____

   b) _____

   _____

   _____

   c) _____

   _____

   _____

   d) _____

   _____

   _____

2. How much weight should a woman gain during the first trimester of pregnancy?

   _____

   _____

   _____

   _____

3. Summarize the general weight gain recommendations for pregnancy using this table.

PREGNANCY WEIGHT GAIN RECOMMENDATIONS		
Pre-Pregnancy BMI (kg/m^2)	Recommended Overall Pregnancy Weight Gain (lbs) [kg]	Average Weekly Weight Gain Recommended in Second and Third Trimesters (lbs) [kg]
Underweight: U.S.: <19.8 Canada: <20.0		
Healthy weight: U.S.: 19.8–26.0 Canada: 20.0–27.0		
Overweight: U.S.: 26.0–29.0 Canada: >27.0		
Obese: U.S.: >29.0 Canada: >30.0		

4. Cassandra is 5′10″ and her pre-pregnancy body weight was 175 lb. How much weight should she gain throughout her pregnancy?

   a) 15 lb   b) 15–25 lb   c) 25–35 lb   d) 28–40 lb   e) 35–45 lb

5. Which statement about the trimesters of pregnancy is **false**?

   a) Most of the fetus' bone calcification and fat deposition occur in the third trimester.
   b) The mother usually starts to notice the fetus' movements during the second trimester.
   c) By the end of the first trimester, the fetus is about 3 inches (7.5 cm) long and weighs approximately 1½ oz (45 g).
   d) During the second trimester, the iron stores increase in the liver of the fetus.
   e) During the first trimester, the internal organs of the fetus start to develop and can be identified.

6. Which micronutrient needs are at risk of not being met in some women during pregnancy?

   _____

   _____

   _____

7. These foods reduce the absorption of nonheme iron, <u>except</u>

   a) whole grain bread   b) yogurt   c) rhubarb   d) legumes   e) tomato

8. Pregnant women should limit their caffeine intake to no more than _____ mg caffeine per day from all sources.

   a) 150   b) 200   c) 250   d) 300   e) 400

9. Women of childbearing age should take a daily supplement containing _____ of folic acid.

   a) 40 μg   b) 60 μg   c) 200 μg   d) 400 μg   e) 600 μg

10. Complete the following DRI recommendations for pregnancy using this table.

Nutrients	Type of DRI Recommendation[Ψ] (EER, RDA, or AI)	Units	Recommendation for Pregnancy
Energy - First Trimester - Second Trimester - Third Trimester			
Protein			
Carbohydrate			
Iron			
Calcium			
Folate			
Vitamin D			
Zinc			
Linoleic Acid			
α-Linolenic Acid			
Total water			
Total fiber			

DRI RECOMMENDATIONS FOR HEALTHY PREGNANT WOMEN*

* Between 19 and 50 years of age.
[Ψ]DRI, Dietary Reference Intake; RDA, Recommended Dietary Allowance; AI, adequate intake; EER, Estimated Energy Requirement.

11. Pregnant women are being screened for gestational diabetes mellitus at _____ weeks' gestation.

   a) 12–16   b) 16–20   c) 20–24   d) 24–28   e) 28–32

UNDERSTAND THE CONCEPTS

1. What are possible nutritional risk factors for pregnant women? List at least 15.

   1- _____

   2- _____

   3- _____

   4- _____

   5- _____

   6- _____

   7- _____

8- _____

9- _____

10- _____

11- _____

12- _____

13- _____

14- _____

15- _____

2. What is the most common nutrient deficiency during pregnancy?

   _____

   _____

3. Define the following pregnancy-related health problems.

   a) Gestational diabetes mellitus (GDM)

   _____

   _____

   b) Preeclampsia

   _____

   _____

   c) Gestational hypertension

   _____

   _____

   d) Hyperemesis gravidarum

   _____

   _____

   e) Placenta previa

   _____

   _____

   f) Preterm membrane rupture

   _____

   _____

   g) Incompetent cervix

   _____

   _____

   h) Hydramnios

   _____

   _____

4. What information should be collected as part of the complete nutritional assessment of pregnant women? *(Note: Classify the information as either **History data** or **A, B, C, or D findings**.)*

History data

_____

_____

_____

_____

_____

_____

_____

_____

_____

_____

A findings

_____

_____

_____

_____

_____

_____

_____

_____

_____

_____

B findings

_____

_____

_____

_____

_____

_____

_____

_____

_____

_____

_____

_____

C findings

_____

_____

_____

_____

_____

_____

_____

_____

_____

_____

_____

_____

D findings

_____

_____

_____

_____

_____

_____

_____

_____

_____

_____

_____

_____

_____

5. What is the weight gain recommended for a mother having a twin pregnancy?

_____

_____

_____

6. What is the weight gain recommended for a triplet pregnancy?

_____

_____

_____

7. What are some of the risks newborns can face in a multifetal pregnancy?

_____

_____

_____

8. What are some of the risks mothers can face with a multifetal pregnancy?

_____

_____

_____

9. Nausea and vomiting may begin around the _____ week of gestation and usually stop at the

_____ week of pregnancy for 80% of women. However, the other 20% of women will suffer from nausea and vomiting for a longer period of time, possibly for the remainder of their pregnancy.

a) 2nd, 6th   b) 4th, 16th   c) 5th, 20th   d) 6th, 12th   e) 8th, 24th

10. About _____% of pregnant women suffer from recurrent nausea of pregnancy.

a) 1   b) 2   c) 3   d) 4   e) 5

11. What is the only safe medication that can be prescribed by physicians to help control excessive nausea and vomiting during pregnancy?

_____

12. What does this medication contain that helps relieve excessive nausea and vomiting during pregnancy?

_____

_____

13. What are the risk factors related to the development of GDM? List at least 10.

1- _____

2- _____

3- _____

4- _____

5- _____

6- _____

7- _____

8- _____

9- _____

10- _____

14. What is the primary treatment for GDM?

_____

15. What are the main nutrition-related goals for women with GDM?

a) _____

_____

b) _____

_____

c) _____

_____

d) _____

16. When the mother has GDM, the fetus is at an increased risk of many complications, <u>except</u>

a) hyperglycemia after birth
b) type 2 diabetes mellitus in the long term
c) macrosomia
d) birth trauma
e) neonatal jaundice

17. What are the recommended preprandial and postprandial glycemic targets for women with GDM that are associated with the best pregnancy outcomes?

_____

_____

_____

18. What more aggressive treatment of GDM is initiated when these glycemic targets are not reached?

_____

_____

19. What are the four main types of hypertensive disorders that can be found in pregnancy? Define each of them.

a) _____

_____

b) _____

_____

c) _____

_____

d) _____

_____

INTEGRATE YOUR LEARNING

1. What is the recommended pregnancy weight gain if the mother's pre-pregnancy BMI is 25.5 kg/m^2 and she is expecting twins?

a) 50 lb (22.5 kg)
b) 35–45 lb (16.0–20.0 kg)
c) 28–40 lb (12.5–18.0 kg)
d) 25–35 lb (11.5–16.0 kg)
e) 15–25 lb (7.0–11.5 kg)

2. Which pregnant women would benefit from iron supplementation? Explain your answer.

_____

_____

_____

_____

_____

_____

3. What is the difference between gestational diabetes mellitus and pre-existing diabetes mellitus in pregnancy?

_____

_____

_____

_____

4. Is there a similarity between gestational diabetes mellitus and type 2 diabetes mellitus? Explain your answer.

_____

_____

_____

_____

5. Is there a similarity between late pregnancy and type 2 diabetes mellitus? Explain your answer.

_____

_____

_____

_____

6. List three main <u>dietary strategies</u> to help women manage their gestational diabetes mellitus.

a) _____

_____

b) _____

_____

c) _____

_____

7. Why are oral antihyperglycemic agents not used during pregnancy?

_____

_____

_____

8. What type of insulin regimen is used to manage GDM?

_____

_____

_____

9. What are the signs and symptoms of preeclampsia?

_____

_____

_____

_____

_____

_____

_____

_____

10. Indicate whether the following statements are TRUE or FALSE, and justify your answer if false.

a) _____ Women with preeclampsia during pregnancy have an increased risk for developing hypertension and acute renal dysfunction.

   Justification: _____

b) _____ Women with preeclampsia during pregnancy have an increased risk for developing GDM or type 2 diabetes mellitus later in life.

   Justification: _____

c) _____ Women with preeclampsia during pregnancy have an increased risk for giving birth to a macrosomic infant.

   Justification: _____

d) _____ Preeclampsia is partly due to insulin resistance in the mother.

   Justification: _____

e) _____ Adequate intake of calcium, vitamin C, and vitamin E during pregnancy may help reduce the incidence of preeclampsia in women at risk.

   Justification: _____

f) _____ A low-sodium diet during pregnancy may help reduce the incidence of preeclampsia in women who are at risk.

   Justification: _____

g) _____ Women with preeclampsia benefit from consuming regular meals and snacks daily and high-glycemic index foods.

   Justification: _____

CHALLENGE YOUR LEARNING

CASE STUDY

Objective

This case will help you integrate your knowledge of nutritional needs during pregnancy and at-risk pregnancies in order to help women manage their health condition(s), meet their nutritional needs using diet therapy as needed, and have the best pregnancy outcome possible.

Description

G.D. is a 35-year-old woman having a singleton pregnancy. Since her blood glucose concentration was 180 mg/dL (10.0 mmol/L) 1 hour after a 50-g glucose-screening test, she was asked to perform a 75-g oral glucose tolerance test (OGTT). The results were as follows: fasting result of 108 mg/dL (6.0 mmol/L); 1-hour result of 229 mg/dL (12.7 mmol/L); and 2-hour result of 160 mg/dL (8.9 mmol/L). Her blood hemoglobin concentration was 10.2 g/dL (102 g/L, 1.58 mmol/L) and her hematocrit 31% (0.31).

She was immediately referred to you for nutrition counseling at 26 weeks' gestation. Here is the information you were able to collect during the nutrition interview, on the afternoon of June 28, 2007.

She lives with her husband and their three daughters (9 months and 7 and 9 years old). They are recent immigrants from Mexico. They have been in the city for 2 months and are living on a minimal income. They speak Spanish and very little English. The only social support they have is from G.D.'s aunt, who owns a Mexican restaurant in town. G.D.'s husband has been working there as many hours as possible since they arrived.

G.D. is able to answer simple questions in English. She is very tired all the time and has no energy to go for a walk. Her height is 5′5″ and her current weight is 186 lb. Her pre-pregnancy body weight was 176 lb. She is not taking prenatal supplements.

The obstetric history of G.D. indicates that this is her sixth pregnancy. She had her first daughter (9 lb, 4100 g) in 1998, her second daughter (9 lb 6 oz, 4250 g) in 2000, a 37-week stillborn infant in 2003, a miscarriage in 2004, and her third daughter (10 lb 2 oz, 4600 g) in 2006, whom she is still breastfeeding full time. Other than that, G.D. has limited information about her previous pregnancies. She says that her mother and older sister are overweight and have diabetes mellitus.

G.D. does not smoke cigarettes or drink alcohol. She informs you that she is lactose intolerant and avoids all milk products. She reports being very thirsty since the beginning of her pregnancy and urinating often, including two to three times a night.

In the last 2 months, her dietary intake has been about the following:

Breakfast:	2 slices of white, enriched sandwich bread toasted (1 oz, 28 g each) butter, salted (4 tsp, 20 mL) 1 large egg (1.8 oz, 50 g), fried with vegetable oil (1 tsp, 5 mL) 1 cup (8 fluid oz, 237 mL) vanilla-flavored, enriched soy milk 1 medium fresh orange (2⅝ inches diameter, 4⅔ oz, 131 g)
Lunch:	1 cup (237 mL, 6⅔ oz, 186 g) cooked white rice (medium grain), with 1 Tbsp (15 mL) corn oil ½ cup (118 mL, 4⅔ oz, 120 g) homemade baked beans 2 cups (474 mL) chopped fried vegetables (½ cup or 118 mL green bell peppers, ½ cup or 118 mL red bell peppers, ½ cup or 118 mL red sweet onions, ½ cup or 118 mL zucchini), with 1 Tbsp (15 mL) corn oil 1 can (1½ cups, 16 fluid oz, 355 mL) of ginger ale soda 2 chocolate chip cookies (½ oz or 14 g each)
Afternoon snack:	3 cups (36 fluid oz, 711 mL) peach drink medium fresh banana (7½ inches long, 4.2 oz, 118 g, ¾ cup, 178 mL)
Dinner:	1 cup (237 mL, 242 g, 8⅔ oz) lentil soup 2 slices of white, enriched sandwich bread (1 oz or 28 g each) butter, salted (4 tsp, 20 mL) 1 cup (237 mL) shredded iceberg lettuce 1 slice (¼ inch thick) of a medium tomato (½ oz, 14 g) 2 Tbsp (30 mL) Caesar salad dressing 1 medium fresh avocado (6.2 oz, 173 g, ¾ cup, 178 mL) 1 can (1½ cups, 16 fluid oz, 355 mL) of iced tea drink
Evening snack:	1 can (1½ cups, 16 fluid oz, 355 mL) of ginger ale soda

1. Why is G.D. at risk of complications during this pregnancy?

2. What is G.D.'s pre-pregnancy BMI?

3. What is your interpretation of G.D.'s pre-pregnancy BMI?

4. What is the recommended pregnancy weight gain for her pre-pregnancy BMI?

5. What do you think about her weight gain so far?

6. What weekly weight gain do you recommend for G.D. for the remainder of her pregnancy?

7. What are G.D.'s risk factors for developing GDM?

8. What is the interpretation of G.D.'s 50-g glucose screening test (glucose challenge test) result?

9. What are the GDM diagnosis criteria based on a 75-g oral glucose tolerance test?

10. What are the implications of G.D.'s oral glucose tolerance test results?

11. When is screening performed on women with multiple GDM risk factors?

12. Is it possible for a woman to develop GDM without having any of the known risk factors? Explain.

13. What is the incidence of GDM?

14. What are the *short-term* risks for the *offspring* when the mother has GDM?

15. What are the *long-term* risks for the *offspring* when the mother has GDM?

16. What are the *short-term* risks for the *mothers* having GDM?

17. What are the *long-term* risks for the *mothers* having GDM?

18. If a woman had GDM, does it mean that she will definitely develop GDM in subsequent pregnancies? Explain your answer and give an example.

19. What do her blood hemoglobin concentration and hematocrit tell you?

20. Identify, for each trimester, what blood hemoglobin and hematocrit values are used when screening pregnant women for anemia.

21. Is G.D.'s usual dietary intake meeting the recommendations of MyPyramid (or Canada's Food Guide)? Explain.

22. Determine the energy and nutrient content of G.D.'s usual dietary intake using a nutrient analysis software program.

23. Estimate G.D.'s pregnancy EER at 26 weeks of pregnancy and keep in mind that she is still breastfeeding full time.

    Adult women EER

    $$= 354 - (6.91 \times \text{Age in years}) + \{\text{PA} \times [(9.36 \times \text{Weight in kg}) + (726 \times \text{Height in meters})]\}$$

24. What are G.D.'s daily protein needs at 26 weeks of pregnancy?

25. What is your assessment of her usual dietary intake?

26. What are the nutritional objectives for G.D.?

27. What are some *dietary strategies* to help G.D. meet the nutritional objectives set and manage her health condition?

28. Write an initial nutrition care plan (in the SOAP or DAP note format) to insert in G.D.'s medical record.

29. Prepare a 1-day menu that G.D. could follow, taking into consideration her energy, protein, and nutrient needs during pregnancy and lactation.

30. Is the 1-day menu you prepared for G.D. meeting the recommendations of MyPyramid (or Canada's Food Guide)? Justify.

31. Determine the energy and nutrient composition of your 1-day menu using a nutrient analysis software-program.

32. Is the 1-day sample menu you prepared for G.D. meeting her energy and micronutrient needs for pregnancy and lactation? Justify.

33. Determine the total carbohydrate and *available carbohydrate* content of each meal and snack of the 1-day menu you prepared for G.D.

Case Follow-up

Following her meeting with the obstetrician at diagnosis of her GDM and the nutrition education session with you 2 weeks ago, G.D. has been able to make a few significant improvements to her eating pattern and lifestyle, which have helped her normalize her glycemia. As a result, she will not require insulin injections at the present time.

During her weekly meetings with Dr. S. Gordon, her obstetrician, G.D. reported that she now drinks water instead of sweetened beverages, is taking a daily prenatal multivitamin and mineral supplement, and has started to walk every day to a nearby park with her children. She feels better and is less tired. Her capillary blood glucose monitoring indicates that her preprandial glycemia is presently about 88 mg/dL (4.9 mmol/L) and her postprandial glycemia is about 133 mg/dL (7.4 mmol/L) 1 hour postmeal.

Dr. Gordon forwards you more detailed blood work results for G.D., with a request for more nutrition education in the coming days:

- serum ferritin concentration: 64 ng/mL (64 μg/L)
- serum iron concentration: 39 μg/dL (7.0 μmol/L)
- serum folate concentration: 6.7 ng/mL (15.0 nmol/L)
- serum vitamin B_{12} concentration: 101 pg/mL (75 pmol/L)

She prescribes G.D. 60 mg elemental iron daily for the coming month, until her blood work is reassessed. This is in addition to the recommendation she was already given to take a daily prenatal multivitamin and mineral supplement for the rest of her pregnancy.

G.D. has contacted you by phone on Tuesday, July 12, 2007, in the afternoon to make an appointment and you have asked her to bring a 3-day food intake record when she comes next week.

34. What are normal serum ferritin, iron, folate, and vitamin B_{12} concentrations for pregnancy?

35. What is your interpretation of G.D.'s serum ferritin, iron, folate, and vitamin B_{12} concentrations?

36. Prepare a brief nutrition progress note (in the SOAP or DAP note format) to insert in G.D.'s medical record.

7.2 Diseases in Infancy and Childhood

REVIEW THE INFORMATION

1. Newborns may lose a small amount of weight after birth as they adapt to their new environment and learn to nurse or be bottle-fed, but they should be at their birth weight or over their birth weight by _____ days of life.

2. An infant's birth weight is usually _____ by 5–6 months and _____ by 12 months.

3. Premature infants are born before _____ weeks of gestation.

4. What is the weight classification (in pounds/ounces or grams) for the following infants?

   a) Macrosomic infants: _____

   b) Normal weight infants: _____

   c) Low-birth-weight infants: _____

   d) Very low-birth-weight infants: _____

   e) Extremely low-birth-weight infants: _____

   f) Extreme extremely low-birth-weight infants or micro-preemies: _____

5. Small-for-gestational-age infants are born weighing less than the _____ percentile for gestational age.

6. What do the following abbreviations stand for?

   a) CF: _____

   b) PKU: _____

   c) LBW: _____

   d) VLBW: _____

   e) ELBW: _____

   f) SGA: _____

   g) DOB: _____

   h) PHE: _____

   i) TYR: _____

   j) EN: _____

   k) TPN: _____

   l) NICU: _____

   m) FTT: _____

7. What are phenylalanine and tyrosine?

   _____

8. Describe the composition of pancreatic digestive juice.

   _____

   _____

9. Explain in detail the process of protein digestion.

   _____

   _____

   _____

   _____

   _____

   _____

   _____

   _____

10. Explain in detail the process of fat (long-chain triglyceride) digestion.

_____

_____

_____

_____

_____

_____

_____

_____

11. Explain in detail the process of complex carbohydrate digestion.

_____

_____

_____

_____

_____

_____

_____

UNDERSTAND THE CONCEPTS

1. What are the causes of iron deficiency anemia in infants? Explain why/how.

_____

_____

_____

_____

_____

_____

_____

_____

_____

_____

_____

_____

2. How many inherited metabolic disorders are there in which toxic expression is due to overproduction, accumulation, or deficiency of normal metabolic substrates and products in the body?

a) >25   b) >50   c) >100   d) >200   e) >300

3. What are some of the inherited disorders that benefit from diet therapy? Briefly indicate the main diet therapy approach used in the treatment of each disorder.

   a) Disorder: _____

      Diet therapy: _____

      _____

   b) Disorder: _____

      Diet therapy: _____

      _____

   c) Disorder: _____

      Diet therapy: _____

      _____

   d) Disorder: _____

      Diet therapy: _____

      _____

   e) Disorder: _____

      Diet therapy: _____

      _____

   f) Disorder: _____

      Diet therapy: _____

      _____

   g) Disorder: _____

      Diet therapy: _____

      _____

   h) Disorder: _____

      Diet therapy: _____

      _____

   i) Disorder: _____

      Diet therapy: _____

      _____

4. What is galactosemia?

   _____

   _____

   _____

5. Describe the nutritional management for infants with galactosemia.

   _____

   _____

   _____

   _____

6. What is phenylketonuria?

7. What is the only treatment for phenylketonuria?

8. What are the different forms of phenylketonuria?

9. PKU is the most common disorder of amino acid metabolism. What is its prevalence?

   a) 1 in 120–150 live births
   b) 1 in 1200–1500 live births
   c) 1 in 12,000–15,000 live births
   d) 1 in 120,000–150,000 live births
   e) 1 in 1,200,000–1,500,000 live births

10. What are the nutritional goals for infants with phenylketonuria?

_____

_____

_____

11. How are newborns fed after PKU diagnosis? Can they be breastfed?

_____

_____

_____

12. What is the approximate phenylalanine content of natural protein?

    a) 2.4–9 mg/100 g (or about 3½ oz)   d) 2.4–9 g/100 g (or about 3½ oz)
    b) 24–90 mg/100 g (or about 3½ oz)   e) 24–90 g/100 g (or about 3½ oz)
    c) 0.24–0.9 g/100 g (or about 3½ oz)

13. Estimate the average phenylalanine content of the natural protein sources listed in this table. (You can use food composition tables or a computerized food analysis software program.)

PHENYLALANINE CONTENT OF SOME COMMON PROTEIN FOOD SOURCES

Foods	Serving Size	Average Phenylalanine Content (g)	Percent Phenylalanine Content by Weight (g/100 g food)
Whole cow's milk (3.3% fat)	1 cup, 8 fluid oz, 237 mL (244 g)		
Plain yogurt (whole milk)	1 cup, 237 mL (245 g)		
Cheddar cheese (regular)	1 oz, ¼ cup, 59 mL (28 g)		
Cooked soybeans	3 oz, ½ cup, 118 mL (86 g)		
Hard cooked egg	1 medium, 1.8 oz (50 g)		
Macaroni noodles (enriched, cooked)	5 oz, 1 cup, 237 mL (140 g)		
Oatmeal (cooked)	8½ oz, 1 cup, 237 mL (234 g)		
Haddock filet (baked)	1 filet, 5⅓ oz (150 g)		
Ground beef (21% fat, broiled)	3 oz (85 g)		
Chicken breast (roasted, no skin)	1 medium, about 6 oz (172 g)		
Corn tortilla	6-inch tortilla, about 1 oz (26 g)		
White rice, long grain (enriched, cooked)	About 3 oz, ½ cup, 118 mL (88 g)		

14. What is cystic fibrosis?

_____

_____

_____

_____

_____

15. What are the signs and symptoms of cystic fibrosis?

_____

_____

_____

_____

_____

_____

_____

_____

_____

_____

_____

_____

_____

16. What is the overall incidence of cystic fibrosis, one of the most common fatal genetic disorders in Caucasians?

a) 1 in 150–200 live births   c) 1 in 15,000–20,000 live births   e) 1 in 1,500,000–2,000,000 live births
b) 1 in 1500–2000 live births   d) 1 in 150,000–200,000 live births

17. What are the goals of nutritional intervention for clients with cystic fibrosis?

_____

_____

_____

_____

_____

_____

_____

_____

_____

_____

_____

_____

18. Define the following terms.

    a) Azotorrhea: _____

    _____

    b) Steatorrhea: _____

    _____

    c) Bronchiectasis: _____

    _____

    d) Emphysema: _____

    _____

19. What is the nutrition goal or *gold standard* for preterm infants?

    _____

    _____

20. Preterm infants usually have a weak or absent sucking reflex and are unable to coordinate sucking-swal-lowing-breathing until _____ weeks of gestational age.

    a) 32–34　　b) 34–36　　c) 36–38　　d) 38–40　　e) 40–42

21. How do you feed premature infants before they can coordinate their sucking-swallowing-breathing and can suck strongly enough to meet their nutritional needs via oral feeding (nursing or bottle-feeding)?

    _____

    _____

    _____

    _____

    _____

    _____

    _____

    _____

22. What is the maximum energy concentration of preterm infant formulas and to which breast milk can be fortified?

    a) 16 kcal/oz or 2.2 kJ/mL　　c) 20 kcal/oz or 2.8 kJ/mL　　e) 24 kcal/oz or 3.3 kJ/mL
    b) 18 kcal/oz or 2.5 kJ/mL　　d) 22 kcal/oz or 3.1 kJ/mL

23. Why is a multinutrient human milk fortifier (powder or liquid) used for premature infants?

    _____

    _____

    _____

    _____

24. Parenteral nutrition is required for infants of < _____ at birth.

    a) 1 lb 10½ oz or 750 g　　c) 3 lb 5 oz or 1500 g　　e) 5 lb 8 oz or 2500 g
    b) 2 lb 3 oz or 1000 g　　d) 4 lb 6½ oz or 2000 g

25. What should be included in the nutrition assessment of infants? Give a detailed description.

_____
_____
_____
_____
_____
_____

26. Up to 2 years of age, the *corrected age* is determined for the follow-up of premature infants. It is utilized in the assessment of growth using growth curves, as well as in the evaluation of the language, psychosocial, and motor development.

    Knowing that the corrected age of a premature infant is *chronologic age (months) − number of months of prematurity,*

    determine the corrected age of a toddler who is presently 14 months old and who was born at 30 weeks' gestation.

_____
_____
_____
_____
_____
_____
_____
_____
_____
_____
_____
_____
_____

INTEGRATE YOUR LEARNING

1. Can infants with galactosemia be breastfed? Explain.

_____
_____

2. Why can't lactose-free infant formula be given to infants with galactosemia?

_____
_____
_____

3. Draw the overall biochemical reaction that occurs when phenylalanine is converted into tyrosine.

4. Approximately how much protein <u>and</u> phenylalanine does a thin slice (25 g; 60 kcal, 250 kJ) of whole wheat bread contain?

   a) 0.3 g; 12 mg   b) 3 g; 12 mg   c) 3 g; 120 mg   d) 6 g; 120 mg   e) 6 g; 1.2 g

5. Circle all of the foods that would be included in the regular diet of children with PKU.

Cheese	Bread	Low-protein bread	Chicken	Fruits
Cow's milk	Rice	Low-protein pasta	Beef	Tofu
Vegetables	Nuts	Phenylalanine-free formula	Oil	Honey
Margarine	Pudding	Phenylalanine-free bars	Eggs	Yogurt
Brown sugar	Sausage	Low-protein bakery foods	Fish	Tomato juice
Shellfish	Seeds	Breakfast cereals	Ham	Soy beverage
Pancake	Potatoes	Low-protein cereals	Popcorn	Fruit jelly
Fruit juice	Ice-cream	Low-protein cheese	Crackers	Legumes

6. How does cystic fibrosis affect digestion of food?

_____

_____

_____

_____

_____

_____

7. How does cystic fibrosis affect the absorption of different nutrients?

_____

_____

_____

_____

8. What type of diet is recommended for the management of cystic fibrosis in children?

_____

_____

_____

_____

_____

_____

9. Which children with CF may require EN?

_____

_____

_____

_____

_____

_____

_____

10. Give six reasons why premature infants are at nutritional risk and explain each reason.

    1- _____

    _____

    _____

    2- _____

    _____

    _____

    3- _____

    _____

    _____

    4- _____

    _____

    _____

    5- _____

    _____

    _____

    6- _____

    _____

    _____

11. What are sepsis and septicemia?

    _____

    _____

    _____

    _____

12. In addition to energy and protein, list six key micronutrients for which premature infants have increased needs.

    1) _____

    2) _____

    3) _____

    4) _____

    5) _____

    6) _____

13. _a)_____ feeds are minimal-volume feeds given through an enteral feeding tube to preterm newborns in the NICU to stimulate their gut to mature. These very small feeds are given in addition to TPN, and are usually initiated during the transition period between birth and 10 days of life. Ideally, the preferred feeding choice for these feeds is _b)_____.

14. Which micronutrient is not included in multinutrient human milk fortifier and for which supplementation is critical to prevent poor growth, decreased brain development, and lethargy in premature infants exclusively given fortified expressed breast milk? _____

    Why? _____

15. Why does the PKU screening test have to be repeated after discontinuation of TPN in neonates requiring TPN?

    _____

    _____

    _____

    _____

16. Many disease states are associated with increased energy needs in children, <u>except</u>

    a) cerebral palsy with rigidity, renal disease, and congenital heart disease
    b) phenylketonuria and conditions requiring artificial ventilation
    c) cystic fibrosis and short bowel
    d) Down syndrome and spina bifida
    e) b and d

CHALLENGE YOUR LEARNING

CASE STUDY

Objective

Here is an opportunity to use diet therapy and your client-centered approach to help a client with an inborn error of protein metabolism. Some clients, like D.O., require lifelong diet therapy to manage their inherited disease. Diet therapy needs to be tailored to the specific type of disease, but also to the stage of life cycle the client is currently going through as well as the monitoring and status (e.g., stability, progression) of the disease condition.

Description

D.O. is a Caucasian female born at 38 weeks' gestation on July 3, 1983. Her birth weight was 5 lb 7 oz and she measured 18 inches long. Her head circumference was 12.6 inches (32 cm) at birth. Her Apgar scores at 1 and 5 minutes after birth were 5 and 6, respectively. The delivery was complicated due to the fact that D.O. had the umbilical cord wrapped around her neck and body three times. When the obstetrician realized that the mother's uterine contractions were no longer effective at pushing D.O. through the birthing canal, he suspected that the umbilical cord was strangling D.O. and performed an episiotomy to unravel the cord. D.O. was very pale and was breathing weakly. After a few seconds on her mother's stomach, she received some oxygen and was quickly placed in an incubator for 2 days.

Her mother was very sad that she was not able to hold D.O. and breastfeed her right away, but a nurse explained that D.O. was too weak to nurse right now and that her vital signs had to be monitored closely. D.O.'s mother expressed her colostrum using an electric pump and fed D.O. in the nursery using a bottle. Although D.O. was only taking a few milliliters of colostrum each time, she became progressively stronger and did not need to be placed in the incubator any longer.

The pediatrician requested that D.O. be kept under observation at the children's hospital a little while longer. On her third day of life, she was able to room with her mother and was successful at nursing for the first time. Her mother was overjoyed. Although she was 7 oz lighter than at birth, D.O.'s body weight was starting to increase. Her father, two brothers (3 and 6 years of age), and grandparents finally got to hold her.

Unfortunately, the first Guthrie screening test result came back positive for PKU on day 4, just as they were getting ready to go home the next day. Her plasma phenylalanine concentration was 8.5 mg/dL or 508 μmol/L. D.O.'s mother agreed to stay longer and D.O.'s blood was retested immediately. The second Guthrie test turned out to also be positive on day 6, with 22.0 mg/dL or 1321 μmol phenylalanine/L plasma.

At 6 days of life, D.O.'s body weight was 5 lb 4 oz. Her plasma phenylalanine concentration was 26.4 mg/dL or 1585 μmol/L. Her plasma tyrosine concentration was 0.55 mg/dL or 30 μmol/L. She had normal urinary tetrahydrobiopterin concentration and erythrocyte dihydropteridine reductase activity. She was diagnosed with phenylketonuria. No one else in the family had phenylketonuria to their knowledge, but D.O.'s mother had been adopted, and it turned out that she was a carrier of the PKU gene. At 4 p.m. that day, the pediatrician ordered a PKU diet, paged the neonatal unit registered dietitian, and requested an initial nutrition counseling session.

1. What is an episiotomy?

2. What is your interpretation of D.O.'s birth weight? Refer to U.S. Centers for Disease Control and Prevention (CDC) growth charts and World Health Organization (WHO) growth standards.

3. What is your interpretation of D.O.'s birth length? Refer to the CDC growth charts and WHO growth standards.

4. What is your interpretation of D.O.'s birth weight-for-length? Refer to the CDC growth charts and WHO growth standards.

5. What is your interpretation of D.O.'s head circumference at birth? Refer to the CDC growth charts.

6. What is your interpretation of D.O.'s Apgar scores?

7. What is the usual plasma phenylalanine concentration of healthy infants?

8. What plasma phenylalanine concentrations are seen in infants with classic phenylketonuria?

9. What plasma phenylalanine concentrations are seen in infants with atypical phenylketonuria?

10. What is tetrahydrobiopterin?

11. What is dihydropteridine reductase?

12. What form of PKU do you think D.O. has? Explain.

13. What is the plasma phenylalanine recommended target/treatment range for infants and children with PKU?

14. When is it preferable to screen and diagnose for PKU?

15. When is it preferable to start PKU management?

16. Explain the PKU screening process, including the Guthrie test (Guthrie bacterial inhibition assay).

17. Why is the first blood sample for PKU screening taken after the child is 48 hours old?

18. Should phenylalanine be completely eliminated from the diet of infants with PKU? Explain.

19. What are the nutritional goals for D.O.?

20. What are the dietary recommendations for small infants like D.O. with PKU?

21. How long does it take for plasma phenylalanine concentrations to reach the recommended concentration range after diet therapy is initiated in newborns with PKU? Explain.

22. How often should plasma phenylalanine concentration be tested during infancy and childhood?

23. Give some examples of infant formulas available on the market for infants with PKU. Low- or no-phenylalanine commercial infant formulas include and are not limited to:

24. Which ethnic groups have higher incidence of PKU?

Case Follow-up

Following the recommendations of the pediatrician and dietitian, D.O. was started on the PKU diet therapy at 7 days of life and was able to reach her birth weight by 14 days of life. Along with her PKU dietary management, her mother continued to partially breastfeed her up to 11 months of age. D.O. adapted well to the PKU diet therapy and her parents ensured that she had excellent dietary compliance and metabolic control. D.O.'s mental development and physical growth were perfectly normal.

At about 13 months old, however, D.O. started to have elevated blood phenylalanine concentrations at her weekly visits. At 15 months of age, her pediatrician and parents were puzzled by her apparently random and unexplained moderately elevated blood phenylalanine concentrations. The pediatrician asked D.O.'s parents to pay special attention to her dietary phenylalanine intake and to bring a weekly food record to the dietitian. He also asked for biweekly blood phenylalanine measurements until her blood phenylalanine concentration could hopefully be stabilized.

The dietitian reviewed the food intake records for D.O. and they seemed to be normal. Then the dietitian asked the parents if some food had been left on the counter that D.O. could reach (e.g., cookie jar), if D.O. could be hiding food from meals/snacks, or if her siblings and relatives were giving her foods that her parents were not aware of. The parents did not think so. "Can the little one open the pantries where food is stored and get some food herself?" asked the dietitian. "It is unlikely; we voluntarily put the phenylalanine-rich foods on the upper shelves of the pantry, where she cannot reach," answered the parents.

The dietitian carried on by asking the parents if there was a domestic animal in the house and where its food was kept. "Yes, we have two cats, a dog, and some goldfish. We keep all the cat and dog food in the basement and the fish food by the aquarium," replied the parents, surprised by the question. The dietitian asked the parents to store the animal food in a place D.O. could not reach and to hide their food bowl after the animals have eaten.

25. What factors can affect the plasma phenylalanine concentration in patients with PKU?

26. Why did the dietitian ask the parents to make sure D.O. could not have access to animal foods?

27. How are solids introduced in the diet of infants with PKU?

28. What are the signs and symptoms of untreated PKU in infants and children?

29. What are the energy needs of infants and children with PKU?

30. What are the protein and phenylalanine needs of infants and children with PKU?

31. What are the dietary recommendations for children with PKU?

32. Explain why the dietary management of PKU is a lifelong treatment that cannot be discontinued after childhood.

33. Which sweetener contains phenylalanine and should therefore be limited in clients with PKU?

Case Follow-up

D.O. is still being teased to this day for eating dog food when she was a toddler! After her parents discovered that, the dog food was well hidden and D.O.'s blood phenylalanine concentration was kept under tight control throughout her childhood. As a teenager, D.O. was responsible and continued to follow her diet therapy fairly well. She is now an adult and is working full time as a veterinary assistant. She just announced to her parents that she and her husband are expecting.

34. What dietary recommendations would you give D.O. during her pregnancy?

35. What is likely to happen to her fetus if D.O. is not following dietary recommendations for the management of PKU during pregnancy?

36. Ideally, when should women with PKU start following pregnancy dietary recommendations for the management of PKU?

37. What is the life expectancy of individuals with PKU?

7.3 Adverse Reactions to Food

REVIEW THE INFORMATION

1. What are the most common food allergies?

   _____

   _____

   _____

2. Is there a difference between celiac disease and gluten-sensitive enteropathy? Explain.

   _____

   _____

3. Milk intolerance could be due to the following reasons, <u>except</u>

   a) food poisoning or a bacterial intestinal infection (e.g., gastroenteritis)
   b) galactosemia
   c) primary or secondary lactase deficiency
   d) a secondary, temporary reaction following a milk allergy episode
   e) none of the above

4. Which of the following signs and symptoms is lactose intolerance often characterized by?

   a) Eczema or hives   c) Nasal congestion   e) Bloody stools
   b) Vomiting   d) Diarrhea

5. Family history is a strong predictor of the risk of food allergy in young children. The risk of an infant developing an allergy is up to _____% if both parents have the same type of allergy (e.g., a food allergy).

   a) 30   b) 40   c) 50   d) 60   e) 70

6. About _____% of young infants suffer from a milk allergy in North America.

   a) 2–3   b) 4–6   c) 6–9   d) 8–12   e) 10–15

7. What are the main classes or types of white blood cells (leukocytes)?

   _____

   _____

8. Which type of leukocytes produces antibodies?

   _____

9. What are immunoglobulins E (IgEs)?

   _____

   _____

UNDERSTAND THE CONCEPTS

1. What is an adverse food reaction?

   _____

   _____

2. What are the main types of adverse food reactions? For each type of reaction, provide some examples.

   _____

   _____

   _____

   _____

   _____

   _____

   _____

   _____

   _____

   _____

   _____

   _____

   _____

   _____

   _____

   _____

   _____

   _____

   _____

   _____

   _____

3. Define the following terms.

   a) Allergen

   _____

   _____

   b) Allergenic food

   _____

   _____

c) Allergic contact dermatitis

_____

_____

d) Allergic eczema

_____

_____

e) Allergic reaction

_____

_____

f) Allergist

_____

_____

g) Allergy

_____

_____

h) Anaphylactic shock

_____

_____

i) Antigen

_____

_____

j) Atopy

_____

_____

k) Food allergy

_____

_____

l) Hypersensitivity

_____

_____

m) Idiosyncratic reaction

_____

_____

n) Inoculation

_____

_____

o) Intolerance

_____

_____

p) Psychogenic reaction

_____

_____

q) Sensitization

_____

_____

r) Urticaria

_____

_____

4. How long does it take for an allergic reaction to occur after a food allergen has been ingested?

_____

_____

5. What are possible signs and symptoms of allergies?

_____

_____

_____

_____

_____

_____

_____

_____

_____

_____

6. Approximately _____ of children <3 years of age and _____ of adults suffer from food allergy.

   a) 3%–4%; 1%   b) 6%–8%; 2%   c) 9%–12%; 3%   d) 12%–16%; 4%   e) 15%–20%; 5%

7. Indicate whether the following statements are TRUE or FALSE.

   a) _____ Food allergies are more common than food intolerance.

   b) _____ Most food allergies remain lifelong.

   c) _____ Cooking certain foods can help prevent an allergic reaction.

   d) _____ Presently, complete avoidance of the allergen(s) is the only universally successful form of treatment.

   e) _____ The immune system triggers some of the symptoms of food intolerance.

   f) _____ A person must be exposed and sensitized to a food before an allergic reaction to that food can happen.

g) _____ Food allergens are fats. They are absorbed and enter the bloodstream after digestion. They go to target organs where they cause allergic reactions.

h) _____ Eggs and fish allergies are the leading causes of deadly food allergic reactions or anaphylaxis.

i) _____ Peanuts are part of the legume family (like soybeans and other beans, chickpeas, peas, and lentils) and are a type of seed. Peanuts are not actually part of the tree-nut family (which includes almonds, cashews, pecans, walnuts, and others).

j) _____ An anaphylactic reaction is not likely to be serious if it begins with mild symptoms like tingling or itching in the mouth.

k) _____ Children are more likely to outgrow an allergy to peanuts or shrimp than an allergy to milk or soy.

l) _____ Certain medications can be taken before eating an allergenic food to prevent the allergic reaction.

m) _____ Young infants are vulnerable to an allergy of cow's milk because their immune and digestive systems are immature.

n) _____ One quarter of all infants that are allergic to cow's milk–based infant formula are also allergic to soy-based infant formula. Therefore, infants that have an atopic family history are given a hydrolyzed protein infant formula to manage cow's milk allergy instead of soy-based infant formula.

o) _____ Lactose intolerance is a common type of food intolerance. It affects at least 10% of all people.

p) _____ Cow's milk is the most common allergen in North American infants and 2%–3% of infants suffer from milk protein allergy.

q) _____ Goat milk is recommended for children who are allergic to cow's milk.

r) _____ Breastfeeding helps prevent allergies, especially in the first months of life.

s) _____ Food allergies are predominantly mediated by immunoglobulins G.

8. What are the three most common food allergens in children?

_____

9. What are the four most common food allergens in adults?

_____

10. What diagnostic procedure is used to identify adverse food reactions? Explain each step of the procedure.

_____

_____

_____

_____

_____

_____

_____

_____

_____

_____

_____

_____
_____
_____
_____
_____
_____
_____
_____
_____
_____
_____
_____
_____
_____
_____
_____
_____

11. What treatments are available to manage food allergies? Explain.

_____
_____
_____
_____
_____
_____
_____
_____
_____
_____
_____
_____

12. According to the American Academy of Pediatrics, eggs should not be introduced in the diet of children

until _____ months of age, especially if there is a family history of allergies. In addition, the introduction

to peanuts, tree nuts, and fish should be delayed until _____ months of age in order to reduce the risk
of an allergy.

a) 6; 12   b) 12; 18   c) 18; 24   d) 24; 36   e) 30; 40

INTEGRATE YOUR LEARNING

1. Antihistamines are used to relieve the following allergic symptoms, <u>except</u>

   a) gastrointestinal symptoms   c) hives   e) sneezing
   b) asthma symptoms   d) runny nose

2. Why do allergic reactions to food occur in some people?

   _____

   _____

   _____

   _____

   _____

   _____

   _____

3. What is MSG and where is it found?

   _____

   _____

   _____

   _____

   _____

4. What are some common MSG sensitivity signs and symptoms?

   _____

   _____

   _____

   _____

5. What are sulfites and where are they found?

   _____

   _____

   _____

   _____

6. In individuals with asthma, ingestion of a large quantity of sulfites may elicit

   a) nausea   b) bronchospasm   c) vomiting   d) diarrhea   e) flushing

7. How can some food intolerances be due to a psychologic cause?

   _____

   _____

   _____

   _____

8. How can the following adverse food reactions be managed? Explain your answers in detail.

a) Wheat allergy

_____
_____
_____
_____
_____
_____
_____
_____
_____
_____
_____

b) Milk protein allergy in a 2-week-old infant fed with cow's milk–based infant formula

_____
_____
_____
_____
_____
_____
_____
_____
_____
_____
_____
_____

c) Egg allergy in a 12-month-old

_____
_____
_____
_____
_____
_____
_____
_____
_____

d) Celiac disease

_____

_____

_____

_____

_____

_____

_____

_____

_____

_____

e) Peanut allergy in a 5-month-old breastfed infant

_____

_____

_____

_____

_____

_____

_____

_____

_____

_____

_____

f) Soy allergy

_____

_____

_____

_____

_____

_____

_____

_____

_____

_____

g) Primary lactase deficiency

_____

_____

_____

_____

_____

_____

_____

_____

_____

_____

h) "Hamburger disease" (hemorrhagic colitis)

_____

_____

_____

_____

_____

_____

_____

_____

_____

_____

_____

i) Intolerance to MSG

_____

_____

_____

_____

_____

_____

_____

_____

_____

_____

CHALLENGE YOUR LEARNING

CASE STUDY

Objectives

This case will help you realize how adverse food reactions can be traumatic for young children and how important it is for their caregivers to protect them from the food-specific allergens threatening their health and possibly their life.

It will also help you understand how important diet therapy recommendations are for the prevention of adverse food reactions in atopic children.

Description

A.C. is a happy and healthy 5-year-old little girl, who lives in your neighborhood. She is very lively and has started junior kindergarten this year. She loves helping her parents in the kitchen. She tells her grandparents that she wants to be a fairy princess or a ballerina when she grows up.

Last fall, A.C. collected lots of candy at Halloween just like the other little children in the neighborhood. It was lots of fun and exciting for A.C. However, back at home, she ended up having a very bad reaction to some chocolate containing peanut butter. Immediately after the ingestion of a piece of peanut butter–containing chocolate, her mouth, lips, and face started to get red and swell up. Her eyes were watery and she was constantly rubbing them. She started to get itchy hives on her hands and face. She felt nauseated and dizzy and complained of stomach cramps. She had trouble breathing and was short of breath. She cried for help in a panic. Her parents quickly realized something was very wrong with her and took her directly to the car, where she vomited. They raced to the nearby children's hospital emergency room, as A.C. was losing consciousness and wheezing. She was immediately given an injection of epinephrine and a mask of oxygen. She also received antihistamines and a bronchodilator.

1. What type of adverse food reaction does A.C. have?

2. What are the dietary recommendations for managing A.C.'s adverse food reaction?

3. What are the main goals of nutrition care for A.C.?

4. What else can A.C.'s parents do to manage her allergy and protect her?

Case Follow-up

A few months later, A.C. was invited to a birthday party for a child in her class. Many other children were present at the party. Two other friends had adverse food reactions, one to eggs and the other to tartrazine. A.C.'s parents were contacted an hour after the party started. A.C. was having another adverse food reaction after consuming some maple ice cream and was rapidly taken to the emergency room. The ice cream was home made and was purchased at a nearby food market.

5. What types of adverse food reactions do A.C.'s friends have?

6. What is tartrazine?

7. Which foods are likely to contain tartrazine?

8. What type of diet is required to manage an adverse reaction to eggs?

9. Why do you think the maple ice cream triggered an allergic reaction in A.C.?

10. Should a lemon cake have been served at that party, given that three children present have adverse reactions to food? Explain why.

7.4 Obesity and Eating Disorders

REVIEW THE INFORMATION

1. How are the following conditions defined?

   a) Malnutrition

   _____

   _____

   _____

   b) Failure to thrive

   _____

   _____

   _____

   c) Stunting

   _____

   _____

   _____

   d) Wasting

   _____

   _____

   _____

   e) Amenorrhea

   _____

   _____

   _____

   f) Underweight in children and teenagers

   _____

   _____

   _____

   g) Underweight in adults

   _____

   _____

   _____

   h) Healthy body weight in children and teenagers

   _____

   _____

   _____

i) Healthy body weight in adults

_____

_____

_____

j) Overweight in children and teenagers

_____

_____

_____

k) Overweight in adults

_____

_____

_____

l) Obesity in children and teenagers

_____

_____

_____

m) Obesity in adults

_____

_____

_____

n) Pica

_____

_____

_____

o) Geophagia

_____

_____

_____

2. _____ is not a direct measure of body fat, but that index is the most useful indicator, to date, of health risks associated with being overweight and underweight.

3. These disease conditions are associated with being overweight or obese, <u>except</u>

a) type 2 DM   c) hyperlipidemia   e) type 1 DM
b) hypertension   d) coronary heart disease

4. Which measurement is an indicator of the health risks associated with excess abdominal fat accumulation?

a) Head circumference   c) Wrist circumference   e) Mid-upper-arm circumference
b) Waist circumference   d) Hip circumference

5. Define metabolic syndrome.

_____

_____

_____

_____

6. BMI is an appropriate tool to use with the following individuals, <u>except</u>

   a) infants and toddlers   c) individuals with an illness   e) c and d
   b) teenagers   d) pregnant women

7. Compared to women of healthy body weight, obese women have a higher incidence of the following conditions, <u>except</u>

   a) complications during pregnancy   d) microsomic infant
   b) GDM   e) infertility
   c) Polycystic ovary (PCO) syndrome

8. What are the limitations of using the BMI as a tool to determine if the body weight of an adult is healthy for his or her height?

_____

_____

_____

_____

_____

9. The following problems may be consequences of being underweight, <u>except</u>

   a) type 1 DM   c) infertility   e) malnutrition
   b) impaired immunity   d) osteoporosis

10. What are the three components of the *female athlete triad*?

   a) _____

   b) _____

   c) _____

UNDERSTAND THE CONCEPTS

1. What are eating disorders?

_____

_____

_____

2. Give some examples of eating disorders.

_____

_____

_____

_____

3. Explain the following statement: "Eating disorders have multifactorial etiologies."

_____

_____

_____

_____

_____

_____

_____

_____

_____

_____

4. What factors or conditions may cause individuals to be underweight?

_____

_____

_____

_____

_____

_____

_____

_____

_____

5. What different lifestyle factors can contribute to the development of overweight and obesity?

_____

_____

_____

_____

_____

_____

_____

_____

_____

_____

6. According to the National Health and Nutrition Examination Survey 1999–2000, what percentage of the population was overweight or obese in the United States?

a) 24   b) 34   c) 44   d) 54   e) 64

7. In 2001, just over _____% of Canadian adults were overweight or obese and almost _____% were obese.

a) 20; 2   b) 30; 5   c) 40; 10   d) 50; 15   e) 60; 20

8. What factors have contributed to the development of the obesity pandemic, and especially the increased incidence of obesity in North Americans? Explain your answer.

_____

_____

_____

_____

_____

_____

_____

_____

_____

_____

_____

_____

_____

_____

_____

_____

_____

_____

_____

_____

_____

_____

_____

_____

_____

_____

_____

_____

_____

_____

_____

9. What health risks are associated with being overweight or obese?

_____

_____

_____

_____

_____

_____

_____

_____

_____

_____

_____

10. What is the *weight management* approach to overweight and obesity treatment?

_____

_____

_____

_____

_____

_____

_____

_____

_____

_____

_____

_____

_____

_____

11. Define the following terms.

a) Binge eating

_____

_____

b) Anorexia nervosa

_____

_____

c) Bulimia nervosa

_____

_____

d) Binge eating disorder

_____

_____

_____

e) Eating disorders not otherwise specified (EDNOS)

_____

_____

_____

f) Alcoholism

_____

_____

_____

12. What are some of the signs of anorexia nervosa for each of these organ systems?

a) Alimentary tract

_____

_____

_____

b) Skin

_____

_____

_____

c) Cardiovascular system

_____

_____

_____

d) Muscles, bones and adipose tissue

_____

_____

_____

13. These strategies are likely to help an obese client, <u>except</u>

a) emphasis on gradual changes to healthy eating
b) emphasis on weight management, through which weight loss may result
c) primary focus on achieving and maintaining healthy lifestyle habits
d) primary focus on body weight and fat losses
e) emphasis on physical, psychological, and emotional well-being

14. These strategies are likely to help an obese client, <u>except</u>

a) eating slowly, chewing well, and eating small portions at a time
b) establishing a routine for meals
c) eating frequent small meals/snacks
d) gradually increasing the intake of whole grain products, fruits, and vegetables
e) taking control of eating by listening to hunger cues

15. What drug approved for use in weight management can prevent the absorption of up to 30% of ingested fat?

    a) Sibutramine   b) Resin   c) Niacin   d) Xenical   e) Fibrate

16. It has been shown that very low-energy diets are usually inadequate in nutrients. To ensure that a well-balanced controlled-energy diet is nutritionally adequate, how many kilocalories or kilojoules should it minimally contain?

    a) 250 kcal or 1050 kJ   c) 750 kcal or 3140 kJ   e) 1250 kcal or 5230 kJ
    b) 500 kcal or 2090 kJ   d) 1000 kcal or 4180 kJ

17. To ensure a gradual body weight loss, overweight or obese people should <u>not</u> lose more than how many pound(s) or kilogram(s) per week?

    a) 1–2 lb or 0.5–0.9 kg   c) 5–6 lb or 2.3–2.7 kg   e) 9–10 lb or 4.1–4.5 kg
    b) 3–4 lb or 1.4–1.8 kg   d) 7–8 lb or 3.2–3.6 kg

INTEGRATE YOUR LEARNING

1. Episodes of anorexia nervosa can be of the *restricting type* or *binge-purging type*. How can these two types of anorexia episodes be distinguished?

    _____

    _____

    _____

    _____

    _____

2. Episodes of bulimia nervosa can be of the *purging type* or *nonpurging type*. How can these two types of bulimia episodes be distinguished?

    _____

    _____

    _____

    _____

    _____

3. Give some examples of eating disorders not otherwise specified (EDNOS).

    _____

    _____

    _____

    _____

    _____

    _____

    _____

4. What are the main goals of nutrition care in clients with eating disorders?

    _____

    _____

    _____

    _____

_____
_____
_____
_____
_____
_____
_____
_____
_____
_____

5. What is the maximum weekly weight loss goal for overweight individuals who need to progressively lose weight to reach a healthy body weight?

   a) 0.5–1.0 lb (0.2–0.5 kg)   c) 1.5–2.5 lb (0.7–1.1 kg)   e) 2.5–3.5 lb (1.1–1.6 kg)
   b) 1.0–2.0 lb (0.5–0.9 kg)   d) 2.0–3.0 lb (0.9–1.4 kg)

6. How can overweight and obesity be prevented?

   _____
   _____
   _____
   _____
   _____
   _____
   _____
   _____
   _____
   _____
   _____
   _____

7. Describe the following medications and indicate what side effects may be seen when individuals with eating disorders misuse them.

   a) **Laxatives**

      Description: _____

      Side effects: _____

   b) **Diuretics**

      Description: _____

      Side effects: _____

   c) **Enemas**

      Description: _____

      Side effects: _____

d) **Ipecac syrup**

Description: _____

Side effects: _____

8. What medications may be used in the treatment of eating disorders?

_____

_____

_____

_____

_____

_____

9. A malnourished client with an eating disorder (e.g., anorexia nervosa) may be at risk of refeeding syndrome. What is the refeeding syndrome?

_____

_____

_____

_____

_____

_____

10. Define the following.

a) Bradycardia

_____

b) Arrhythmia

_____

c) Hypotension

_____

d) Hemolysis

_____

e) Stamina

_____

f) Lanugo

_____

11. What types of surgeries are sometimes performed when other medical treatments have failed to help morbidly obese adults with life-threatening morbidity?

_____

_____

_____

_____

12. An obese man is trying to reach a healthy body weight by adopting a healthier lifestyle. He is eating fruits and vegetables for snacks instead of junk food. He is drinking water instead of regular soft drinks when he is thirsty. He is also taking the stairs instead of using elevators at work. He is 6'2″ and his body weight is presently 235 lb.

a) Determine his current BMI.

_____

_____

b) What energy deficit will allow this man to lose 1 lb of excess body fat per week?

_____

_____

c) How long will it take him to reach a BMI of 24.5 kg/m^2 if he loses 1 lb a week? Explain.

_____

_____

_____

_____

_____

_____

_____

CHALLENGE YOUR LEARNING

CASE STUDY

Objective

This case will help you realize that the development of obesity and eating disorders is progressive, complex, and multifactorial, and that a multidisciplinary approach is necessary for its management.

Description

A.E. was an extremely desired infant cherished by her parents and family. Her mother was a particularly patient and kind caregiver working part time in a daycare. Her father was an experienced high school teacher. Her mother had obesity class II and her father had obesity class I. They had tried for many years to have a child, but they concluded that they were probably infertile. They were both very sad not to have children. A few years after giving up any hopes of becoming pregnant, A.E.'s mother lost a significant amount of weight due to illness and unexpectedly became pregnant shortly after recovery. A.E.'s mother stopped working when she became pregnant and never worked afterward. She gained weight rapidly during pregnancy and was diagnosed with gestational diabetes mellitus in early pregnancy. She required diet therapy and insulin injections to manage her blood glucose concentrations. Fortunately, A.E. was a healthy 9-lb term baby. She was 20½ inches long. Her mother and father fed her infant formula.

A.E. was a unique and lonely young child. A.E. did not have many opportunities to play with younger children, as the only other children in the area were older boys. A.E. played with her parents and sometimes they would take her to visit her cousin who was around the same age. At 5½ years old, A.E. was still sucking her thumb and loved to eat. She spent most of her time coloring, making art crafts, playing computer games, and snacking while watching television. She measured 44 inches and weighed 54 lb at the age of 5 ½ years.

A.E. was shy, so she had a hard time making friends in school. She felt rejected when others would occasionally have prejudice against her and call her "the fat ugly girl." She rarely played outside and did not like sports. She learned piano and turned out to be an excellent seamstress. She also enjoyed cooking and regularly eating out with her parents.

As an older child, food was A.E.'s best friend and comfort. When she was lonely or sad, she would eat her favorite foods to make herself feel better, such as ice cream. When she was happy, she would celebrate with a candy treat. Her parents would frequently reward her for good grades at school by taking her out to restaurants.

During her teenage years, A.E. blamed her parents for her obesity. She did not feel attractive and she could not control the fact that she did not have a boyfriend. However, food was something she decided she was going to control. She was constantly on a new very restrictive fad diet to lose weight, but it was without success, as her weight continued to increase. She was desperate to be thin to pursue her dream of becoming a fashion designer. She kept telling her mother that a fashion designer could not be both obese and successful and that everyone would laugh at her if she tried.

Her many attempts at losing weight led her to develop very restricted eating patterns, interrupted by bouts of binging episodes, during which she would lose control and quickly eat a large amount of food. Her binging episodes were mostly triggered by her frustrations related to her unsuccessful attempts to make friends, especially male friends.

At 21 years old, she was successful at designing a line of young children's clothes, which was produced and sold in a reputable downtown store. Her clothes were popular. However, she was still very unhappy with her body weight, which was 217 lb, while her height was only 5′5″.

At 28 years old, she started a business and met a man who became her life partner. She decided to consult a physician for weight loss purposes. She weighed 245 lb. After a medical assessment, she was diagnosed with impaired glucose tolerance, hypertension, hyperlipidemia, and atherosclerosis.

1. What was the weight-for-length and sex percentile of A.E. at birth? Refer to U.S. Centers for Disease Control and Prevention (CDC) growth charts and World Health Organization (WHO) growth standards and give your interpretation.

2. What was the height-for-age and sex percentile of A.E. at 5½ years old? Refer to CDC growth charts and give your interpretation.

3. What was the BMI of A.E. at 5½ years old?

4. What was the BMI-for-age and sex percentile of A.E. at 5½ years old? Refer to CDC growth charts and give your interpretation.

5. What could have been done to help A.E. with her obesity when she was a child?

6. Did A.E. develop an eating disorder during adolescence? Explain.

7. What was A.E.'s BMI when she was 21 years old? Give your interpretation.

8. What factors may have contributed to A.E.'s obesity?

9. What was A.E.'s BMI when she was 28 years old? Give your interpretation.

10. Explain why very low-energy diets make it even harder to lose weight afterward.

11. What are the main goals of nutrition treatment for A.E.?

12. Determine A.E.'s adjusted body weight, which can be used to estimate her daily energy needs.

Case Follow-up

A couple of years later, A.E. is diagnosed with type II diabetes mellitus. At 38 years old, she has a myocardial infarction. A year later, A.E. weighs 258 pounds and is seriously considering bariatric surgery as a weight loss option.

13. Which clients are eligible for bariatric surgery? Is A.E. a ///candidate for bariatric surgery? Explain.

7.5 Cardiovascular Disease

REVIEW THE INFORMATION

1. Define these medical nutrition abbreviations.

1- CAD _____	12- UL _____
2- CVD _____	13- SFA _____
3- CHD _____	14- MUFA _____
4- CVA _____	15- PUFA _____
5- HF _____	16- EPA _____
6- MI _____	17- DHA _____
7- HT _____	18- Chol _____
8- BP _____	19- TG _____
9- HBP _____	20- ApoB _____
10- AMDR _____	21- LDL _____
11- AI _____	22- HDL _____

2. Coronary heart disease is the _____ cause of death among North American women and men.

   a) first   b) second   c) third   d) forth   e) fifth

3. Fill in the blank spaces with one choice from the following list.

long-chain triglycerides	linoleic acid	unsaturated fatty acids
hyperlipidemias	atheroma	liver
α-linolenic acid	saturated fatty acids	lipoproteins
cholesterol	trans-fatty acids	fat
monounsaturated fatty acids	glycerol	hydrogenation

   a) _____ are mostly found in animal products, such as butter, meat, and cheese, as well as in coconut and palm oil.

   b) _____ of vegetable oils result in the formation of trans-fatty acids.

   c) Plant products such as vegetable oils, nuts, and seeds are the main source of

   _____ .

   d) _____ are the main constituents of dietary fats.

   e) _____ are present in shortening, hard margarines, and baked goods, such as snack foods, crackers, cookies, and fried items.

f) Linoleic acid and _____ are essential fatty acids.

g) _____ can be found in safflower, corn, soybean, cottonseed, sesame, and sunflower seed oils.

h) Canola oil and olive oil are good sources of _____.

i) Triglycerides consist of fatty acids and _____.

j) _____ is a fat-soluble component synthesized by the liver and also found in food from animal sources (e.g., milk products, eggs, meat, fish, poultry, shrimp, butter).

k) _____ is the macronutrient most often associated with the development of obesity and cardiovascular disease.

l) _____ transport lipids and cholesterol in the blood.

m) Cholesterol is mainly stored in the _____.

n) _____ are chronic disease conditions associated with elevated blood lipid and lipoprotein concentrations.

o) Long-term consequences of a diet high in fat, saturated and *trans*-fatty acids, and cholesterol include the development of _____ plaques, which impair arterial blood flow and lead to the development of coronary heart disease.

4. Indicate what the AMDR recommendations are for fat, protein, and carbohydrates.

_____

_____

_____

5. Explain the following cardiovascular conditions.

a) Cardiovascular diseases

_____

_____

b) Heart disease

_____

_____

c) Atherosclerosis

_____

_____

d) Heart failure

_____

_____

e) Coronary heart disease

_____

_____

UNDERSTAND THE CONCEPTS

1. What are lipoproteins and what is their structure?

_____

_____

_____

_____

_____

_____

_____

_____

2. How are lipoproteins classified and differentiated?

_____

_____

_____

_____

_____

_____

_____

3. Describe each main group (or class) of lipoproteins.

a) Chylomicrons

_____

_____

b) HDL

_____

_____

c) VLDL

_____

_____

d) IDL

_____

_____

e) LDL

_____

_____

4. What are apolipoproteins and what are their principal functions?

_____

_____

_____

_____

_____

_____

_____

_____

_____

_____

5. Where are the different apolipoproteins found?

_____

_____

_____

_____

_____

_____

_____

_____

_____

_____

_____

_____

_____

6. Do lipoproteins have the same metabolism and functions? Explain.

_____

_____

_____

_____

_____

_____

_____

_____

_____

7. Explain the metabolism of chylomicrons. (You can refer to the figure illustrating the metabolism of lipoproteins below to help you.)

_____

_____

_____

_____

_____

_____

_____

_____

_____

_____

_____

_____

Metabolism of Lipoproteins

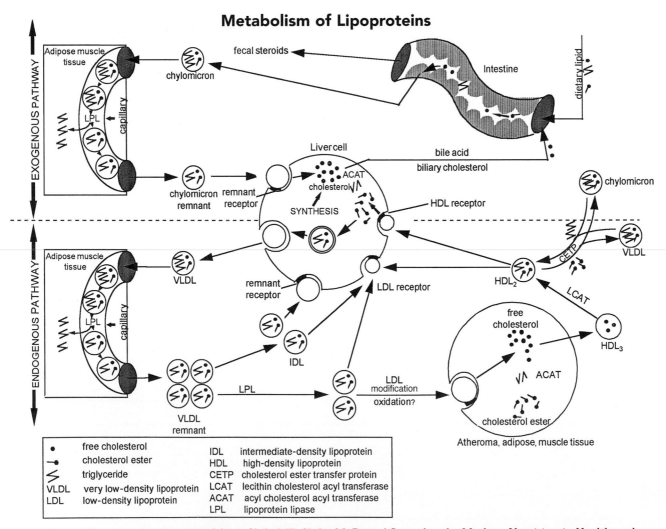

Metabolism of lipoproteins. Reprinted from Shils ME, Shike M, Ross AC, et al., eds. Modern Nutrition in Health and Disease. 10th Ed. Baltimore: Lippincott Williams & Wilkins, 2006:100.

8. Explain the metabolism of VLDLs, IDLs, and LDLs. (You can refer to the figure illustrating the metabolism of lipoproteins above to help you.)

_____

_____

_____

_____

_____

_____

_____

_____

_____

_____

_____

_____

_____

_____

_____

9. Explain the metabolism of HDLs. (You can refer to the figure illustrating the metabolism of lipoproteins above to help you.)

_____

_____

_____

_____

_____

_____

_____

_____

_____

_____

_____

_____

_____

_____

_____

10. What is the role of the liver in the metabolism of cholesterol and lipoproteins? (You can refer to the figure illustrating the metabolism of lipoproteins to help you.)

_____

_____

_____

_____

_____

11. Explain the metabolism of cholesterol within the liver. (You can refer to the figure illustrating the metabolism of lipoproteins to help you.)

_____

_____

_____

_____

_____

_____

_____

_____

_____

_____

_____

_____

_____

12. Explain what the following medical terms mean.

a) Hypercholesterolemia

_____

_____

b) Hypertriglyceridemia

_____

_____

c) Hyperlipoproteinemias

_____

_____

d) Hypertension

_____

_____

e) Cerebrovascular accident

_____

_____

f) Stroke

_____

_____

g) Ischemia

_____

_____

h) Ischemic stroke

_____

_____

i) Transient ischemic attacks

_____

_____

j) Myocardial ischemia

_____

_____

k) Angina pectoris

_____

_____

l) Congestive heart failure

_____

_____

m) Myocardial infarction

_____

_____

n) Percutaneous transluminal coronary angioplasty

_____

_____

o) Coronary artery bypass graft

_____

_____

p) Xanthomata

_____

_____

13. List 15 risk factors for coronary heart disease.

1- _____   9- _____

2- _____   10- _____

3- _____   11- _____

4- _____   12- _____

5- _____   13- _____

6- _____   14- _____

7- _____   15- _____

8- _____

14. What are the main types of hyperlipidemias?

_____

_____

_____

15. For each one of these types of hyperlipoproteinemias, indicate which lipoproteins are in excess and which blood lipids are increased.

a) Type I

_____

_____

b) Type IIa

_____

_____

c) Type IIb

_____

_____

d) Type III

_____

_____

e) Type IV

_____

_____

f) Type V

_____

_____

16. What is a blood lipid profile or lipid panel?

_____

_____

_____

_____

17. What is the effect of the following dietary components on blood lipid and lipoprotein concentrations, and where are they mainly found in the diet?

    a) **Fat**

       Effect: _____

       _____

       Sources: _____

       _____

    b) **SFA**

       Effect: _____

       _____

       Sources: _____

       _____

    c) *Trans*-**FA**

       Effect: _____

       _____

       Sources: _____

       _____

    d) **MUFA**

       Effect: _____

       _____

       Sources: _____

       _____

    e) **PUFA from ω-6 FA sources**

       Effect: _____

       _____

       Sources: _____

       _____

    f) **PUFA from fish**

       Effect: _____

       _____

       Sources: _____

       _____

    g) **Cholesterol**

       Effect: _____

       _____

       Sources: _____

       _____

h) **Soluble fiber**

Effect: _____

_____

Sources: _____

_____

i) **Insoluble fiber**

Effect: _____

_____

Sources: _____

_____

j) **Plant sterols**

Effect: _____

_____

Sources: _____

_____

k) **Soy protein**

Effect: _____

_____

Sources: _____

_____

18. Which factor(s) may contribute to low serum HDL cholesterol concentrations?

a) Physical inactivity   c) High-sugar diet   e) All of the above
b) Abdominal obesity   d) Cigarette smoking

19. According to the AMDR recommendations, healthy adults should get no more than _____% of the energy intake from fat, whereas healthy young children (1–3 years old) should get _____% of the energy intake from fat, and healthy children and teenagers (4–18 years old) should get _____% of the energy intake from fat.

a) 35; 15–25; 20–30   c) 40; 15–35; 10–20   e) 40; 25–45; 20–40
b) 45; 20–35; 25–40   d) 35; 30–40; 25–35

20. Is there a UL for dietary fat? Explain.

_____

_____

21. Does the Nutrition Board of the U.S. Institute of Medicine of the National Academies have some recommendations about the intake of *trans-* and saturated fatty acids and cholesterol? Explain.

_____

_____

_____

_____

22. What recommendations were included in the *Dietary Guidelines for Americans 2005* about the intake of total, saturated, and *trans*-fat and cholesterol?

_____

_____

_____

23. What is the purpose of nutrition care for clients with hyperlipidemia/hyperlipoproteinemia?

_____

_____

_____

_____

24. What type of diet is recommended for the management of hypercholesterolemia?

_____

_____

_____

_____

25. What are the National Cholesterol Education Program and its Adult Treatment Panel III?

_____

_____

_____

_____

26. Give the current dietary guidelines of the American Heart Association for the general population and the treatment of hypercholesterolemia and cardiovascular disease.

_____

_____

_____

_____

27. What were the American Heart Association Step 1 and Step 2 diets?

_____

_____

_____

_____

_____

_____

28. According to the AHA Dietary Guidelines for Healthy American Adults, diet should provide _____% of the energy intake as saturated fatty acids.

    a) <7   b) ≤8   c) <10   d) ≤15   e) ≤20

29. According to the AHA Therapeutic Lifestyle Change Diet and recommendations revision of 2006 for the treatment of hypercholesterolemia in adults, diet should provide _____% of the energy intake as saturated and _____% as *trans*-fatty acids.

    a) <7; <1   b) ≤8; ≤2   c) <10; <3   d) ≤15; ≤4   e) ≤20; ≤5

30. According to the 2006 Canadian guidelines for the prevention and treatment of hypercholesterolemia in adults, diet should provide _____% of the energy intake as saturated and *trans*-fatty acids.

    a) <7   b) ≤8   c) <10   d) ≤15   e) ≤20

31. The AHA Dietary Guidelines for Healthy American Adults and the Canadian guidelines for the prevention and treatment of hypercholesterolemia in adults state that diet should provide _____ mg cholesterol daily.

    a) <100   b) <200   c) <300   d) <400   e) <500

32. The Therapeutic Lifestyle Change Diet (published in 2001 by the American Heart Association) states that diet should provide _____ mg cholesterol daily.

    a) <100   b) <200   c) <300   d) <400   e) <500

33. What is the percent energy coming from monounsaturated fatty acids recommended as part of the AHA Therapeutic Lifestyle Change Diet?

    a) Up to 7%   c) Up to 10%   e) Up to 20%
    b) Up to 8%   d) Up to 15%

34. Every 1% reduction of energy from saturated fatty acids has been associated with a _____ mg/dL (_____ mmol/L) reduction of blood total cholesterol and LDL cholesterol concentrations.

    a) 0.4; 0.01   b) 0.8; 0.02   c) 1.2; 0.03   d) 1.5; 0.04   e) 1.9; 0.05

35. What are the target values of serum total cholesterol, HDL cholesterol, and LDL cholesterol concentrations for clients in the high level of risk for coronary artery disease in the United States?

    a) <150 mg/dL; ≥40 mg/dL; <70 mg/dL   d) <300 mg/dL; ≥100 mg/dL; <160 mg/dL
    b) <200 mg/dL; ≥60 mg/dL; <100 mg/dL   e) <350 mg/dL; ≥120 mg/dL; <190 mg/dL
    c) <250 mg/dL; ≥80 mg/dL; <130 mg/dL

36. What are the target values of the serum total cholesterol-to-HDL cholesterol ratio and of serum LDL cholesterol concentrations for clients in the high level of risk for coronary artery disease in Canada?

    a) <3.0 and <77 mg/dL (<2.0 mmol/L)   d) <4.0 and <97 mg/dL (<2.5 mmol/L)
    b) <6.0 and <154 mg/dL (<4.0 mmol/L)   e) <5.0 and <135 mg/dL (<3.5 mmol/L)
    c) <2.5 and <116 mg/dL (<3.0 mmol/L)

37. What is the target value of serum ApoB concentration for clients in the high level of risk for coronary artery disease?

    a) <90 mg/dL (<0.9 g/L)   d) <250 mg/dL (<2.5 g/L)
    b) <150 mg/dL (<1.5 g/L)   e) <290 mg/dL (<2.9 g/L)
    c) <190 mg/dL (<1.9 g/L)

38. Blood cholesterol concentrations may be low during

    a) weight loss   c) acute illness   e) none of the above
    b) the 3 months post-MI   d) all of the above

39. What type of diet is recommended for the management of hypertriglyceridemia?

_____

_____

_____

_____

40. What dietary component is used to help decrease elevated serum triglyceride concentrations?

a) ω-6 fatty acids

b) ω-3 fatty acids from fish

c) Monounsaturated fatty acids from olive oil

d) ω-3 fatty acids from egg

e) Plant sterols

41. What is the optimal serum triglyceride concentration?

a) <116 mg/dL (<1.3 mmol/L)

b) <150 mg/dL (<1.7 mmol/L)

c) <222 mg/dL (<2.5 mmol/L)

d) <249 mg/dL (<2.8 mmol/L)

e) <284 mg/dL (<3.2 mmol/L)

42. What medications may be used to manage the following lipid profile abnormalities?

a) High blood LDL cholesterol concentration

_____

b) High blood LDL cholesterol and low HDL cholesterol concentrations

_____

c) High blood LDL cholesterol and moderately high TG concentrations

_____

d) High blood TG concentration

_____

e) Low blood HDL concentration

_____

43. How are the target blood lipid concentrations determined for clients with hyperlipidemias?

_____

_____

_____

44. Every 1% reduction of blood cholesterol concentration has been associated with a _____ % reduction of coronary artery disease risk.

a) 1   b) 2   c) 3   d) 4   e) 5

45. What diet is recommended for the treatment of hyperchylomicronemia?

_____

_____

_____

_____

_____

_____

_____

46. What are the sodium AI and UL for adults?

_____

47. What is the optimal blood pressure in healthy individuals?

_____

48. What blood pressures correspond to high blood pressure (hypertension)?

_____

_____

49. What is the DASH diet? Describe its main recommendations and benefits.

_____

_____

_____

50. What lifestyle modifications are included as part of the current Canadian Hypertension Education Program Recommendations?

_____

_____

_____

_____

_____

_____

_____

51. One teaspoon of table salt contains _____ mg sodium.

    a) 1325   b) 2325   c) 3325   d) 4325   e) 5325

52. What are the treatment targets for clients with hypertension?

_____

_____

_____

_____

_____

53. What are the main medications used for the management of high blood pressure?

_____

_____

_____

_____

_____

_____

54. These factors are associated with an increased risk for developing hypertension, <u>except</u>

    a) Caucasian ethnicity
    b) cigarette smoking
    c) excessive alcohol consumption
    d) diabetes mellitus
    e) stress

INTEGRATE YOUR LEARNING

1. The lipids originating from the diet are absorbed and transported in the lymph to the liver by the

    a) fat micelles   b) VLDL   c) LDL   d) chylomicrons   e) bile salts

2. Knowing the sodium AI and UL, how much salt do you recommend healthy adults include in their diet?

    _____

    _____

    _____

3. List the Dietary Guidelines for Healthy American Adults published in 2001 by the American Heart Association for prevention and treatment of hypercholesterolemia and cardiovascular disease.

    _____

    _____

    _____

    _____

    _____

    _____

    _____

    _____

    _____

    _____

    _____

    _____

    _____

    _____

    _____

    _____

    _____

    _____

    _____

    _____

    _____

    _____

4. What are the recommendations of the Dietary Guidelines for Healthy Children published in 2001 by the American Heart Association?

_____

_____

_____

_____

_____

_____

_____

_____

_____

_____

_____

_____

_____

_____

_____

_____

5. List the recommendations of the Therapeutic Lifestyle Change Diet published in 2001 by the American Heart Association, and indicate what are the main Diet and Lifestyle Recommendations Revision 2006.

_____

_____

_____

_____

_____

_____

_____

_____

_____

_____

_____

_____

6. Summarize and compare the AHA Therapeutic Lifestyle Change Diet with 2006 Recommendations Revision and the Canadian Recommendations for the Management of Dyslipidemia & Prevention of Cardiovascular Disease.

AMERICAN HEART ASSOCIATION AND CANADIAN RECOMMENDATIONS FOR DYSLIPIDEMIA MANAGEMENT		
Composition of Diet	**American Heart Association Therapeutic Lifestyle Change Diet With 2006 Recommendations Revision**	**Canadian Recommendations for the Management of Dyslipidemia & Prevention of CVD**
Total fat		
SFA and *trans*-FA		
PUFA, including ω-3 FA		
MUFA		
Cholesterol		
Carbohydrates		
Added sugar		
Protein		
Energy		
Alcohol		

7. Is regression of atherosclerosis and coronary heart disease possible? Explain your position.

_____

_____

_____

8. One of your clients is a 58-year-old man who smokes cigarettes, has a systolic blood pressure of 140 mm Hg, and blood total and HDL cholesterol concentrations of 251 mg/dL and 37 mg/dL, respectively.

1- What are his blood total and HDL cholesterol concentrations in mmol/L?

_____

_____

2- Determine his 10-year risk for CHD.

_____

_____

_____

_____

3- Determine his risk category for CHD (low, moderate, or high).

_____

4- Determine his target blood lipid values according to his level of risk for CHD.

_____

_____

_____

_____

9. What is the typical effect of type 2 diabetes mellitus on blood lipid concentrations?

   a) ↑ chylomicrons, ↑ LDL cholesterol, ↑ VLDL cholesterol.
   b) ↑ LDL cholesterol, ↑ HDL triglyceride, ↓ total-to-HDL cholesterol ratio.
   c) ↑ VLDL cholesterol, ↑ HDL triglycerides, ↑ total-to-HDL cholesterol ratio.
   d) ↑ LDL cholesterol, ↑ triglycerides, ↓ HDL cholesterol.
   e) ↑ chylomicrons, ↑ LDL cholesterol, ↑ HDL cholesterol

10. What main dietary recommendations would you give to a client with hypertension treated with furosemide?

_____

_____

_____

_____

_____

11. The following effects are cardioprotective effects of EPA and DHA, <u>except</u>

   a) reduced serum triglyceride and VLDL concentrations
   b) improved endothelial relaxation
   c) enhanced endothelial vasodilatation
   d) decreased blood platelet reactivity
   e) reduced serum LDL cholesterol concentrations

12. These food components are cholesterol-lowering food components promoted by the Portfolio Eating Plan, <u>except</u>

   a) viscous fiber   c) plant sterols   e) olive oil
   b) soy protein   d) almonds

13. These sources of dietary fiber help to reduce elevated blood cholesterol concentrations, <u>except</u>

   a) oat   b) guar   c) wheat   d) pectin   e) psyllium

14. What type of diet is recommended for clients with cardiac cachexia?

_____

_____

_____

_____

_____

15. What diet is recommended after a CABG or angioplasty?

_____

_____

_____

_____

16. What diet is recommended after a heart valve surgery?

_____

_____

_____

_____

_____

17. What dietary recommendations are given to clients on Coumadin to limit adverse effects from nutrient–drug interactions?

_____

_____

_____

_____

_____

18. These factors can be secondary causes of dyslipoproteinemias, <u>except</u>

a) sedentary lifestyle   c) stress   e) nephrotic syndrome
b) smoking   d) thiazide diuretics

19. These criteria are used as a basis to calculate the 10-year risk factor for coronary heart disease in the United States and Canada, <u>except</u>

a) saturated fat content of the diet   d) systolic blood pressure
b) total blood cholesterol concentration   e) cigarette smoking
c) blood HDL cholesterol concentration

20. Which type of dyslipoproteinemia is due to excess LDL and VLDL particles?

a) Type I   b) Type IIA   c) Type IIB   d) Type IV   e) Type V

21. What is the drug of choice for the treatment of elevated serum LDL cholesterol concentrations with mildly elevated serum triglyceride concentrations?

a) Niacin   b) Statin   c) Resin   d) Fibrate   e) None of the above

22. What type of lipid-lowering drug primarily acts by increasing the activity of lipoprotein lipase?

a) Niacin   b) Statin   c) Resin   d) Fibrate   e) None of the above

23. Adequate intakes of _____ are recommended, as a deficiency in these vitamins is thought to be associated with the development of hyperhomocysteinemia (high blood concentrations of homocysteine, an atherogenic protein increasing the risk for coronary heart disease), especially in elderly individuals who have suboptimal intake of these vitamins.

a) vitamins A, C, and E   d) β-carotene, pantothenic acid, and vitamin C
b) all B-complex vitamins   e) folate, pyridoxine, and vitamin B_{12}
c) thiamin, riboflavin, and pantothenic acid

24. Which statement is **false** about heart failure?

a) Heart failure is the only major cardiovascular syndrome.
b) It increases blood pressure.
c) It increases filling pressures.
d) It decreases cardiac output.
e) Clients with heart failure do not all have coronary artery disease.

25. These signs or symptoms are usually associated with heart failure, <u>except</u>

    a) weight loss   c) nocturia   e) shortness of breath
    b) liver tenderness   d) increased heart rate

26. These are characteristics associated with chronic heart failure, <u>except</u>

    a) arrhythmia   d) hypernatremia
    b) hypokalemia   e) increased blood urea concentration
    c) increased blood creatinine concentration

27. Which drug type is introduced first in the treatment of heart failure according to consensus guidelines?

    a) Beta-blockers   d) Digoxin
    b) Nitrates   e) Aldosterone antagonists
    c) Angiotensin-converting enzyme inhibitors

28. Which drug type increases the strength of the pumping action of the heart?

    a) Beta-blockers   d) Digoxin
    b) Nitrates   e) Aldosterone antagonists
    c) Angiotensin-converting enzyme inhibitors

29. Which drug type reduces the stress on the heart and also has a weak diuretic effect?

    a) Beta-blockers   d) Digoxin
    b) Nitrates   e) Aldosterone antagonists
    c) Angiotensin-converting enzyme inhibitors

30. Which drug is given as a spray to treat angina episodes?

    a) Calcium channel blocker   d) Thiazide
    b) Nitroglycerine   e) β-Adrenergic blocking agent (beta-blockers)
    c) Angiotensin-converting enzyme inhibitor

31. Which drug is an angiotensin-converting enzyme inhibitor?

    a) Amiloride   b) Captopril   c) Atenolol   d) Felodipine   e) Hydrochlorothiazide

32. Which drug is a potassium-wasting loop diuretic?

    a) Amiloride   b) Captopril   c) Atenolol   d) Felodipine   e) Hydrochlorothiazide

33. Which drug makes the heart beat slower by decreasing the force of the pumping of the heart?

    a) Calcium channel blocker   d) Thiazide
    b) Nitroglycerine   e) β-Adrenergic blocking agent (beta-blockers)
    c) Angiotensin-converting enzyme inhibitor

34. The effect of which drug may be increased by grapefruit juice?

    a) Calcium channel blocker   d) Thiazide
    b) Nitroglycerine   e) β-Adrenergic blocking agent (beta-blockers)
    c) Angiotensin-converting enzyme inhibitor

35. Which drug helps to dilate and open up blood vessels?

    a) Calcium channel blocker   d) Thiazide
    b) Nitroglycerine   e) β-Adrenergic blocking agent (beta-blockers)
    c) Angiotensin-converting enzyme inhibitor

36. Why is aspirin sometimes given to clients with controlled hypertension?

_____

_____

_____

CHALLENGE YOUR LEARNING

CASE STUDY

Objectives

This case will help you understand that cardiovascular disease and complications resulting from it usually develop progressively and that clients often have more than one factor contributing to its development, including their lifestyle.

It will also help you assist clients in preventing or managing cardiovascular disease and its complications by reducing the risk factors contributing to its development. Gradually adopting a healthy lifestyle and, when needed, reaching a healthier body weight through weight management will often help clients significantly reduce their risk of disease and improve or at least maintain their health status and quality of life.

This case will help you realize that even though the dietitian may perceive that many aspects of the lifestyle and diet of a client need improvement, patiently working with the client step by step toward improving the big picture will be more helpful to the client in the long run than attempting a quick "total makeover" of his lifestyle.

Description

J.S. is a 55-year-old father and civil engineer. A nurse recently found his blood pressure to be elevated during an employee health awareness week at work. The nurse repeated the measurement the following day and J.S.'s blood pressure was similarly elevated. When questioned by the nurse, J.S. said that he had not seen his family physician for years and that he did not think about going for yearly check-ups since he was not sick. As a follow-up, the nurse asked J.S. to visit his family physician for a more complete medical assessment and evaluation of his blood pressure.

The family physician diagnosed J.S. with arterial hypertension and obesity, and discussed with him ways he should improve his lifestyle, including smoking cessation. He referred J.S. to you, the dietitian, to start the nutrition intervention in the following days. The family physician prescribed weight management and education about a heart-healthy diet low in salt. The physician also requested to see J.S. again to reassess his blood pressure in a few days, once his fasting blood lipid and glucose concentrations have been determined.

You see J.S. in the nutrition clinic for an initial consultation (40 minutes), on October 15, 2007, at 2:00 p.m. During the nutrition interview, he tells you that he does not have previous history of high blood pressure, but has been told many times to watch his weight by his wife, two children, and family physician. His wife, who was present at the interview, says that his answer to their remarks has always been, "My grandparents lived up to 80 years old and my parents are still alive. There is no history of heart attacks in my family."

You determine that he measures 5'10", currently weighs 252 lb, and has a large frame size. His wife says that he has been gaining weight gradually, about 4 lb every year, since she met him when he was 25 years old. He does not have a family history of cardiovascular disease, but his father is overweight and has been diagnosed with non–insulin-dependent type 2 diabetes mellitus 2 years ago at the age of 77.

He admits that he usually smokes eight cigarettes a day, eats many snacks, and watches television to cope with his life stress. He complains that he does not sleep well. He says that he has a sedentary lifestyle. He tells you that he does not like to exercise and does seated work with little movement involved.

The physical examination performed by the physician revealed the following:
Blood pressure of 170/102 mm Hg
Waist circumference: 41¼ inches (105 cm)

His biochemical laboratory data are now available and indicate the following:
Fasting plasma glucose = 123 mg/dL

Serum total cholesterol = 278 mg/dL
Serum LDL cholesterol = 239 mg/dL
Serum HDL cholesterol = 27 mg/dL
Fasting serum triglycerides = 347 mg/dL
Serum ApoB concentrations = 130 mg/dL (1.3 g/L)

You perform a 24-hour dietary recall and obtain what seems to be his typical daily food intake:

Breakfast: At home
- 1½ cup (12 fluid oz or 355 mL) fruit punch drink (prepared from frozen concentrate with tap water)
- ¾ cup (178 mL) scrambled eggs prepared from 3 large eggs (1.8 oz or 50 g each), 1 fluid oz (30 mL) of 2% fat milk, and 1 tsp (5 mL) salted butter, with a pinch (2 mL, 0.09 oz, 2.4 g) of table salt and a pinch of pepper
- 2 slices of commercial white enriched bread toasted (1 oz or 28 g each) each with 1 tsp (5 mL) salted butter and 1 tsp (5 mL) orange marmalade
- 1 cup (8 fluid oz, 237 mL) coffee, brewed (prepared with tap water) with 2 tsp (10 mL) white sugar and 1 Tbsp (15 mL) cream 18% fat

Morning snack: At work
- 1 cup (8 fluid oz, 237 mL) coffee, brewed (prepared with tap water) with 2 tsp (10 mL) white sugar and 1 Tbsp (15 mL) cream 18% fat
- 1 medium (2.3 oz, 65 g) cinnamon Danish pastry (4¼ inches or 11 cm diameter)

Lunch: At the restaurant
- 1 plain cheeseburger: single ground beef patty (3 oz, 84 g), regular bun/roll (1½ oz, 43 g), and a slice of American cheese (1 oz, 28 g), with 2 pieces (0.6 oz or 16 g) of cooked bacon and 2 tsp (10 mL) of tomato ketchup
- 1 large serving of French fries (30 pieces, 5⅓ oz, 150 g), frozen, restaurant-prepared, in vegetable oil with some table salt (about 2 mL, 0.09 oz, 2.4 g) and 3 Tbsp (45 mL) of ketchup
- 1 piece of cheese cake, commercial, ⅙ of cake (3 oz, 80 g)
- 1 cup (8 fluid oz, 237 mL) orange soda, soft drink

Afternoon snack: At work
- 1 medium Mars Almond chocolate candy bar (1.8 oz, 50 g)
- 1 cup (8 fluid oz, 237 mL) coffee, brewed (prepared with tap water) with 2 tsp (10 mL) white sugar and 1 Tbsp (15 mL) cream 18% fat

Dinner: At home
- 1 chicken breast, broiled, meat and skin (3½ oz, 100 g)
- 1 medium (2¼ inches or 5.7 cm diameter, 6.2 oz, 173 g) oven-baked potato, flesh and skin with 1 Tbsp (15 mL) regular sour cream 14% fat and some table salt (1 mL, 0.04 oz, 1.2 g) and pepper
- 1 cup (237 mL) rich vanilla ice cream
- 1 large (2 oz, 56 g) commercial brownie square (2¾ × ¾ inches thick or 7 × 2 cm thick)
- 1 cup (8 fluid oz, 237 mL) tea, brewed (prepared with tap water) with 2 tsp (10 mL) white sugar

Snack during the evening: At home
- 1 medium bag of plain, salted potato chips (about 60 chips, 4¼ oz, 120 g)
- 4 cups (32 fluid oz, 950 mL) cola, soft drink

Afterward, you ask J.S. how he thinks he could reduce his salt intake and he says he will try to avoid adding salt to his foods. You go on to discuss ways he could reduce his intake of high-salt and high-energy foods with J.S. and his wife. His wife, who buys foods and does the cooking at home, is willing to help. You ask J.S. to bring a 3-day food record to the next visit in 3 weeks. Before leaving, he says he might consider your suggestion of popcorn and diet pop instead of chips and regular cola in the evening.

1. What are J.S.'s main health concerns or problems?

2. Since J.S. has a large bone frame, do you agree with the physician that he is obese? Explain why.

3. What type of obesity does J.S. have?

4. Do you think J.S. was obese as a young adult? Explain.

5. Why was J.S. diagnosed with arterial hypertension?

6. What are his blood lipid and glucose values in mmol/L?

7. Is J.S. at low, moderate, or high risk for cardiovascular disease? Explain why.

8. What are his target blood lipid values according to his level of risk for CHD?

9. How does his blood lipid profile compare to the target blood lipid values recommended according to his level of risk for CHD?

10. Does J.S. have hyperlipidemia? If so, what type?

11. Does J.S. suffer from the metabolic syndrome? Justify your answer.

12. What CVD risk factors are associated with the metabolic syndrome?

13. What is your interpretation of J.S.'s fasting plasma glucose concentration? What is to be done about it?

14. Explain and justify each component of the nutrition prescription.

15. Analyze the 24-hour dietary recall of J.S. using a table of nutrient content of foods. Afterward, complete the table below with the breakdown of his dietary intake and compare it to the DRI recommendations for healthy individuals.

DIETARY INTAKE OF J.S. AND COMPARISON TO DRI RECOMMENDATIONS		
Energy, Nutrients, and Other Dietary Components	Intake of J.S. Over 24 Hours	Comparison to DRI Daily Recommendations for Healthy Individuals (EER, RDA, or AI)
Energy (kcal) [kJ]		
Protein (g)		
Energy from protein (%)		
Total fat (g)		
Energy from fat (%)		
Saturated fat (g)		
Energy from saturated fat (%)		
Monounsaturated fat (g)		
Energy from monounsaturated fat (%)		
Polyunsaturated fat (g)		
Energy from polyunsaturated fat (%)		
Carbohydrate (g)		
Energy from carbohydrate (%)		

DIETARY INTAKE OF J.S. AND COMPARISON TO DRI RECOMMENDATIONS *(continued)*

Energy, Nutrients, and Other Dietary Components	Intake of J.S. Over 24 Hours	Comparison to DRI Daily Recommendations for Healthy Individuals (EER, RDA, or AI)
Sugars (g)		
Energy from sugars (%)		
Cholesterol (mg)		
Sodium (mg)		
Total dietary fiber (g)		
Iron (mg)		
Calcium (mg)		
Vitamin C (mg)		
Vitamin D (μg)		
Vitamin A – RAE* (μg)		
Total Water (fluid oz) [L]		
Caffeine (mg)		

*RAE, retinol activity equivalents.

16. Compare the daily intake of J.S. to the recommendations of MyPyramid or Canada's Food Guide to Healthy Eating using this table.

DIETARY INTAKE OF J.S. COMPARED TO THE RECOMMENDATIONS OF MY PYRAMID OR CANADA'S FOOD GUIDE TO HEALTHY EATING

Food Groups	Intake of J.S. Over 24 hours (Quantity Consumed)	Comparison to the Recommendations of MyPyramid or Canada's Food Guide to Healthy Eating
Grains		
Vegetables		
Fruits		
Meat and beans		
Milk		
Also: Fat/oil, sugars, salt		

17. Use this table to compare the dietary intake of J.S. to the American Heart Association Therapeutic Lifestyle Change Diet with 2006 Recommendations Revision and the Canadian Recommendations for the Management of Dyslipidemia & Prevention of Cardiovascular Disease.

DIETARY INTAKE OF J.S. COMPARED TO AHA AND CANADIAN RECOMMENDATIONS FOR DYSLIPIDEMIA MANAGEMENT

Composition of Diet	Daily Intake of J.S.	Canadian Recommendations for Dyslipidemia Management	AHA Therapeutic Lifestyle Change Diet with 2006 Recommendations Revision
Total fat			
SFA and *trans*-FA			
PUFA, including ω-3 FA			
MUFA			
Cholesterol			
Fiber			
Carbohydrate			
Protein			
Alcohol			
Refined carbohydrates and added sugar			
Energy			
Alcohol			

18. List the major differences between the nutrition prescription and the reported usual daily intake.

19. Do you perceive J.S. as being ready and motivated to change? Why? How would you help J.S. at this point?

20. Summarize the data, observations, assessment, and plan of action in an initial nutrition care plan, using the SOAP or DAP charting format. Include a Nutrition Diagnosis Statement (in PES format [problem—etiology—signs and symptoms]) as part of your charted note.

Case Follow-up

When J.S. returns to see his family physician the following week, he receives the additional diagnosis of hyperlipidemia, impaired fasting glucose, and metabolic syndrome. J.S.'s blood pressure is still elevated. The physician prescribes an ACE inhibitor and a statin. He also recommends J.S. eat fish twice a week.

21. What is an ACE inhibitor?

_____

_____

_____

22. Give some examples of ACE inhibitors on the North American market. Provide their generic name.

_____

_____

_____

23. What is a statin?

_____

_____

_____

24. Give some examples of statins on the North American market. Provide their generic name.

_____

_____

_____

25. Why did the physician recommend that he eat fish twice a week?

_____

_____

_____

Case Follow-up

After 5 months of counseling, J.S. has made some significant improvements to his lifestyle and dietary habits. He is following your dietary recommendations fairly well and his wife is helping him. He has lost 21 lb, is walking 40 minutes most evenings, and is smoking only on rare occasions.

26. Prepare an example of a well-balanced **menu day** that you will give J.S. as a handout to help him.

   - Your menu should meet his dietary needs and be in agreement with the heart-healthy diet low in sodium prescribed by his physician. Be practical and realistic, and consider J.S.'s individual preferences!

   - The handout sheet should be clear, concise, and attractive.

27. Analyze the menu day you prepared for J.S. using a food analysis software program. Compile the information in this table and justify that your menu is appropriate for J.S.

DIETARY ANALYSIS OF MENU DAY PREPARED FOR J.S.	
Energy, Nutrients, and Other Dietary Components	Menu Day for J.S.
Energy (kcal) [kJ]	
Protein (g)	
Energy from protein (%)	
Total fat (g)	
Energy from fat (%)	
Saturated fat (g)	

(continued)

DIETARY ANALYSIS OF MENU DAY PREPARED FOR J.S. *(continued)*	
Energy, Nutrients, and Other Dietary Components	**Menu Day for J.S.**
Energy from saturated fat (%)	
Monounsaturated fat (g)	
Energy from monounsaturated fat (%)	
Polyunsaturated fat (g)	
Energy from polyunsaturated fat (%)	
Carbohydrate (g)	
Energy from carbohydrate (%)	
Sugars (g)	
Energy from sugars (%)	
Cholesterol (mg)	
Sodium (mg)	
Total dietary fiber (g)	
Iron (mg)	
Calcium (mg)	
Vitamin C (mg)	
Vitamin D (μg)	
Vitamin A – RAE* (μg)	
Total Water (fluid oz) [L]	
Caffeine (mg)	

*RAE, retinol activity equivalents.

7.6 Diabetes Mellitus

REVIEW THE INFORMATION

1. Define these medical abbreviations:

   BG _____

   2hPG _____

   IFG _____

   IGT _____

BGC _____

bgm _____

A_{1C} _____

DM _____

GDM _____

IDDM _____

CDE _____

CHO _____

FBS _____

gluc _____

Hb or Hgb _____

GTT _____

OGTT _____

H/O _____

meds. _____

p.c. _____

q.3h _____

i.c. _____

a.c. _____

b.i.d. _____

t.i.d.a.c. _____

2. Which organ produces insulin? _____

3. Where is insulin secreted? _____

4. Define the following.

   a) Diabetes mellitus

   _____

   _____

   b) Type 1 diabetes mellitus

   _____

   _____

   c) Type 2 diabetes mellitus

   _____

   _____

   d) Gestational diabetes mellitus

   _____

   _____

5. How is GDM diagnosed?

_____

_____

_____

_____

_____

_____

_____

_____

_____

_____

6. What are the blood glucose targets for the management of GDM?

_____

_____

_____

7. List 12 risk factors for type 2 diabetes mellitus.

1- _____

2- _____

3- _____

4- _____

5- _____

6- _____

7- _____

8- _____

9- _____

10- _____

11- _____

12- _____

8. Which foods contain carbohydrates?

_____

_____

_____

_____

_____

UNDERSTAND THE CONCEPTS

1. Use this grid to help you fill in the following text with appropriate words relating to glucose metabolism and diabetes mellitus.

Terms Related to Glucose Metabolism and Diabetes Mellitus

a) The concentration of glucose in the blood is _____ (*word of 6 letters*) controlled by the body, to make sure that it is maintained within a healthy range.

b) Blood glucose mainly enters the body _____ (*word of 5 letters*) by facilitated diffusion, using facilitative-diffusion glucose transporter (GLUT) proteins.

c) The pancreatic _____ (*word of 4 letters*) cells of the islets of Langerhans produce insulin, which is very important in the regulation of blood glucose concentration.

d) Insulin is a _____ (*word of 7 letters*) secreted in reaction to an increase in blood glucose concentration over the normal range causing hyperglycemia.

e) Insulin binds to a _____ (*word of 8 letters*) on body cells and promotes transport of blood glucose into these cells using glucose transporters and cotransporters.

f) Some glucose transporters, such as those in _____ (*word of 7 letters*) tissue and muscles, are insulin dependent. These tissues are called insulin sensitive.

g) When insulin binds to the insulin receptor at the surface of the cells, glucose transporters migrate from

the inside to the _____ (*word of 7 letters*) of the cells to increase glucose transport into the cells.

h) The _____ (*word of 7 letters*) -stimulated glucose transporter located in skeletal muscle cells and adipocytes is GLUT 4.

i) In the _____ (*word of 5 letters*), insulin has a different action. It increases glucose metabolism or glucose storage as glycogen.

j) Glucagon and adrenaline are some of _____ (*word of 3 letters*) other hormones involved in the close regulation of blood glucose concentrations.

k) _____ (*word of 8 letters*) is a hormone secreted by the pancreatic A cells in reaction to hypoglycemia.

l) _____ (*word of 11 letters*) refers to abnormal blood glucose concentrations.

m) In addition to hyperglycemia, other classic symptoms of uncontrolled diabetes mellitus include polyuria, _____ (*word of 10 letters*), and weight loss.

n) Clients with diabetes mellitus should self- _____ (*word of 7 letters*) their blood glucose concentration to avoid both hyperglycemia and hypoglycemia.

o) Euglycemia refers to _____ (*word of 6 letters*) blood glucose concentration.

p) _____ (*word of 11 letters*) qualifies a condition of impaired glucose tolerance and/or impaired fasting glucose, which increases the risk of developing diabetes mellitus.

q) Clients with type 1 diabetes mellitus lack insulin. It makes them prone to hyperglycemia and

_____ (*word of 12 letters*), the latter resulting from elevated levels of ketone bodies in the blood.

r) The insulin _____ (*word of 10 letters*) seen in clients with type 2 diabetes mellitus refers to insulin being less effective in reducing blood glucose concentration. This can be caused by abnormal insulin cell receptors or the presence of antibodies binding insulin.

s) _____ (*word of 16 letters*) is the presence of a high insulin concentration in the blood. It is a reaction to compensate for a reduced efficiency of insulin.

t) Clients with type 2 diabetes mellitus _____ (*word of 3 letters*) require insulin injections if their pancreas has exhausted the capacity to produce a sufficient amount of insulin.

u) LADA stands for latent _____ (*word of 10 letters*) diabetes in adults.

v) MODY is another term used in the field of diabetes, which stands for _____ (*word of 8 letters*) onset diabetes of the young.

2. What are the diagnostic criteria for diabetes mellitus?

_____

_____

_____

_____

_____

_____

_____

3. What are the diagnostic criteria for prediabetes?

_____

_____

_____

_____

_____

_____

_____

4. What are *acute* complications of diabetes mellitus?

_____

_____

_____

_____

_____

5. What are symptoms associated with hyperglycemia that clients with diabetes mellitus might experience?

_____

_____

_____

6. What are long-term complications of diabetes mellitus?

_____

_____

_____

_____

_____

7. What may cause hyperglycemia in clients with diabetes mellitus?

_____

_____

_____

_____

_____

8. Define hypoglycemia.

_____

_____

_____

9. What are symptoms associated with hypoglycemia that clients with diabetes mellitus might experience?

_____

_____

_____

_____

_____

10. How are mild to moderate hypoglycemic episodes treated in adults?

_____

_____

_____

_____

11. What may cause hypoglycemia in clients with diabetes mellitus?

_____

_____

_____

_____

12. What are blood glucose targets for most adults with diabetes mellitus?

_____

_____

_____

_____

13. Explain briefly how type 1 diabetes mellitus is managed.

_____

_____

_____

_____

14. Explain briefly how type 2 diabetes mellitus is managed.

_____

_____

_____

_____

15. What are the main goals of nutrition care for clients with diabetes mellitus?

_____

_____

_____

_____

_____

_____

16. What are *basic* healthy eating recommendations for clients with diabetes mellitus?

_____

_____

_____

_____

_____

_____

_____

_____

_____

_____

_____

_____

_____

_____

17. Who are certified diabetes educators?

_____

_____

_____

_____

_____

18. What is A_{1C}, and why is it useful to measure its blood concentration?

_____

_____

_____

_____

_____

_____

_____

19. Give the target A_{1C} values used to monitor glycemic control in most adults with diabetes mellitus.

_____

_____

_____

_____

_____

20. Provide the main nutrient recommendations for clients with diabetes mellitus.

_____

_____

_____

_____

_____

_____

_____

_____

_____

_____

_____

_____

_____

_____

_____

_____

21. Provide the recommendations concerning alcohol consumption for clients with diabetes mellitus.

_____

_____

_____

_____

_____

22. What is carbohydrate counting, and why is it useful?

_____

_____

_____

_____

_____

_____

_____

_____

23. Where are the values used for carbohydrate counting found?

_____

_____

_____

24. Give the National Diabetes Association food exchange system used for carbohydrate counting.

Exchange List Food Groups	Size of One Serving or Choice or Exchange	Carbohydrate (g)	Protein (g)	Fat (g)	Energy (kcal) [kJ]
NATIONAL DIABETES ASSOCIATION FOOD EXCHANGE LIST VALUES					

25. What are *available carbohydrates*?

_____

_____

_____

26. Explain the glycemic index of food.

_____

_____

_____

_____

27. Why is the glycemic index of food helpful?

_____

_____

_____

_____

28. What are the target lipid concentrations for most adults with diabetes mellitus?

_____

_____

_____

_____

_____

_____

_____

29. What are the target systolic and diastolic blood pressures for most clients with diabetes mellitus?

_____

_____

_____

30. What instructions should be given to clients in order to ensure that their OGTT is valid?

_____

_____

_____

_____

_____

31. How are the different types of insulin used in the management of diabetes mellitus classified?

_____

_____

_____

32. What types of insulin are used in the management of diabetes mellitus?

_____

_____

_____

_____

_____

_____

_____

33. What types of antihyperglycemic agents are used in the management of type 2 diabetes mellitus?

_____

_____

_____

_____

_____

_____

_____

34. Recent guidelines for the treatment of diabetes mellitus promote the prescription by physicians of the
_____ type of insulin more often because it gives a better postmeal blood glucose
control and is associated with lower risk of hypoglycemia, especially overnight.

35. According to the latest diabetes mellitus screening recommendations, people of _____ years and older should have a fasting plasma glucose test every 3 years, and those at high risk should be tested every year.

   a) 40   b) 45   c) 50   d) 55   e) 60

36. Where is insulin injected?

   a) Immediately under the skin   c) Into the subcutaneous tissue   e) Into a vein
   b) Into the fat layer under the skin   d) Into a skeletal muscle

37. Blood ketone concentration should be tested in clients with diabetes mellitus when they have a prepran-dial blood glucose concentration of _____ mg/dL or _____ mmol/L.

   a) ≤72; ≤4.0   b) >144; >8.0   c) >180; >10.0   d) >200; >11.1   e) >252; >14.0

38. Which of the following is a neurogenic (autonomic) symptom of hypoglycemia?

   a) Nausea   b) Headache   c) Confusion   d) Dizziness   e) Drowsiness

39. Which statement about hypoglycemia is **false**?

   a) Neuroglycopenic symptoms of hypoglycemia are lost over time.
   b) Blood glucose concentration ≤50 mg/dL (≤2.8 mmol/L) denotes severe hypoglycemia.
   c) Symptoms of moderate hypoglycemia include autonomic and neuroglycopenic symptoms.
   d) Speech impairment and visual changes are neuroglycopenic hypoglycemia symptoms.
   e) Mild hypoglycemia symptoms are autonomic-mediated symptoms.

40. What is the treatment of severe hypoglycemia in an unconscious client?

   a) Glucagon injection   b) 20 g carbohydrate in glucose tablets
   c) 15 g carbohydrate in glucose solution   d) Insulin injection
   e) Adrenaline injection

41. For each food, give the related American or Canadian Diabetes Association food group and the size of a serving.

NATIONAL DIABETES ASSOCIATION FOOD GROUPS AND SERVINGS		
Food	Exchange List Food Group	Size of One Serving or Choice or Exchange
Plain, nonfat yogurt		
Lean meat/poultry		
Baked potato		
Green peas		
Egg		
Soy beverage, flavored		
Corn kernels		
Hot cereals		
Unsweetened, ready-to-eat cereals		

NATIONAL DIABETES ASSOCIATION FOOD GROUPS AND SERVINGS   *(continued)*

Food	Exchange List Food Group	Size of One Serving or Choice or Exchange
Apple or pear or orange		
Milk (skim, low-fat, or whole)		
Banana		
Bagel		
Oatmeal granola bar		
Tomato juice		
Margarine or butter or oil		
Sweet potato, mashed		
Nuts or seeds		
Milk pudding, skim, no sugar added		
Regular salad dressing		
Cooked rice (white or brown)		
Grapefruit		
Fresh tomato		
Broccoli/cabbage/cauliflower		
Cooked pasta or barley or couscous		
Celery/cucumber/lettuce		
Sugar, honey, or jelly		
Lemon juice		
Melon		
Beans (pinto, garbanzo, kidney)		
Popcorn, air popped, low-fat		
Strawberries		
Squash		
Chocolate milk		
Soy beverage, plain		
Cheddar cheese		
Slice of bread (white or whole wheat)		
Apple juice		
Peanut butter		

INTEGRATE YOUR LEARNING

1. What is the place of nutrition therapy in diabetes mellitus management?

    _____

    _____

    _____

    _____

2. What is the profile of clients with type 1 diabetes mellitus?

    _____

    _____

    _____

    _____

3. What is the profile of clients with type 2 diabetes mellitus?

    _____

    _____

    _____

    _____

    _____

4. Why is it preferable to say "clients with diabetes mellitus," rather than "diabetic clients"?

    _____

    _____

    _____

    _____

5. Sonia is a pregnant woman with diabetes mellitus. She has been referred to you for nutrition assessment and counseling. What type of diabetes mellitus do you think she might have?

    _____

    _____

    _____

    _____

6. Give six examples of 15 g of easily absorbed carbohydrates that can be used for the treatment of hypoglycemia.

    1- _____

    2- _____

    3- _____

    4- _____

    5- _____

    6- _____

7. Circle the foods with a low (≤55) glycemic index and underline the foods with a medium (56–69) glycemic index.

Oatmeal	Popcorn	Pita bread	Chickpeas	Rice cake
Couscous	Waffles	Corn	Cheerios	Oat bran cereal
Barley	Soda crackers	Muffin	Basmati rice	Converted rice
Pretzels	Lentils	Cake	White bagel	Bran flakes
Pasta	Yam	White bread	Cookies	Whole wheat bread
Rice Krispies	Baked beans	Sweet potato	Pie	Pancakes
Rye bread	Kaiser roll	French fries	Pumpernickel bread	Black bean soup
White potato	Corn Flakes	All bran cereal	Short-grain rice	Chocolate bar

8. The following are symptoms of type 1 diabetes mellitus, <u>except</u>

   a) fatigue   b) weakness   c) unexplained weight loss   d) blurred vision   e) oliguria

9. Which of the following is a diagnostic criterion for diabetes mellitus?

   a) Fasting plasma glucose >108 mg/dL (>6.0 mmol/L)
   b) Symptoms of diabetes mellitus plus a casual plasma glucose >162 mg/dL (>9.0 mmol/L)
   c) Fasting plasma glucose ≥72 mg/dL (≥4.0 mmol/L)
   d) Plasma glucose 2 hours following a 75-g glucose load ≥146 mg/dL (≥8.1 mmol/L)
   e) Symptoms of diabetes mellitus plus a casual plasma glucose ≥200 mg/dL (≥11.1 mmol/L)

10. The main cause of death in people with diabetes mellitus is

   a) hyperosmolar coma   c) heart disease and stroke   e) nephropathy
   b) ketoacidosis   d) pancreatic failure

11. Intolerance to fat and fiber in a client with diabetes mellitus may indicate the presence of

   _____.

12. Which statement about people with type 1 diabetes mellitus is **false**?

   a) Ketoacidosis is the acute complication of hypoglycemia in these people.
   b) They tend to have a normal body weight or to be a little underweight.
   c) They require lifelong insulin injections.
   d) Insulin resistance is not the cause of their diabetes mellitus.
   e) They represent about 10% of people with diabetes mellitus.

13. Which statement about people with type 2 diabetes mellitus is true?

   a) Some of them are on oral antihyperglycemic agent(s) and/or insulin injections.
   b) They tend to have a normal body weight or to be a little overweight.
   c) They usually have reduced hepatic glucose output and glucose resistance.
   d) Most of the individuals are diagnosed before they are 45 years old.
   e) They represent about 60% of people with diabetes mellitus.

14. One diagnostic criterion for diabetes mellitus is fasting plasma glucose levels ≥

   a) 90 mg/dL or 5.0 mmol/L   c) 162 mg/dL or 9.0 mmol/L   e) 234 mg/dL or 13.0 mmol/L
   b) 126 mg/dL or 7.0 mmol/L   d) 198 mg/dL or 11.0 mmol/L

15. Approximately how many grams of carbohydrate are present in 1 cup (8 fluid oz, 237 mL) of milk, according to the National Diabetes Association carbohydrate counting system?

   a) U.S.: 12 (Canada: 15)   c) U.S.: 32 (Canada: 35)   e) U.S.: 52 (Canada: 55)
   b) U.S.: 22 (Canada: 25)   d) U.S.: 42 (Canada: 45)

16. Approximately how many grams of carbohydrate are present in 1 cup (237 mL) of mashed potatoes, according to the National Diabetes Association carbohydrate counting system?

    a) 10   b) 15   c) 20   d) 25   e) 30

17. According to the present guidelines for the dietary management of diabetes mellitus, about _____ % of the energy intake should be from carbohydrates.

    a) U.S.: 50–70 (Canada: 55–60)   c) U.S.: 40–60 (Canada: 45–50)   e) U.S.: 30–35 (Canada: 30–35)
    b) U.S.: 45–65 (Canada: 50–55)   d) U.S.: 35–45 (Canada: 40–45)

18. Which statement about sweeteners is **false**?

    a) Up to 60 g of added fructose per day is acceptable.
    b) Ingesting more than 10 g sugar alcohols per day can result in gastrointestinal side effects.
    c) Those suffering from phenylketonuria should limit their intake of aspartame.
    d) Sucralose loses its sweetness during heating.
    e) Cyclamate and saccharin are not recommended during pregnancy and lactation.

19. What are the serum LDL and HDL cholesterol concentration targets for most adult clients with diabetes mellitus, according to the 2006 American Diabetes Association Clinical Practice Recommendations?

    a) <90 mg/dL (<2.3 mmol/L) and >30 mg/dL (>0.8 mmol/L)
    b) <100 mg/dL (<2.6 mmol/L) and >40 mg/dL (>1.1 mmol/L)
    c) <110 mg/dL (<2.8 mmol/L) and >50 mg/dL (>1.3 mmol/L)
    d) <120 mg/dL (<3.1 mmol/L) and >60 mg/dL (>1.6 mmol/L)
    e) <130 mg/dL (<3.4 mmol/L) and >70 mg/dL (>1.8 mmol/L)

20. What is the target serum total-to-HDL cholesterol ratio for most adult clients with diabetes mellitus, according to the 2003 Canadian Diabetes Association Clinical Practice Guidelines?

    a) <2.5   b) <3.0   c) <3.5   d) <4.0   e) <4.5

21. What is the target blood pressure for clients with diabetes mellitus?

    a) <120/75 mm Hg   b) <130/80 mm Hg   c) <135/85 mm Hg   d) <140/90 mm Hg   e) <145/95 mm Hg

22. Which of the following foods has the lowest glycemic index?

    a) Sweet potato   c) White bread   e) Rice Krispies
    b) White potato   d) Whole wheat bread

23. The recommendation to treat a mild to moderate hypoglycemic episode in a conscious adult with diabetes mellitus is to take _____ g of fast-absorbed carbohydrate and test blood glucose levels _____ minutes later.

    a) 10; 10   b) 15; 15   c) 20; 20   d) 25; 25   e) 30; 30

24. Which outcome marker is a measure of blood glucose control over the past 3 months reflecting long-term control of blood glucose and that can be used to partly evaluate the success of diabetes mellitus care and education? _____

25. These conditions are associated with a high risk of developing diabetes mellitus, except

    a) acanthosis nigricans   d) dermatitis herpetiformis
    b) polycystic ovarian syndrome   e) history of delivery of a macrosomal infant
    c) schizophrenia

26. These are signs and symptoms of diabetic ketoacidosis, except

    a) vomiting   c) abdominal pain   e) ketone breath
    b) dehydration   d) hypoglycemia

27. How much sugar is there in a can (1½ cup, 12 fluid oz, 355 mL) of regular cola pop?

    a) 40 g (8 tsp)   c) 50 g (10 tsp)   e) 60 g (12 tsp)
    b) 45 g (9 tsp)   d) 55 g (11 tsp)

28. Which statement about short-acting insulin is true?

    a) Inject rapid insulin 20 minutes before eating.
    b) Individuals on regular insulin have to eat every 2½ hours during the day.
    c) Regular insulin can be injected right after a meal.
    d) Individuals on rapid insulin are encouraged to have regular daytime snacks.
    e) The injections of rapid insulin should be 2½ to 5 hours apart.

29. Which statement is **false** about the long-acting insulin glargine?

    a) Its peak time is unique to each person.
    b) It is helpful in overweight clients.
    c) It cannot be mixed.
    d) It cannot be injected at the same site as short-acting insulin.
    e) It does not require daytime snacks.

30. These are long-term complications of diabetes mellitus, <u>except</u>

    a) enteropathy   c) cerebrovascular disease   e) retinopathy
    b) neuropathy   d) nephropathy

31. What are the targets for glycemic control for most clients (over age 12) with diabetes mellitus?

    a) Capillary plasma glucose between 90 and 146 mg/dL (5.0 and 8.1 mmol/L) before meals
    b) Capillary plasma glucose <180 mg/dL (10.0 mmol/L) 2 hours after meals
    c) Capillary plasma glucose <98 mg/dL (11.0 mmol/L) before bed
    d) Capillary plasma glucose between 54 and 92 mg/dL (3.0 and 5.1 mmol/L) before meals
    e) Capillary plasma glucose <162 mg/dL (9.0 mmol/L) in the early morning

32. What is the A_{1C} target for most clients with diabetes mellitus?

    a) <5.0%   b) <6.0%   c) <7.0%   d) <8.0%   e) <9.0%

33. What is the A_{1C} target to prevent macrovascular complications of diabetes mellitus and that corresponds to a normal (nondiabetic) A_{1C}?

    a) <5.0%   b) <6.0%   c) <7.0%   d) <8.0%   e) <9.0%

34. What is the blood pressure threshold to initiate antihypertensive drug treatment in clients with diabetes mellitus?

    a) >120/75 mm Hg   c) >135/85 mm Hg   e) >145/95 mm Hg
    b) >130/80 mm Hg   d) >140/90 mm Hg

35. Clients with diabetes mellitus (especially those with type 1 diabetes mellitus) should **not** get

    <_____ g of carbohydrate per kilogram body weight per day, and their carbohydrate needs increase with their level of physical activity.

    a) 2   b) 3   c) 4   d) 6   e) 7

36. What would you recommend for adults with diabetes mellitus to treat a mild to moderate episode of hypoglycemia?

    a) Drink 1 cup (8 fluid oz, 237 mL) Gatorade.
    b) Drink ½ cup (4 fluid oz, 118 mL) milk.
    c) Drink ½ cup (4 fluid oz, 118 mL) orange juice.
    d) Put three glucose gels in the mouth.
    e) Eat a chocolate bar.

37. To prevent dangerous situations from arising when people with diabetes mellitus have a hypoglycemic episode while driving, individuals must have a blood glucose concentration of at least _____ mg/dL or _____ mmol/L to drive.

    a) 72; 4.0   b) 90; 5.0   c) 108; 6.0   d) 126; 7.0   e) 144; 8.0

38. Which sweetener may cause diarrhea and gastric distress, especially in clients taking metformin?

   a) Fructose   b) Xylitol   c) Aspartame   d) Sucralose   e) Saccharin

39. Which sweetener should be avoided during pregnancy?

   a) Fructose   b) Xylitol   c) Aspartame   d) Sucralose   e) Saccharin

40. What type of insulin may justify or require a bedtime snack if it is peaking through the night?

   a) Rapid-acting insulin
   b) Regular-acting insulin
   c) Intermediate-acting insulin
   d) Long-acting insulin
   e) Extended long-acting insulin

41. Which statement about insulin premixes is **false**?

   a) Dietary carbohydrate targets are "locked in" when premixed insulin is used.
   b) Insulin premixes contain intermediate-acting insulin.
   c) Premixed insulin is an easy-to-use and less demanding insulin regimen.
   d) Insulin premixes contain short- or rapid-acting insulin.
   e) Premixed insulin is generally best suited for clients with type 1 diabetes mellitus.

42. Which statement is true about alcohol consumption in clients with diabetes mellitus using insulin or insulin secretagogues?

   a) They should wait 2–3 hours after the evening meal to consume alcohol.
   b) They should eat a fat-containing food when drinking alcohol to prevent hyperglycemia.
   c) Clients on insulin injections should skip their insulin injection when drinking alcohol.
   d) They should limit alcohol consumption to 15% of the energy intake or two drinks per day, whichever is most.
   e) Alcohol can cause a delayed hypoglycemic episode up to 14 hours after its consumption.

43. Which statement about clients with type 1 diabetes mellitus is **false**?

   a) Once insulin treatment is started, a weight gain of about 9 lb (4 kg) within 7–10 days is not unusual.
   b) Insulin needs may drop dramatically anytime within the first 2 years after diagnosis.
   c) At any time in poor metabolic control, they tend to gain weight.
   d) Stress tends to increase their blood glucose levels.
   e) They can manipulate their weight via "purging" by withholding insulin injections.

44. Which statement is **false** about the management of sick days in clients with type 1 diabetes mellitus?

   a) Very low blood glucose levels and dehydration will lead to ketoacidosis.
   b) If water cannot be kept down, they need to get to an emergency room and an intravenous fluid solution will be started.
   c) The insulin needs are increased.
   d) They need to take 10–15 g of carbohydrates per hour in juices, ginger ale, gelatin, and/or popsicles.
   e) They must beware of the increased likelihood of hypoglycemia on recovery due to reduced glycogen stores.

45. Which of the following is a diagnostic criterion for **prediabetes**?

   a) Fasting plasma glucose between 110 and 125 mg/dL (6.1 and 6.9 mmol/L)
   b) Casual plasma glucose >144 mg/dL (>8.0 mmol/L)
   c) Fasting plasma glucose ≥90 mg/dL (≥5.0 mmol/L)
   d) Plasma glucose between 105 and 144 mg/dL (5.8 and 8.0 mmol/L) 2 hours following a 75-g glucose load
   e) Casual plasma glucose ≥128 mg/dL (≥7.1 mmol/L)

46. These conditions are often associated with insulin resistance, <u>except</u>

   a) hypertension
   b) hyperuricemia
   c) polycystic ovarian syndrome
   d) impaired glucose tolerance
   e) type 1 diabetes mellitus

47. Which statement referring to insulin resistance is **false**?

    a) There is increased insulin production and secretion.
    b) There is decreased glucose production by the liver.
    c) The liver is the major organ affected by insulin resistance.
    d) It is associated with defects in several intracellular enzymes responsible for the uptake and metabolism of glucose.
    e) Hyperinsulinemia and hyperglycemia are complications that can lead eventually to type 2 diabetes mellitus.

48. Which statement about clients with type 2 diabetes mellitus is **false**?

    a) There is a correlation between their blood glucose monitoring values and their blood A_{1C} concentration.
    b) They are prone to ketoacidosis.
    c) At diagnosis, the ability of their pancreas to produce insulin is already decreased.
    d) If they fall asleep after meals, it might be a sign of excess energy intake.
    e) If they feel tired, it might be due to elevated blood glucose levels.

49. What is the onset time of rapid insulin?

    a) 1–2 minutes   d) 10–15 minutes
    b) 2–5 minutes   e) 15–30 minutes
    c) 5–10 minutes

50. These population groups are at high risk for developing type 2 diabetes mellitus, <u>except</u>

    a) Asian   d) African
    b) Aboriginal (First Nations, Native)   e) European
    c) Hispanic

51. Which statement about type 2 diabetes mellitus is **false**?

    a) Insulin resistance decreases the action of lipoprotein lipase.
    b) Insulin promotes the conversion of glucose to glycerol, which combines with free fatty acids to form triglycerides.
    c) Clients with type 2 diabetes mellitus and dyslipoproteinemia have up to three times greater risk of myocardial infarction.
    d) Hypertension is a primary risk factor for cardiovascular disease and, in clients with type 2 diabetes mellitus, it increases the likelihood of kidney damage.
    e) Impaired fasting glucose and impaired glucose tolerance are now considered prediabetes.

52. Which statement about type 2 diabetes mellitus is **false**?

    a) Most clients are expected to eventually need a drug treatment and ultimately insulin injections.
    b) If individuals are significantly overweight at diagnosis, they tend to progress faster to needing more medications.
    c) An overweight client who loses weight early in the course of his or her diabetes mellitus may go off medications.
    d) In overweight clients, a weight loss of 5%–10% is recommended at diagnosis.
    e) Dietary messages and medication needs change over time for each client.

53. Which of the following is presently the oral agent of choice for the treatment of overweight or obese clients with type 2 diabetes mellitus?

    a) Thiazolidinedione   d) α-Glucosidase inhibitor
    b) Sulfonylurea   e) Meglitinide
    c) Metformin

54. If a client wants to avoid insulin injections, which drug has relatively low efficacy and is often the last drug added prior to starting insulin?

    a) Insulin sensitizer   d) Metformin
    b) Sulfonylurea   e) α-Glucosidase inhibitor
    c) Meglitinide

55. Which statement is **false** about sulfonylureas?

a) Sulfonylureas are insulin secretagogues that increase insulin production and secretion by the pancreas.
b) Snacks are important for clients on sulfonylureas, especially in the afternoon.
c) Increasing frequency of hypoglycemia may signal the need to decrease dosage.
d) Sulfonylureas are associated with decreased appetite and weight loss.
e) One important diet message with sulfonylureas is that the clients must not skip meals.

56. Which statement is true about biguanide?

a) It is used to treat poor hepatic glucose release and insulin resistance.
b) It is contraindicated in the presence of hypercholesterolemia or hypertriglyceridemia.
c) It is inexpensive and does not cause hypoglycemia.
d) The main side effects are constipation, gas, and bloating.
e) It should not be combined with other oral agents.

57. For which drug treatment should the pill (dosage) be skipped if a meal or snack is missed?

a) Meglitinide   d) Biguanide
b) Sulfonylurea   e) α-Glucosidase inhibitor
c) Thiazolidinedione

58. Which statement is **false** about thiazolidinediones?

a) They increase glucose and fatty acid uptake and metabolism by muscles and adipose tissue.
b) They take 4–6 days to start to work and up to 12 days for full effect.
c) They can be combined with other oral agents and insulin.
d) They do not promote hypoglycemia, but cause weight gain.
e) They are a relatively more recent classification of drugs and are expensive.

59. Which type of eating style is indicated for clients on insulin premixes?

a) Flexible eating style
b) Rigid eating style
c) Eating style with a carbohydrate load limit
d) Very flexible eating style
e) Eating style flexible to a certain limit

60. Which description about clients with type 2 diabetes mellitus is **false**?

a) They may not feel unwell and they are generally overweight and sedentary.
b) Often, if they eat fewer carbohydrates than usual at a meal, they feel less hungry.
c) Significant improvements in blood glucose, lipids, and pressure can occur with modest weight loss.
d) They may have been insulin resistant for years before diagnosis.
e) High circulating insulin promotes overeating of fatty foods.

61. What could explain a normal A_{1C} in a client having poor blood glucose control?

_____

_____

_____

_____

_____

_____

_____

_____

_____

CHALLENGE YOUR LEARNING

CASE STUDY

Objective:

This case will help you recognize that diabetes mellitus is a complex disease and be able to see its impact on all aspects of the life of clients.

It will also help you get a good grasp of the multidisciplinary approach to diabetes mellitus management and realize how each component of the treatment has to be coordinated.

Description

Mr. B.T. is a 42-year-old computer programmer diagnosed with type 2 diabetes mellitus, essential hypertension, and hyperlipidemia. The physician of the endocrinology clinic prescribed lifestyle changes, NPH intermediate-acting insulin at bedtime, metformin, atenolol, simvastatin, and smoking cessation. The physician has referred Mr. B.T. to you for diabetes mellitus education and counseling on a low-fat, low-cholesterol diet, sodium restriction (3 g/day), and weight management.

At the first interview with B.T. this morning, you find out that his mother was from Aboriginal descent and his father was Hispanic. His mother suffered from type 2 diabetes mellitus most of her life and his father had a myocardial infarction. They both passed away in their late 50s. B.T. has two teenage boys under his care.

He currently weights 276 lb and is 6'2" tall. He is sedentary and highly stressed due to a recent divorce, which keeps him awake at night. He smokes a pack of cigarettes a day, and especially at night while watching television. Since his divorce last month, he eats at a popular coffee shop in the morning, skips lunch, and has a big dinner at a fast food restaurant with his sons. He drinks cola throughout the day to stay awake at work, sometimes up to six cans a day, and nibbles on pretzels or peanuts. He says that he is lactose intolerant like his mother and does not consume milk products. He drinks alcohol on social occasions, but says that he does not keep any at home to set a good example for his teenagers. He does not like the taste of water from the tap and does not cook. He says that he has been very thirsty in the last month and has been drinking a lot of soda pop. He gained 20 lb in the last year. He tells you, "I always feel so tired and sleepy, especially after eating dinner, so I have a 2-hour nap around 6 p.m."

His blood pressure was 155/94 mm Hg at diagnosis.

His labs were the following:
Casual blood glucose = 324 mg/dL (18.0 mmol/L)
A_{1C} = 9.1 %
Serum total cholesterol level = 320 mg/dL (8.3 mmol/L)
Serum LDL cholesterol level = 259 mg/dL (6.7 mmol/L)
Serum HDL cholesterol level = 19 mg/dL (0.5 mmol/L)
Serum TG level = 311 mg/dL (3.5 mmol/L)
Serum ApoB levels = 200 mg/dL (2.0 g/L)

1. What is your interpretation of B.T.'s body weight?

2. What is the basis on which B.T. was diagnosed with diabetes mellitus?

3. What is the basis on which B.T. was diagnosed with type 2 diabetes mellitus?

4. What is your interpretation of B.T.'s blood pressure?

5. What is B.T.'s blood pressure target?

6. What is your interpretation of B.T.'s blood lipid profile?

7. What is B.T.'s CHD risk category?

8. What are the target blood lipid concentrations for B.T.?

9. What is your interpretation of B.T.'s A_{1C}?

Case Follow-up

After his diabetes mellitus diagnosis, B.T. started to monitor his capillary blood glucose levels daily, and you notice that his capillary plasma glucose levels are around 153 mg/dL (8.5 mmol/L) before breakfast. He tells you that since he started to take NPH insulin, he feels weak and faint in the middle of the night. He also says, "Some of these pills are giving me diarrhea."

10. Write a SOAP or DAP note for B.T.'s medical record with the information provided. Make sure to include a nutrition diagnosis statement (in PES format [problem—etiology—signs and symptoms]) and a detailed nutrition care plan.

7.7 Gastroesophageal Reflux Disease

REVIEW THE INFORMATION

1. What do the following abbreviations stand for?

   a) GER _____

   b) GERD _____

   c) LES _____

   d) IBW _____

   e) Hx _____

   f) PHx _____

   g) FH _____

   h) meds _____

   i) Pt.Ed. _____

   j) S&S _____

   k) Tx _____

   l) Sgx _____

   m) WNL _____

2. Define these terms.

   a) Dysphagia: _____

   _____

   b) Aspiration: _____

   _____

   c) Reflux aspiration: _____

   _____

   d) Aspiration pneumonia: _____

   _____

e) Mucosa: _____

_____

f) Mucus: _____

_____

3. Draw a sketch of the stomach and adjacent organs from memory in the space below. Then, identify the following anatomic structures on the sketch.

Pylorus of stomach	Lesser omentum	Lesser curvature	Fundus of stomach
Pyloric sphincter	Pyloric orifice	LES	Body of stomach
Cardiac orifice	Greater curvature	Greater omentum	

4. Which endocrine hormone released by the stomach stimulates hydrochloric acid secretion?

_____

5. What diets are indicated for the management of dysphagia?

_____

_____

_____

_____

_____

_____

UNDERSTAND THE CONCEPTS

1. Define the following terminology.

a) GERD: _____

_____

b) Reflux esophagitis: _____

_____

c) Eructation: _____

_____

d) Odynophagia: _____

_____

e) Stricture: _____

_____

f) Ulcer: _____

_____

g) Scar: _____

_____

h) Metaplasia: _____

_____

i) Dysplasia: _____

_____

j) Endoscopy: _____

_____

k) Adenocarcinoma: _____

_____

2. What type of mucosa covers the lower esophagus?

_____

_____

3. What type of mucosa covers the gastric cardia?

_____

_____

4. What type of mucosa covers the fundus and body of the stomach?

_____

_____

5. Explain the difference between GER and GERD.

_____

_____

_____
_____
_____
_____
_____

6. What are the protection and defense mechanisms against GER injury? Explain how/why.

_____
_____
_____
_____
_____
_____
_____
_____
_____

7. What are the signs and symptoms of GERD?

_____
_____
_____
_____
_____
_____
_____
_____
_____

8. Give some complications that can result from GERD.

_____
_____
_____
_____
_____
_____
_____
_____
_____

9. List some of the many etiologic factors and conditions that can contribute to the development of GERD.

_____

_____

_____

_____

_____

_____

_____

_____

_____

_____

10. Indicate the types of treatment available for GERD.

_____

_____

_____

_____

_____

_____

11. Which foods would <u>not</u> be recommended for clients with GERD?

Skim milk	Spaghetti sauce	Broccoli	Chocolate	Low-fat yogurt
Doughnuts	Fried bologna	Mint	Grapefruit	Pear
Breakfast cereals	Wheat bread	Tea	Pasta	Low-fat ice cream
Potatoes	Brownies	Soda pop	Banana	Apple
Black pepper	French fries	Rice	Wieners	Cucumber
Refried beans	Whipped cream	Coffee	Cola pop	Carrot
Low-fat bran muffin	Lentil soup			

INTEGRATE YOUR LEARNING

1. What anatomic structure of the upper alimentary tract is found at the squamocolumnar mucosal junction?

_____

_____

2. Explain the mechanisms by which gastric acid secretion is stimulated.

_____

_____

_____

3. Explain in detail what happens to the esophageal mucosa during the development of **mild to moderate GERD**.

4. Explain in detail what happens to the esophageal mucosa in clients with **prolonged and severe GERD**.

5. What is the purpose of nutrition care for patients suffering from GERD?

6. Describe the dietary and lifestyle recommendations for patients with GERD.

7. What are the types of drugs used for the management of GERD? Why are they used?

8. What is a *gastric fundoplication*?

9. Which food is more likely to be tolerated by a GERD patient with <u>esophageal ulceration</u>?

    a) French fries   b) Coffee   c) Yogurt   d) Orange juice   e) Tomato juice

10. These are appropriate recommendations for patients with GERD, <u>except</u>

    a) have a bedtime snack   d) avoid chocolate
    b) limit carbonated beverages   e) avoid mint
    c) limit cola drinks

11. A client with GERD does not tolerate citrus fruits and their juice. What other dietary sources of ascorbic acid can you recommend he or she consume?

    _____

    _____

    _____

    _____

12. Long-term management of GERD with a proton pump inhibitor, such as omeprazole or lansoprazole, can reduce the absorption of _____, which can result in a reduced status in these micronutrients.

    a) phosphorus and zinc   d) iron and vitamin B_{12}
    b) calcium and potassium   e) folate and magnesium
    c) vitamins C and K

CHALLENGE YOUR LEARNING

CASE STUDY

Objectives

The objectives for this case are to recognize what factors, such as longstanding lifestyle habits, may lead to the development of GERD, and to recognize the different ways to help patients using a respectful and client-centered approach.

As much as health care professionals may know the best treatment to effectively treat clients with cutting-edge technology, one of the most influential ways to start helping clients is by making them feel that you are not judging them and that you will be there to support them.

As a health care provider, you will acquire a lot of useful knowledge pertaining to health, probably work in a fast-paced health care environment, and have the desire to effectively treat people's health problems. As a result, you may sometimes be shocked by clients' ignorance of what seems so obvious to you. Also, many times you may be rushed to get the work done. At times, you might have the impression that you are more important than most with your specialized knowledge and skills. Therefore, you may be tempted to quickly dictate to your clients what to do to fix their health problems before they open their mouths. Do not be surprised if some clients do not follow your directions or do not come back.

If that were to happen, remember that the decision to go ahead with any kind of treatment is that of the client, not of the health care professional. Be as patient, kind, and respectful with patients as you would be with your own parents and loved ones. Listen attentively to what they are expressing, their situation, experience, and feelings (e.g., despair, frustration, anxiety, fears), and you will find the way to understand and help them. Take time to give them explanations and educate them so that they can care for themselves and make the best decisions for themselves. Ask yourself if your clients have learned and retained something from consultations with you, something that significantly helped them in their own life. If you are client centered, you may be surprised that clients who might have been frightened by any sort of changes you were suggesting at first may come back to you asking for help and respect you for your knowledge and skills. If so, you will know that you have truly helped someone and that they will remember you for your kindness, care, and support. You may then humbly and rightfully think about yourself as very important, as you will have gained the trust of others in need.

Description

Mr. B.J. is a 39-year-old Caucasian science-fiction novel writer, who has published a dozen books, many of which have been very well read and translated into other languages. Mr. B.J. is a lonely man with a peculiar lifestyle and schedule. He tells his parents that he does not want a family by choice because of his career, so he can spend most of his time writing novels. Besides, he says, "I can enjoy the many children of my siblings when I feel like it and I still have the freedom to write whenever I want!" Writing is his passion and success. His most successful books have been written in the middle of the night, in his peaceful and quiet bungalow by the lake, when the moon and stars are the only lights to be seen.

When he is working on a book, which is most of the time, Mr. B.J.'s schedule is roughly the same. He wakes up around 11 a.m. and has a coffee with cream while reading the morning newspapers. He gets ready around noon and drives to a nearby restaurant for a brunch-type all-you-can-eat meal. He is usually very hungry by that time and gobbles down two fried eggs and ham, bacon, a croissant with butter, pancakes and sausage with syrup, and a dessert-type pastry, while sipping a few cups of coffee with cream. Back at home a couple hours later, he lies down on his cozy couch to watch television and often falls asleep for the rest of the afternoon.

When he wakes up around 6 or 7 o'clock, he often orders in dinner and slowly gets started on whichever novel he is writing at the time while waiting for his food delivery. One of his favorites is the extra-cheese large pizza with lots of jalapeno peppers. He also likes the spicy fried chicken wings with curried rice or French fries. He drinks cola pop and/or guarana soft drink throughout the night as he writes his novels by the dim glow of the stars, the moon, and his computer screen. When he has good inspiration and writes avidly all night, he often gets cravings for double-fudge-swirl ice cream or mint chocolate. By early morning, he is satisfied with his prolific night and goes quickly to sleep, dreaming about the next part of the extraordinary story he is writing. "It's just like you live in another world!" teases his oldest sister, who has always been looking out for him since he was a child.

Mr. B.J.'s lifestyle has led him to be very sedentary and gain weight regularly since he started to be a professional writer 11 years ago. He is aware of his lifestyle, but he refuses to exercise, claims to be allergic to sunlight, and prefers quiet indoor occupations. He once told his family physician that he does not smoke or drink alcohol, and that therefore, things could be worse. This was 8 years ago and he has not seen a physician since. He is now 238 lb (108.0 kg) and has never attempted to modify his lifestyle habits. When his mother voices her worries to him, he reassures her that he is rarely sick and feels healthy as can be.

Last Sunday, however, he did not feel so well, as he started to suffer from odynophagia. Heartburn and frequent belching disrupted his sleep during the following days. By Wednesday afternoon, he was exhausted and had the drugstore deliver him some Tums, under the caring advice of his oldest sister. He felt better after taking the Tums, so he continued taking them when he suffered from the pain (which was up to 12 times a day), thinking he had just gotten a bad flu. Meanwhile, he went back to his regular writing schedule, intending to finish his latest novel by the deadline fixed with his editor. On Saturday, he was not paying much attention to his heartburn anymore, but after his usual large brunch, he had an acute thoracic pain attack radiating to his neck and back while napping on the couch. He was scared when he saw some blood coming out of his mouth as he was regurgitating and contacted his parents. Over the phone his parents panicked, because they believed he had suffered a heart attack. In no time his oldest sister was at the door to take him to the nearest emergency room. Once there, he was quickly diagnosed with GERD by a resident after an endoscopy of the upper GI tract and kept overnight for observation and some more tests, including barium radiology studies.

1. What is a guarana soft drink?

2. What are Tums, and what is their action?

3. If Mr. B.J. measures 5'8", what is his BMI?

4. What is your interpretation of his BMI?

5. What factors may have contributed to the development of GERD in Mr. B.J.?

6. What tests are performed to diagnose GERD?

7. Why is it important to screen clients diagnosed with GERD, like Mr. B.J., to determine if they are at nutritional risk?

8. What laboratory tests are you going to take a look at for the biochemical assessment of his nutrition status? Why?

Case Follow-up

The next afternoon, Mr. B.J. met with a gastroenterologist, Dr. Jacobson, who told him that he suffers from severe GERD with complications, caused by cardiac sphincter looseness and delayed gastric emptying, secondary to his chronic obesity and lifestyle. The complications he is experiencing from GERD include short-segment Barrett's esophagus with bleeding ulceration and stricture causing slight dysphagia to solids. Dr. Jacobson cautioned Mr. B.J. that his ulcer may perforate and his Barrett's esophagus may worsen if he continues with the same eating and lifestyle pattern and does not lose weight. She gave him a Prilosec prescription to start immediately and asked to see him in 2 weeks to monitor his health status. She also signed a consultation order for a registered dietitian to see him before he leaves the hospital. The referral is for nutrition assessment, GERD diet therapy, and lifestyle changes for weight management.

Meanwhile, the following lab test results came back and were WNL: serum albumin, prealbumin, transferrin, and ferritin concentrations. However, his blood lipid profile showed elevated blood LDL cholesterol levels and TG concentrations.

9. What is a short-segment Barrett's esophagus?

10. What is Prilosec and why did the physician prescribe it to Mr. B.J.?

11. What goals of nutrition care would be appropriate for Mr. B.J.?

12. What dietary and lifestyle recommendations would you suggest to Mr. B.J. in order for him to manage his GERD?

7.8 Peptic Ulcer Disease

REVIEW THE INFORMATION

1. What do the following medical abbreviations stand for?

   a) PUD: _____

   b) LUQ: _____

   c) N&V: _____

   d) AIDS: _____

   e) DAT: _____

   f) Abd: _____

2. What is the term used for the distal half of the stomach?

   _____

3. Which foods may increase gastric acid secretion?

   _____

   _____

   _____

4. Which one of these medications is used to reduce gastric acid secretion?

   a) Omeprazole   c) Metoclopramide   e) Gastrozepine
   b) Calcium carbonate   d) Magnesium hydroxide

5. Define the term *ischemia*.

   _____

   _____

6. What is somatostatin?

   _____

   _____

   _____

UNDERSTAND THE CONCEPTS

1. Associate the following terms with their definition.

   Gastrectomy   Peptic ulcer   Gastropathy   Gastritis
   Gastroscope   Gastroenterologist   Gastroscopy   Gastrorrhaphy
   Gastrology   Gastroplasty   Gastrostomy   Fistula
   Dyspepsia   Gastrotomy   Gastrorrhagia   Gastrorrhea
   Resection   Enterogastric reflex   Hemigastrectomy   Antrectomy
   Anastomosis   Pyloroplasty   Vagotomy   Zollinger-Ellison syndrome

   a) _____ Disease of the stomach

   b) _____ Excess production of gastric exocrine secretions

   c) _____ Surgical cut (or incision) into the stomach

d) _____ Surgical repair of the stomach or lower esophagus using the stomach wall for the reconstruction

e) _____ Surgical removal of the distal half of the stomach, including the pylorus, antrum, and part of the body of the stomach

f) _____ Specialist in the medical study of the function and disorders of the stomach, intestines, and associated organs

g) _____ Impaired digestion of stomach content with epigastric pain caused by disorders affecting gastric function

h) _____ A break in the mucosa of an organ of the alimentary tract exposed to gastric acid and pepsin (gastric juice)

i) _____ Surgical revision of the pylorus to make it leaky by widening of the pyloric canal

j) _____ Surgical connection of two hollow anatomic structures

k) _____ Peristaltic contraction wave produced in the small intestine when food enters the stomach

l) _____ Instrument used to examine the stomach

m) _____ Inflammation of the stomach, especially the mucosa, with leukocyte infiltration

n) _____ Rare syndrome including diarrhea and severe peptic ulceration due to gastric hypersecretion secondary to excessive gastrin release from an endocrine gastric and pancreatic neoplasm

o) _____ Surgical incision of the vagus nerve

p) _____ Surgical excision or removal of part or all of the stomach

q) _____ Formation of an artificial or surgical opening into the stomach

r) _____ Abnormal opening or connection formed between one epithelial surface and another. The artificial passage can be between two organs or two parts of the same organ.

s) _____ Bleeding of the stomach

t) _____ Suture of the stomach after a perforation

u) _____ Branch of medicine studying the stomach, its function, and its diseases

v) _____ Visual observation and examination of the inner surface of the stomach with an endoscope

w) _____ Excision or procedure performed to remove a part, such as an organ or a section of an organ

x) _____ Surgical removal of the antrum and pyloric antrum of the stomach

2. Which anatomic structure(s) is(are) at risk for peptic ulceration?

_____

_____

3. What are the causal agents of peptic ulceration?

_____

_____

_____

_____

_____

4. Which factors or conditions may increase gastric acid secretion?

_____

_____

_____

_____

5. Which factors or conditions may impair the integrity of gastric and duodenal mucosa?

_____

_____

_____

_____

_____

_____

_____

6. Which factors or conditions may reduce blood flow to the gastric and duodenal mucosa?

_____

_____

_____

_____

7. What may trigger pain in patients with PUD?

_____

_____

_____

8. Outline the treatment options for clients with peptic ulcers.

_____

_____

_____

_____

_____

_____

_____

9. What symptoms are usually associated with the following peptic ulcer locations?

   a) Esophagus

   _____

   b) Stomach

   _____

   c) Duodenum

   _____

   d) Jejunum

   _____

10. Outline the main goals of nutrition care for clients with PUD.

   _____

   _____

   _____

   _____

   _____

   _____

   _____

   _____

   _____

   _____

11. What are the usual dietary recommendations for clients with PUD?

   _____

   _____

   _____

   _____

   _____

   _____

   _____

   _____

   _____

   _____

   _____

   _____

12. What are the complications of peptic ulcer disease?

   _____

   _____

   _____

   _____

INTEGRATE YOUR LEARNING

1. What is the difference between gastropathy and gastritis?

_____

_____

_____

_____

_____

_____

2. Explain in detail the process of developing peptic ulcer disease.

_____

_____

_____

_____

_____

_____

_____

_____

_____

_____

_____

_____

_____

_____

_____

_____

3. Indicate whether the following statements are TRUE or FALSE, and justify your answer.

a) _____ *Helicobacter pylori* is the major causal agent in the development of gastric and duodenal ulcers.

  Justification:_____

  _____

b) _____ Individuals infected with *Helicobacter pylori* all develop a gastric and/or duodenal ulcer.

  Justification:_____

  _____

c) _____ *Helicobacter pylori* is a curved or S-shaped bacterium, which is a Gram-positive rod with four to seven flagella at one pole. Acute infection with this bacterium is characterized by sudden onset of epigastric pain, nausea, and vomiting.

  Justification:_____

  _____

d) _____ Many factors may be involved in the pathogenesis of a gastric ulcer. *Helicobacter pylori* infection and NSAID usage are the most frequent conditions resulting in impaired mucosal defense. Ulcers form when damaging factors are not counterbalanced by protective factors.

Justification:_____

_____

e) _____ Chronic active *Helicobacter pylori* gastritis can be asymptomatic or lead to the appearance of peptic ulcers (gastric and/or duodenal), gastric MALT (mucosa-associated lymphoid tissue) lymphoma, environmental metaplastic atrophic gastritis, or gastric carcinoma.

Justification:_____

_____

f) _____ Gastric acid secretion is always increased in clients with gastric ulcers.

Justification:_____

_____

g) _____ Dietary and lifestyle habits have an impact on the incidence of duodenal ulcers.

Justification:_____

_____

4. What is the treatment for a *Helicobacter pylori* infection–induced peptic ulcer?

_____

_____

_____

_____

_____

_____

_____

_____

5. Why may PUD put clients at risk for malnutrition?

_____

_____

_____

_____

_____

6. A connection has been found between _____ bacterial infection and the pathogenesis of peptic ulcer disease, as well as an increased risk of developing of gastric and duodenal cancers.

7. What is the effect of salicylates on the mucosa of the stomach?

_____

_____

8. What surgical procedure(s) may have to be used for the treatment of severe PUD?

_____

_____

_____

_____

_____

_____

_____

_____

_____

_____

CHALLENGE YOUR LEARNING

CASE STUDY

Objective

This case will help you understand how disease progression influences diet therapy. As you will realize with this case, the dietary recommendations appropriate for a client may change significantly over time according to disease progression and management. It is a concept that is sometimes confusing for the clients and that may cause frustration and lack of compliance. Clients may not understand why their dietary recommendations have changed and they may tell you that your recommendations are contradicting previous recommendations from yourself or other dietitian(s). It is therefore important to spend time explaining to clients that monitoring of the disease state is necessary and that adjustments to their dietary recommendations may be required over time.

Description

N.K. is a 23-year-old assertive young woman of Ukrainian descent. She performed exceptionally well in her two first undergraduate university years, applied to law school, and was accepted to a very reputable program. She is now finishing her second year of law school. Next year will be her final year of university and she cannot wait to finally start working as a lawyer. She is doing really well in her program of study so far, but she feels under constant pressure. This year was especially hard and she had a couple of nervous breakdowns. She says that she has to achieve a high academic standing because it is a competitive program. She is determined and pushes herself to maintain outstanding grades to ensure the renewal of her yearly undergraduate financial aid, in order to pay her tuition until the end of the university program.

N.K.'s parents are extremely proud of her, their only child. Unfortunately, they live out of town, 3 hours from the university. They cannot afford to support her financially either. N.K. sees them rarely, but keeps good contact.

N.K. lives in a student residence. She is very independent and takes care of herself. She works on weekends at a clothing store to pay for part of her living expenses.

N.K. and her boyfriend are motivating one another to work really hard to obtain superior grades, which will allow them to apply for national scholarships. Her boyfriend is doing a master's degree in engineering. They hope that later on they will be able to attain key positions in the work force and become successful professionals in their chosen careers.

They call themselves "driven workaholics," as they study until late at night and on weekdays, nibbling on junk food and sipping coffee. To help reduce her anxiety and sleep better, N.K. has developed the habit of taking a couple extra-strength aspirins before bed with a glass of chocolate milk. In the morning, N.K. often wakes up with an upset stomach and only has hot tea. However, she brings some food along and snacks all afternoon while attending course lectures.

On Saturday nights, after working all day, they are out and about in the city bars having fun with their friends. They smoke cigarettes and drink beer until the early morning. N.K. takes extra-strength aspirins to help her deal with the hangover she has on Sundays. By Sunday evening, she is back to her studies, preparing herself for another challenging week.

One week, during the spring final examination period, N.K. started to feel more severe and more frequent episodes of epigastric pain. She was very stressed and afraid that she might not be able to finish her exams or that she would not do well. A close friend convinced her to try the bland diet her mother was following for her chronic heartburn. It did not seem to help N.K.

In the beginning, her gastric pain episodes lasted only a few minutes, but they became worse, lasting hours and causing her to vomit some blood. Although she was trying to hold on and hide her pain, she started to feel so weak and anemic that she phoned her boyfriend and told him what was happening to her. He brought her immediately to the Student Health Services on campus. The physician said to N.K.: "I suspect you may have a peptic ulcer." He gave her a referral to see a gastroenterologist at the university hospital right away for diagnostic studies.

1. What are the signs and symptoms that lead you to believe that N.K. might have a peptic ulcer?

2. Which factor(s) from the case description may have initially contributed to N.K. developing a peptic ulcer?

3. Which factor(s) from the case description could have aggravated N.K.'s peptic ulcer?

4. What are NSAIDs?

5. Give some examples of NSAIDs.

6. Why was the *bland diet* not helpful in the treatment of N.K.'s peptic ulcer?

7. What dietary recommendations would have been more useful to manage N.K.'s peptic ulcer?

8. Are medical history and physical examinations reliable diagnostic tools in order to diagnose a peptic ulcer? Explain why.

9. What diagnostic procedure(s) is(are) required for the diagnosis of a peptic ulcer?

10. What diagnostic procedure(s) is(are) required to determine if there is *Helicobacter pylori* infection?

Case Follow-up

The gastroenterologist diagnosed N.K. with acute *Helicobacter pylori* gastritis with gastrorrhagia and severe peptic ulceration. She was hospitalized and started on a 14-day antibiotic regimen and a prescription of omeprazole. She also received a blood transfusion to help treat her anemia and hypovolemia.

However, to make things worse, N.K.'s peptic ulcer perforated that night and she required emergency surgery the following morning. The gastroenterologist performed a truncal vagotomy with antrectomy, followed by a Billroth I anastomosis procedure. He also noticed that N.K. had mild duodenitis.

Finally, the gastroenterologist ordered the diet progression appropriate for postgastrectomy for N.K. and asked the dietitian to perform a nutrition assessment and some *postgastrectomy diet* counseling.

11. What is a truncal vagotomy?

12. What is a highly selective vagotomy?

13. What is a Billroth I?

14. How is a Billroth I different from a Billroth II?

15. Explain in detail the role of *Helicobacter pylori* in the pathogenesis of peptic duodenal ulcer disease.

16. What diet is recommended in the days following a gastrectomy?

17. Describe the *postgastrectomy diet*.

18. What are the goals of nutrition care postgastrectomy?

19. What are the complications resulting from gastric surgeries?

20. What is dumping syndrome?

21. What are the signs and symptoms of dumping syndrome?

22. What are the main dietary recommendations to help treat dumping syndrome?

23. Why are clients who have had a gastrectomy at risk of impaired iron and calcium status?

7.9 Inflammatory Bowel Disease

REVIEW THE INFORMATION

1. What is inflammatory bowel disease?

_____

_____

2. What are the two main inflammatory bowel diseases?

a) _____

b) _____

3. Where does the majority of digestion of food and absorption of nutrients take place?

a) Esophagus   b) Stomach   c) Small intestine   d) Colon   e) Pancreas

4. Which anatomic structure is located below the pancreas?

a) Stomach   b) Liver   c) Transverse colon   d) Ileum   e) Gallbladder

5. The cecum and ileocecal valve are located in which abdominopelvic quadrant?

a) RLQ   b) LLQ   c) RUQ   d) LUQ   e) None of the above

6. What is the composition of intestinal juice?

_____

_____

_____

7. Beneficial bacteria that colonize in the ileum produce

   a) thiamin   b) riboflavin   c) folate   d) vitamin K_2 e) vitamin B_{12}

8. Highlight the nutrients absorbed in the **duodenum**, underline those absorbed in the <u>jejunum</u>, circle those absorbed in the (ileum), and box those absorbed in the [colon].

Zinc	Calcium	Glucose	Fatty acids	Amino acids	Cobalamin
Magnesium	Folate	Water	Sodium	Iron	Vitamin K
Riboflavin	Galactose	Vitamin A	Cholesterol		

9. Where are bile acids reabsorbed?

   a) Duodenum   b) Jejunum   c) Proximal ileum   d) Distal ileum   e) Colon

10. Secretion of the endocrine gastrointestinal regulatory peptide _____ by the duodenum and jejunum is stimulated by the presence of glucose, amino acids, and fatty acids. It causes a reduction of gastric acid secretion and an increase of insulin release by the pancreas.

11. The ileal brake slows the bowel transit due to the release of _____ from the ileal mucosa.

12. Overall, about _____ of the water present in the gastrointestinal tract is being absorbed by the jejunum and ileum, and about _____ by the colon.

    a) 85%; 13%   b) 65%; 33%   c) 45%; 53%   d) 25%; 73%   e) 5%; 93%

13. About _____ of the water present in the colon is absorbed.

    a) 95%   b) 90%   c) 85%   d) 80%   e) 75%

14. Vitamin B_{12} is absorbed bound to the

    a) gastric-binding protein   d) intrinsic factor
    b) cobalamin complex   e) intestinal brush border–binding protein
    c) pancreatic protease

15. Define the term *ulcer*.

    _____

    _____

16. Define *endoscopy*.

    _____

    _____

17. How much dietary fiber is included in a fiber-restricted diet and a high-fiber diet?

    _____

    _____

    _____

UNDERSTAND THE CONCEPTS

1. In adults, the length of the jejunum is about _____ meter(s) or _____ yard(s).

   a) 1.4; 1.6   b) 2.4; 2.7   c) 3.4; 3.8   d) 4.4; 4.9   e) 5.4; 6.0

2. In adults, the length of the ileum is about _____ meter(s) or _____ yard(s).

   a) 0.6; 0.7   b) 1.6; 1.8   c) 2.6; 2.9   d) 3.6; 4.0   e) 4.6; 5.1

3. In adults, the length of the colon is about _____ cm or _____ inches.

    a) 50–100; 20–39   d) 200–250; 79–98

    b) 100–150; 39–59   e) 250–300; 98–118

    c) 150–200; 59–79

4. How are the jejunum and the ileum differentiated anatomically?

_____

_____

_____

_____

5. Define the following disorders.

    a) Ulcerative colitis

_____

_____

_____

    b) Crohn's disease

_____

_____

_____

    c) Irritable bowel syndrome (IBS)

_____

_____

_____

6. Explain what the following medical terms mean.

    a) Inflammation

_____

_____

    b) Transmural inflammation

_____

_____

    c) Fistula

_____

_____

    d) Toxic megacolon

_____

_____

    e) Proctocolitis

_____

_____

f) Erythema nodosum

_____

_____

g) Pyoderma

_____

_____

h) Pyoderma gangrenosum

_____

_____

i) Cholangitis

_____

_____

j) Sclerosing cholangitis

_____

_____

k) Exsanguinating hemorrhage

_____

_____

l) Aphthous stomatitis

_____

_____

m) Uveitis

_____

_____

n) Hydronephrosis

_____

_____

o) Amyloidosis

_____

_____

p) Colostomy

_____

_____

q) Malignant stricture

_____

_____

r) Peritonitis

_____

_____

s) Tenesmus

_____

_____

t) Colonoscopy

_____

_____

u) Intractable disease

_____

_____

v) Acute disease

_____

_____

w) Chronic disease

_____

_____

7. How does ulcerative colitis present clinically? Give the signs and symptoms.

_____

_____

_____

_____

_____

_____

_____

_____

8. What are the complications of ulcerative colitis?

_____

_____

_____

_____

_____

_____

_____

_____

9. How is ulcerative colitis diagnosed?

10. Which parts of the gastrointestinal tract are more frequently affected in Crohn's disease?

11. How does Crohn's disease present clinically? Give the signs and symptoms.

12. What are the complications of Crohn's disease?

13. What tests assist in the diagnosis of Crohn's disease?

_____

_____

_____

_____

_____

_____

_____

_____

_____

14. Define the following types of fistulas.

a) Enterocutaneous fistula _____

_____

b) Mesenteric fistula _____

_____

c) Enteroenteric fistula _____

_____

d) Enterovesical fistula _____

_____

e) Enterovaginal fistula _____

_____

f) Retroperitoneal fistula _____

_____

15. What can cause a fistula?

_____

_____

_____

16. Give five reasons why a client may have developed a proctocolitis.

a) _____

b) _____

c) _____

d) _____

e) _____

17. In what part of the world is inflammatory bowel disease most prevalent?

_____

_____

18. Which ethno-racial groups have the highest and lowest incidence of inflammatory bowel disease?

_____

_____

_____

19. What is the incidence of ulcerative colitis by sex and age of onset?

_____

_____

20. What is the incidence of Crohn's disease by sex and age of onset?

_____

_____

21. What is the purpose of nutrition therapy for clients with inflammatory bowel disease?

_____

_____

_____

_____

_____

_____

_____

22. What are the dietary recommendations for clients with inflammatory bowel disease?

_____

_____

_____

_____

_____

_____

_____

_____

_____

_____

_____

_____

_____

_____

23. How does irritable bowel syndrome present clinically? Give the signs and symptoms.

_____

_____

_____

_____

_____

_____

_____

_____

_____

INTEGRATE YOUR LEARNING

1. Why are individuals with inflammatory bowel disease at high risk of malnutrition?

_____

_____

_____

_____

_____

_____

_____

_____

_____

_____

2. The intake and absorption of which nutrients are at risk of not being adequate in clients with inflammatory bowel disease? For each nutrient, explain why.

_____

_____

_____

_____

_____

_____

_____

_____

_____

_____

_____

_____

3. Give four main differences between Crohn's disease and ulcerative colitis.

   a) _____

   _____

   b) _____

   _____

   c) _____

   _____

   d) _____

   _____

4. Give four similarities between Crohn's disease and ulcerative colitis.

   a) _____

   _____

   b) _____

   _____

   c) _____

   _____

   d) _____

   _____

5. What are some of the theories used to explain the etiology of inflammatory bowel disease?

   _____

   _____

   _____

   _____

   _____

   _____

   _____

   _____

   _____

   _____

6. What drugs are typically used in the treatment of ulcerative colitis?

   _____

   _____

   _____

_____

_____

_____

_____

_____

_____

7. What drugs are typically used in the treatment of Crohn's disease?

_____

_____

_____

_____

_____

_____

_____

_____

8. What surgical procedures may need to be performed for the management of ulcerative colitis?

_____

_____

_____

_____

9. What surgical procedures may need to be performed for the management of Crohn's disease?

_____

_____

_____

_____

10. When do clients with ulcerative colitis require surgery? List seven indications.

a) _____

b) _____

c) _____

d) _____

e) _____

f) _____

g) _____

11. Comment on postoperative recurrence of Crohn's disease compared with that of ulcerative colitis.

_____

_____

_____

_____

_____

12. Which statement relating to the bowel physiology is **false**?

a) Most of the fluid that passes through the intestine daily is absorbed, except about 3⅓ fluid oz (100 mL).

b) The maximum daily absorptive capacity of the small intestine is 12.7 quarts (12 liters) and that of the colon is 5.3 quarts (5 liters).

c) Bacteria in the colon metabolize insoluble fiber to short-chain fatty acids and gas.

d) Of the 9 quarts (8.5 liters) of fluid that enter the intestine daily, usually about 1.1 quarts (2 liters) are derived from oral intake and the remaining amount is derived from endogenous secretions.

e) Passive permeability in the jejunum is high, which allows rapid adjustment of the luminal osmolality in response to a meal.

CHALLENGE YOUR LEARNING

CASE STUDY

Objectives

This case will help you understand how inflammatory bowel disease impacts the different aspects of life in individuals and how they usually learn to cope with their disease by managing their symptoms.

It will also help you understand how the diet of individuals with inflammatory bowel disease often becomes restrictive and how hard it may be to meet their nutritional needs.

Description

R.G. was a colicky baby, even though she was breastfed. Her mother decided to continue to breastfeed her up to 8 months, because she was accepting very few solids. As a toddler and preschooler, R.G. would fuss and refuse to eat some days for no apparent reason. She grew up to be a beautiful little girl, but she often complained of abdominal pain and cramps. Her parents were trying to help R.G. and identify the reason of her obscure abdominal pain. They figured that she was lactose intolerant like some close relatives. By avoiding milk products, R.G.'s gastrointestinal symptoms seemed to be relieved, so they substituted soy for milk products in her diet. They also gave her a low-fiber diet by limiting whole grain breads and cereals. Although she had no appetite and was rather thin, she was still growing normally. Her parents were Jewish and both were tall and slender.

In her preteen years, R.G. benefited from her thin silhouette and became a promising young ballerina. However, her health seemed to be deteriorating. She started to look fragile and missed many days of school due to intermittent abdominal pain and diarrhea. The family doctor diagnosed her with irritable bowel syndrome and lactose intolerance. He also treated her for iron and vitamin B_{12} deficiency anemia.

In high school, R.G. realized that some of her sporadic diarrhea episodes were triggered by fatty foods or stress during examination periods. However, some other bouts of diarrhea remained unexplained. When she ate some fatty foods with her friends at lunchtime at the school food court, she had to run to the bathroom shortly after. She had painful abdominal cramps, which were partly relieved after a bout of abrupt and intense diarrhea.

R.G. had to stop ballet, which was her favorite activity, because she was too fatigued and developed joint pain. She was very sad as she felt that she could not be with her peers and do what they were able to do. She saw her dream of becoming a professional ballerina crumble and became lonely. Her academic performance plummeted.

The following year, she started to have more frequent episodes of diarrhea, lost even more weight, and felt depressed. R.G.'s situation was progressively worsening month after month. She successively developed red eyes, mouth ulcers, perianal disease, skin rash, and fever. At this point, she had not been eating much of anything for days, restricting her diet for fear of triggering more symptoms. Her daily intake could be summarized as soup and ginger ale, with the occasional plain white pasta or rice. One evening, R.G. complained of unbearable appendicitis-like abdominal pain. R.G.'s parents were extremely worried and took her to see an emergency clinic physician. The physician immediately requested her admission to the hospital, where a gastroenterologist quickly evaluated her status.

1. Do you think R.G. is lactose intolerant? Why?

2. What are some reasons why R.G. may be suffering from lactose intolerance?

3. Why do you think R.G. developed iron and vitamin B$_{12}$ deficiency anemia?

4. Why do you think R.G. was originally diagnosed with irritable bowel syndrome?

5. List other clinical signs and symptoms that R.G. developed during high school.

6. What is your assessment of her clinical condition from the signs and symptoms she had previously and those she developed during high school? Explain why.

7. What diagnostic procedures would you recommend?

8. Justify why you would or would not rule out ulcerative colitis.

9. Was it a good idea to give R.G. a low-fiber diet by limiting her intake of whole grain products when she was a child? Explain your position.

10. Explain the dietary theory used to explain the etiology of inflammatory bowel disease.

11. Analyze the diet R.G. followed in the days prior to admission.

7.10 Diseases of the Liver and Pancreas

REVIEW THE INFORMATION

1. In which abdominopelvic quadrant is the pancreas located?

   a) LLQ   b) LUQ   c) RLQ   d) RUQ   e) None of the above

2. Which vein brings blood full of nutrients from the digestive tract to the liver, before it enters the systemic circulation?

   _____

3. Which organ can regenerate itself?

   a) Stomach   b) Salivary glands   c) Pancreas   d) Liver   e) Small bowel

4. Which organ secretes the enzyme trypsin?

   a) Stomach   b) Pancreas   c) Liver   d) Salivary glands   e) Small bowel

5. These organs secrete digestive enzymes, with the exception of

    a) stomach   b) salivary glands   c) pancreas   d) liver   e) small bowel

6. What organ secretes bile acids?

    a) Stomach   b) Pancreas   c) Liver   d) Salivary glands   e) Small bowel

7. Describe the composition of pancreatic juice.

    _____

    _____

    _____

8. What hormones secreted by the pancreas are involved in blood glucose regulation?

    _____

9. Which endocrine gastrointestinal regulatory peptide stimulates gallbladder contraction and pancreatic secretions in response to peptides, amino acids, and fatty acids in the duodenum and jejunum?

    a) Cholecystokinin   b) Secretin   c) Somatostatin   d) Bombesin   e) Motilin

10. Which endocrine gastrointestinal regulatory peptide stimulates biliary and pancreatic bicarbonate secretion in response to acid in the duodenum?

    a) Cholecystokinin   b) Secretin   c) Somatostatin   d) Bombesin   e) Motilin

11. Which endocrine gastrointestinal regulatory peptide inhibits pancreatic bicarbonate and enzyme secretion?

    a) Cholecystokinin   b) Secretin   c) Somatostatin   d) Bombesin   e) Pancreatic polypeptide

12. Which statement about long-chain triglycerides is **false**?

    a) Most dietary fats are long-chain triglycerides.
    b) Sublingual and gastric lipases start hydrolyzing triglycerides into diglycerides.
    c) Bile salts hydrolyze diglycerides and triglycerides to form fat micelles.
    d) Pancreatic lipase and colipase hydrolyze diglycerides into monoglycerides and free fatty acids.
    e) Intestinal brush border lipase hydrolyzes monoglycerides in glycerol and free fatty acids.

13. What are liver cells called?

    _____

14. Which autosomal recessive congenital metabolic disorder is characterized by progressive decline of lung and pancreas function due to abnormal exocrine body secretions plugging up passageways, such as bronchi, pancreatic and bile ducts, and intestines?

    _____

15. What pancreatic cells are responsible for the secretion of amylase, glucagon, and insulin?

    _____

    _____

    _____

UNDERSTAND THE CONCEPTS

1. What do the following medical terms mean?

    a) Hepatomegaly: _____

    _____

    _____

b) Hepatitis: _____

_____

_____

c) Liver steatosis: _____

_____

_____

d) Cirrhosis: _____

_____

_____

e) Laennec's cirrhosis: _____

_____

_____

f) Bilirubin: _____

_____

_____

g) Jaundice: _____

_____

_____

h) Encephalopathy: _____

_____

_____

i) Wernicke's encephalopathy: _____

_____

_____

j) Lithiasis: _____

_____

_____

k) Cholelithiasis: _____

_____

_____

l) Cholecyst: _____

_____

_____

m) Gallstone: _____

_____

_____

n) Cholelith: _____

_____

_____

o) Cholecystolithiasis: _____

_____

_____

p) Ductus choledochus: _____

_____

_____

q) Choledocholithiasis: _____

_____

_____

r) Cholestasis: _____

_____

_____

s) Cholecystitis: _____

_____

_____

t) Cholecystectomy: _____

_____

_____

u) Hemochromatosis: _____

_____

_____

v) Pancreatitis: _____

_____

_____

w) Pancreatectomy: _____

_____

_____

x) Laparoscopy: _____

_____

_____

y) Laparoscope: _____

_____

_____

z) Lithotomy: _____

_____

_____

aa) Lithotripsy: _____

_____

_____

2. What may trigger the formation of gallstones?

_____

_____

_____

_____

_____

3. What factors and disease conditions are associated with an increased risk for the formation of cholelithiasis?

_____

_____

_____

_____

_____

_____

_____

_____

_____

_____

4. What factors are commonly involved in the pathogenesis of hepatitis?

_____

_____

_____

_____

5. What is the most frequent etiology for chronic liver disease?

_____

6. What are the clinical manifestations of hepatitis?

_____

_____

_____

_____

_____

7. What are the complications of hepatitis?

_____

_____

_____

_____

_____

8. What are the clinical manifestations of cirrhosis?

_____

_____

_____

_____

_____

_____

_____

_____

_____

_____

9. Explain the purpose of nutrition care in liver disease.

_____

_____

_____

_____

_____

10. Why are clients with liver disease at risk of protein-energy malnutrition?

_____

_____

_____

_____

11. What is the best method to determine the energy needs of clients with liver disease?

_____

_____

12. Which biochemical data may help identify the presence of liver disease?

_____

_____

_____

_____

_____

_____

_____

_____

_____

13. What other biochemical measures are useful in assessing the nutritional status of clients with liver disease?

_____

_____

_____

_____

_____

_____

_____

14. How is the liver examined for proper diagnosis when liver disease is suspected from clinical signs and symptoms and biochemical tests?

_____

_____

_____

_____

_____

15. What is the main dietary recommendation postcholecystectomy?

_____

_____

16. How is alcoholic liver disease managed?

_____

_____

_____

_____

17. What diet is recommended for liver disorders such as hepatitis, cirrhosis, and biliary disease?

_____

_____

_____

_____

_____

_____

18. Which clients with liver disease are especially susceptible to fat maldigestion and, therefore, may require a fat-restricted diet?

_____

_____

_____

_____

_____

19. When are fluid and sodium restrictions necessary in clients with liver disease?

_____

_____

_____

_____

_____

20. Which vitamins and minerals may need to be supplemented in clients with liver disease due to a suboptimal status and possible deficiency?

_____

_____

_____

_____

_____

_____

21. _____ is a synthetic nonabsorbable disaccharide used in the treatment of hepatic encephalopathy. It acts as a nonabsorbable fiber and is metabolized to lactate by bacteria in the colon. It acts as a laxative and favors ammonia and nitrogen excretion in the feces.

22. What are the most frequent causes of acute and chronic pancreatitis?

_____

_____

23. Give the signs and symptoms of acute pancreatitis.

24. Describe the most severe complication of acute pancreatitis.

25. What is the medical nutrition therapy for clients with chronic pancreatitis?

26. What is the medical nutrition therapy for clients with acute pancreatitis?

_____

_____

_____

_____

_____

_____

INTEGRATE YOUR LEARNING

1. Recurrent insults followed by repair of the liver tissue can cause fibrosis and scarring known as

   _____, which involves an irreversible distortion of hepatocyte structure, usually occurring after long-term liver dysfunction.

2. What is the effect of long-term alcohol abuse on the liver?

   _____

   _____

3. Describe how hepatic steatosis may progress to cirrhosis.

   _____

   _____

   _____

   _____

   _____

4. Differentiate between hepatitis A, B, C, D, and E.

   _____

   _____

   _____

   _____

   _____

   _____

   _____

   _____

   _____

   _____

   _____

   _____

   _____

5. What is a biliary cirrhosis?

_____

_____

6. Explain how advanced liver disease alters the metabolism of each macronutrient.

   a) Carbohydrate metabolism

   _____

   _____

   b) Lipids

   _____

   _____

   c) Proteins

   _____

   _____

7. How is hepatic encephalopathy treated?

_____

_____

_____

_____

_____

_____

8. What are clinical manifestations of severe alcoholism?

_____

_____

_____

_____

_____

_____

_____

_____

_____

9. What diet therapy is recommended for the management of cystic fibrosis?

_____

_____

_____

_____

10. Fill in each blank space with one appropriate word.

    a) _____ is synthesized by the liver and is the main blood protein. Therefore, blood

    concentration of this protein can be used as a marker of liver *b)* _____ .

    A *c)* _____ in its blood concentration is seen in liver disease. However, it is not a

    sensitive marker as its *d)* _____ is 12 to 18 days. In addition, it is not

    e) _____ , as many other factors can alter its blood concentration, including

    f) _____ , fluid status, inflammation, and pregnancy.

11. These complications are associated with alcoholic cirrhosis, <u>except</u>

    a) impaired glucose tolerance   c) steatorrhea   e) insulin resistance
    b) encephalopathy   d) hyperinsulinemia

12. These conditions are associated with an increased risk of cholelithiasis formation, <u>except</u>

    a) cystic fibrosis   c) rapid weight loss   e) prolonged fasting
    b) menopause   d) ileal resection

13. Which statement related to the nutrition guidelines for liver disease is **false**?

    a) Sodium restriction may be necessary to alleviate fluid retention associated with edema or ascites.
    b) Because resting energy expenditure is variable in liver disease, it is recommended to estimate energy requirements regularly using the modified Harris-Benedict formulas.
    c) The recommended amount of protein intake to ensure nitrogen balance is 0.5–0.7 g/lb (1.2–1.5 g/kg)/day, unless there is severe encephalopathy.
    d) Hyperglycemia is usually controlled with insulin rather than by restricting dietary sugars.
    e) Fat intake is not routinely restricted, unless there is fat malabsorption.

14. Disease-specific nutrition support formulas like Nutrihep and other hepatology formulas are usually lower in

    a) aromatic amino acids   c) energy   e) phosphorus
    b) potassium   d) branched-chain amino acids

15. What are the dietary recommendations for clients with mild chronic cholecystitis with symptomatic gallstones?

    _____

    _____

    _____

    _____

    _____

16. What are the dietary recommendations for clients with acute cholecystitis with symptomatic gallstones awaiting an emergency cholecystectomy by laparoscopy?

    _____

    _____

    _____

    _____

    _____

    _____

CHALLENGE YOUR LEARNING

CASE STUDY

Objectives

This case will help you realize how critical the liver and pancreas are for the normal digestion of foods. It will also help you use critical thinking in the analysis and interpretation of data related to clients with liver and/or pancreatic disease.

Description

F.V. is a 27-year-old Caucasian woman and mother of two preschool children. She consulted her family physician today due to chronic abdominal pain, loose stools, and unintentional weight loss. F.V. says that her abdominal pain was worsened by food intake, which made it hard for her to tolerate food, even her favorite foods. She suspected that she might have had a gastrointestinal infection, so she avoided milk products, because they seemed to trigger more diarrhea. F.V. said that she usually has two servings of milk a day and has no problem digesting it.

F.V. has been suffering from anorexia, nausea, and vomiting for the last 2 weeks. She has had no stamina to take care of her young children. She took the last few days off work due to illness. She realized that her feces were oily and foul smelling, so her husband convinced her to consult her family physician.

When asked by the physician about her alcohol consumption, F.V. replied that she is a social drinker. Although she enjoys going out and having a few alcoholic drinks with her husband or friends, she has not had the opportunity to do it more than once a month on average in the last 5 years. She has shared an occasional bottle of wine with her husband at home when they had company.

F.V. lost 3 lb in the last week and presently weighs 162 lb. She is 5′7″ tall. Her body temperature is only slightly elevated.

Her blood work indicates the following:

Blood ALP concentration:	136 units/L (2.3 μkat/L, i.e., 2.3 microkatal per liter)
Blood AST concentration:	56 units/L (0.93 μkat/L)
Blood ALT concentration:	37 units/L (0.63 μkat/L)
Blood GGT concentration:	27 units/L (0.41 μkat/L)
Blood amylase concentration:	276 units/L (4.70 μkat/L)
Blood lipase concentration:	220 units/L (3.7 μkat/L)
Blood albumin concentration:	3.7 g/dL (37 g/L)
Blood WBC count:	$12 \times 10^3/\mu L$ ($12 \times 10^9/L$)
Fasting serum glucose concentration:	114 mg/dL (6.3 mmol/L)
Fasting blood A_{1C} concentration:	6.3% (0.063)
Serum osmolality:	303 mOsm/kg (303 mmol/kg)
Serum sodium concentration:	133 mEq/L (133 mmol/L)
Fasting serum TG concentration:	53 mg/dL (0.6 mmol/L)

1. What is your interpretation of F.V.'s clinical data?

2. What is your interpretation of her usual BMI?

3. What is your interpretation of her percent weight change?

4. What is your interpretation of F.V.'s blood test results?

5. What disease condition(s) do you think F.V. has, based on the above data? Justify your answer.

6. Does F.V. suffer from viral hepatitis? Why or why not?

7. Is F.V.'s disease condition caused by alcohol abuse? Explain your position.

8. Describe the medical nutrition therapy appropriate to help F.V. manage her disease condition.

Case Follow-up

F.V.'s disease has been fairly well controlled by diet and drug therapy for the past 12 years. However, her chronic disease has progressed and she is now experiencing dehydration, weight loss, and polyuria. Her physician recommends a reassessment of her disease condition.

This is what her blood work is presently showing:

Blood ALP concentration:	129 units/L (2.2 μkat/L)
Blood AST concentration:	49 units/L (0.81 μkat/L)
Blood ALT concentration:	28 units/L (0.48 μkat/L)
Blood GGT concentration:	27 units/L (0.41 μkat/L)
Blood amylase concentration:	24 units/L (0.41 μkat/L)
Blood lipase concentration:	45 units/L (0.8 μkat/L)
Blood albumin concentration:	4.2 g/dL (42 g/L)
Blood WBC count:	$11 \times 10^3/\mu L$ ($11 \times 10^9/L$)
Fasting serum glucose concentration:	324 mg/dL (18.0 mmol/L)
Postprandial serum glucose concentration (2 hours post–75-g glucose load):	508 mg/dL (28.2 mmol/L)
Urine glucose concentration:	955 mg/dL (53 mmol/L)
Fasting blood A_{1C} concentration:	17.4% (0.174)
Serum osmolality:	306 mOsm/kg (306 mmol/kg)
Serum sodium concentration:	138 mEq/L (138 mmol/L)
Fasting serum TG concentration:	107 mg/dL (1.2 mmol/L)

9. What is your interpretation of F.V.'s more recent clinical and biochemical data?

10. What disease condition(s) do you think F.V. now has, based on the new data? Justify your answer.

11. How should F.V. manage her condition at this point?

7.11 Gastrointestinal Surgery and Short Bowel Syndrome

REVIEW THE INFORMATION

1. By what cellular transport mechanism are most nutrients absorbed in the gastrointestinal tract?

   _____

2. By what main cellular transport mechanism is water absorbed in the gastrointestinal tract?

   _____

3. By what cellular transport mechanism is fructose absorbed in the gastrointestinal tract?

   _____

4. Where are the following nutrients absorbed?

   a) Folate: _____

   b) Iron: _____

   c) Magnesium: _____

   d) Fatty acids: _____

   e) Calcium: _____

f) Vitamin B_{12}: _____

g) Amino acids: _____

h) Glucose: _____

i) Short-chain fatty acids produced by bacterial fermentation of unabsorbed carbohydrates:

_____

j) Galactose: _____

k) Cholesterol: _____

l) Vitamin C: _____

m) Water: _____

n) Sodium: _____

o) Potassium: _____

p) Zinc: _____

q) Vitamin D: _____

5. What nutrient is required for the absorption of folate in the small bowel?

_____

6. What are the clinical manifestations of the following micronutrient deficiencies?

a) Zinc: _____

b) Iron: _____

c) Calcium: _____

d) Magnesium: _____

e) Vitamin A: _____

f) Vitamin D: _____

g) Vitamin E: _____

h) Vitamin K: _____

i) Folate: _____

j) Vitamin B_{12}: _____

7. Describe the different fluids entering the gastrointestinal tract on a daily basis.

_____

_____

_____

_____

8. Which organ secretes the enzyme lactase?

a) Stomach   b) Salivary glands   c) Pancreas   d) Liver   e) Small bowel

9. These body structures secrete lipase, except

a) stomach   b) pancreas   c) liver   d) gland under the tongue   e) small bowel

10. Which endocrine gastrointestinal regulatory peptide reduces motility in the ileum in the presence of fatty acids and glucose in the ileum?

a) Peptide YY   b) Secretin   c) Somatostatin   d) Bombesin   e) Motilin

11. Which paracrine gastrointestinal regulatory peptide inhibits gastrin release, gastric acid secretion, and pancreatic enzyme and hormone secretions?

    a) Cholecystokinin   b) Secretin   c) Somatostatin   d) Bombesin   e) Motilin

12. Which statement about the physiology of gastrointestinal regulatory peptides is true?

    a) Vasoactive intestinal polypeptide relaxes sphincters and gut circular muscle.
    b) Gastrin is released by the fundus of the stomach and it increases gastric acid secretion.
    c) Secretin is released in the jejunum and increases gastric acid secretion.
    d) Bombesin decreases gastrin release.
    e) Pancreatic polypeptide increases pancreatic bicarbonate and enzyme secretions.

13. Which statement about the digestion and absorption of vitamin B_{12} is true?

    a) Vitamin B_{12} is absorbed complexed with a gastric-binding protein.
    b) Vitamin B_{12} is absorbed by facilitated diffusion in the jejunum.
    c) Vitamin B_{12} binds to the gastric intrinsic factor in the stomach.
    d) Vitamin B_{12} is absorbed at the distal ileum complexed with the intrinsic factor.
    e) Vitamin B_{12} is absorbed in the duodenum by active transport.

14. The following are consequences of a standard truncal vagotomy, <u>except</u>

    a) there is an increase in relaxation of the pylorus
    b) there is less antral contraction and no neural stimulation of gastric acid secretion
    c) there is no vagal stimulation of pancreas and gallbladder
    d) there is no vagal stimulation of small intestine
    e) there is delayed emptying of solids

15. Which statement about the antrectomy procedure is **false**?

    a) There is rapid emptying of liquids.
    b) There is resection of the antrum of the stomach.
    c) There is delayed emptying of solids after eating.
    d) It is usually performed with a standard truncal vagatomy procedure.
    e) In Billroth I, the gastric remnant is anastomosed to the duodenum.

16. The absorption of which nutrients is especially reduced after gastric surgery?

    a) Zinc, thiamin, magnesium, vitamin K   d) Vitamin C, zinc, cholesterol, fat
    b) Iron, vitamin B_{12}, folate, calcium   e) Vitamin D, vitamin K, folate, zinc
    c) Magnesium, vitamin D, vitamin B_{12}

17. These symptoms characterize the dumping syndrome, <u>except</u>

    a) diaphoresis   b) hyperglycemia   c) diarrhea   d) abdominal pain   e) nausea

18. Define the following medical terms.

    a) Stoma: _____

    _____

    b) Stomy: _____

    _____

    c) Ostomy: _____

    _____

    d) Gastrostomy: _____

    _____

    e) Enterostomy: _____

    _____

    f) Duodenostomy: _____

_____

    g) Jejunostomy: _____

_____

    h) Ileostomy: _____

_____

    i) Colostomy: _____

_____

19. Candidates considering bariatric surgery as a weight loss option should be carefully screened and usually must have a BMI over _____ with comorbid condition(s) or over _____ in the absence of comorbid conditions to be eligible.

    a) 30.0; 25.0   b) 35.0; 30.0   c) 40.0; 35.0   d) 45.0; 40.0   e) 50.0; 45.0

UNDERSTAND THE CONCEPTS

1. What is short bowel syndrome?

_____

_____

_____

2. List five determinants of the capacity for fluid absorption in the intestine.

    a) _____

    b) _____

    c) _____

    d) _____

    e) _____

3. Who are ostomates?

_____

_____

4. Compare the permeability to water and electrolytes of the different parts of the intestine.

_____

_____

_____

_____

5. Describe the structural and functional adaptations that usually occur after intestinal resection.

_____

_____

_____

_____
_____

6. What underlying conditions may lead to short bowel syndrome?

_____
_____
_____
_____

7. Which factors (such as nutrients, hormones, etc.) are taught to stimulate <u>or</u> inhibit intestinal adaptation after resection?

_____
_____
_____
_____

8. What may cause maldigestion and malabsorption in an individual with small bowel syndrome?

_____
_____
_____
_____

9. Give five main clinical consequences of short bowel syndrome.

a) _____

b) _____

c) _____

d) _____

e) _____

10. Diarrhea causes increased _____ losses in the stool, and in those with a short bowel and high fecal outputs, _____ deficiency may also contribute to diarrhea, creating a vicious circle.

a) magnesium, magnesium   d) zinc, zinc
b) iron, iron   e) calcium, calcium
c) selenium, selenium

11. The following are clinical manifestations of vitamin B_{12} deficiency, <u>with the exception of</u>

a) ataxia   b) diarrhea   c) anemia   d) paresthesias   e) alopecia

12. The large bowel absorbs about _____ kcal (_____ kJ)/day through the carbohydrate salvage pathway.

a) 250; 1050   b) 500; 2090   c) 750; 3140   d) 1000; 4180   e) 1250; 5230

13. The absorption of which components would be compromised after resection of the terminal ileum?

    a) Riboflavin, cholesterol, and short-chain fatty acids
    b) Vitamin B_{12}, vitamin K, and bile salts
    c) Soluble fibers, fatty acids, and vitamins A, D and E
    d) Pyridoxine, cholesterol, and bile acids
    e) Fatty acids, cholesterol, and liposoluble vitamins.

14. There are a number of adaptive structural changes occurring in the remaining intestine following

resection, including _____, which is an increase in the number of absorptive epithelial cells. The presence of nutrients in the intestinal lumen stimulates this process of adaptation.

15. _____ refers to the process by which carbohydrates not absorbed in the small intestine are fermented by bacteria in the colon, resulting in the production of short-chain fatty acids, which are then absorbed by the colon.

16. In cases of a) _____ resection of >39 inches (100 cm), foods high in b) _____ such as rhubarb, spinach, strawberries, chocolate, and tea should be avoided, because the presence of fat and bile salts in the colon increases the absorption of this substance from food and results in high levels in the blood and urine, increasing the risk of renal stones.

17. Why are ostomies created?

_____

_____

_____

18. Give common reasons why clients may require an ileostomy or colostomy placement.

_____

_____

_____

_____

_____

19. What are the goals of medical nutrition therapy for clients with an ileostomy or colostomy?

_____

_____

_____

_____

_____

_____

_____

_____

20. Provide dietary recommendations appropriate for clients to follow in the weeks after the creation by surgery of their ileostomy or colostomy.

_____

_____

_____

_____

_____

_____

_____

_____

_____

_____

_____

_____

_____

21. Give examples of foods to avoid in the first couple of months after the creation of an ileostomy (especially) or colostomy, as these foods are incompletely digested and increase the risk of stoma obstruction.

a) _____

b) _____

c) _____

d) _____

e) _____

f) _____

g) _____

h) _____

i) _____

j) _____

k) _____

l) _____

m) _____

n) _____

o) _____

p) _____

q) _____

r) _____

s) _____

t) _____

22. Give examples of foods to limit, at least in the first couple of months after the creation of an ileostomy or colostomy, as they may contribute to fast intestinal transit and diarrhea.

a) _____

b) _____

c) _____

d) _____

e) _____

f) _____

g) _____

h) _____

i) _____

j) _____

k) _____

l) _____

m) _____

n) _____

o) _____

23. Give examples of foods that may cause gas in clients with an ileostomy or colostomy.

a) _____

b) _____

c) _____

d) _____

e) _____

f) _____

g) _____

h) _____

i) _____

j) _____

k) _____

l) _____

m) _____

n) _____

o) _____

p) _____

q) _____

r) _____

s) _____

t) _____

24. Give examples of foods that may cause odors in clients with an ileostomy or colostomy.

a) _____

b) _____

c) _____

d) _____

e) _____

f) _____

g) _____

h) _____

i) _____

j) _____

25. Give examples of foods that may help to slow intestinal transit time and control diarrhea in clients with an ileostomy or colostomy.

a) _____

b) _____

c) _____

d) _____

e) _____

f) _____

g) _____

h) _____

i) _____

j) _____

k) _____

l) _____

26. Give examples of foods that may help ostomates control gas and odors.

_____

_____

27. Octreotide is a long-lasting analog of the gastrointestinal regulatory peptide called _____. It inhibits all gastrointestinal secretions and at high doses slows small bowel transit.

28. Give five factors affecting the severity of short bowel syndrome.

a) _____

b) _____

c) _____

d) _____

e) _____

29. Explain how the rest of the intestine adapts after the following resections and comment on the ability of the remaining intestine to absorb nutrients.

a) Partial jejunectomy

_____

_____

_____

_____

_____

b) Partial ileectomy with preserved ileocecal valve

_____

_____

_____

_____

_____

c) Total ileectomy with resection of the ileocecal valve

_____

_____

_____

_____

_____

_____

d) Extensive jejunoileectomy with total colectomy

_____

_____

_____

_____

_____

_____

30. Nonhealing skin ulcers are sometimes linked to _____ deficiency.

   a) folate   b) vitamin C   c) vitamin K   d) vitamin A   e) magnesium

31. Intestinal adaptation after bowel resection is stimulated by many factors, <u>except</u>

   a) soluble fibers   b) short-chain fatty acids   c) glutamine   d) nucleotides   e) somatostatin

32. _____ of enterocutaneous fistulas arise after surgical procedure.

   a) 30%   b) 45%   c) 60%   d) 75%   e) 90%

33. The mortality rate in high-output, postoperative enterocutaneous fistulas is _____.

   a) 13%   b) 21%   c) 37%   d) 49%   e) 61%

34. High-output fistulas produce over _____ of output per 24 hour.

   a) 200 mL (6⅔ fluid oz)   c) 600 mL (20 fluid oz)   e) 1000 mL (33⅓ fluid oz)
   b) 400 mL (13⅓ fluid oz)   d) 800 mL (26⅔ fluid oz)

35. A lysis of _____ must sometimes be performed to remove the excessive scar tissue formed after a surgery.

36. Give five factors that are important to consider when choosing the type of nutrition support for a patient with a fistula.

   a) _____

   b) _____

   c) _____

d) _____

e) _____

37. What are current surgical options to help manage morbid obesity? Describe each option.

_____

_____

_____

_____

_____

_____

_____

_____

_____

_____

_____

_____

_____

INTEGRATE YOUR LEARNING

1. The most frequent underlying condition leading to the small bowel syndrome is

   a) radiation therapy   c) strangulated bowel   e) Crohn's disease
   b) ulcerative colitis   d) bowel ischemia

2. Draw how the intestinal villi look in these four situations:

   a) Intestinal villi of a well-nourished individual

   b) Intestinal villi of a chronically, severely malnourished individual

c) Gut atrophy during prolonged TPN without enteral stimulation

d) Villi hyperplasia after intestinal resection, followed by stimulation by some oral intake

3. Provide the appropriate medical term corresponding to each definition.

Paresthesia   Stomatitis   Cheilosis   Necrotizing enterocolitis
Glossitis   Tetany   Cheilitis   Polyp
Aerophagia   Volvulus   Ataxia   Atresia
Ileus

a) Excessive swallowing of air _____

b) The absence of a normal luminal opening at birth _____

c) An intestinal intertwine or twist that can obstruct intestinal transit and blood flow _____

d) Considerable ulceration of the ileocolon with necrosis in some infants born prematurely

   _____

e) Intermittent muscle spasm and cramps _____

f) Aberrant or abnormal tactile sensation _____

g) A mass of tissue bulging from a normal body surface or structure _____

h) Lack of coordination of muscle contraction resulting in ineffective voluntary movements

   _____

i) An inflammation of the mouth _____

j) An inflammation of the tongue _____

k) An inflammation of the lip(s) _____

l) Dry, fissuring lips and corners of the mouth due to riboflavin deficiency _____

m) Lack of intestinal peristalsis with abdominal cramps _____

4. What are the long-term complications of the short bowel syndrome?

   _____

   _____

   _____

_____
_____
_____
_____
_____
_____
_____
_____
_____
_____
_____
_____

5. These descriptions are in agreement with the dietary recommendations for clients with an ostomy, <u>except</u>

   a) foods should be chewed well
   b) addition of foods high in water-soluble fiber may help to reduce fluid losses
   c) serve small portions of well-cooked foods at regular intervals
   d) progression to a well-balanced, regular diet is usually achieved by 5 days postsurgery
   e) concentrated fruit juices may need to be diluted to prevent osmotic diarrhea

6. Which statement about the dietary recommendations for patients with ostomy is **false**?

   a) Foods that may cause gas include cucumber and celery.
   b) Foods that may produce odor include eggs, fish, asparagus, and turnips.
   c) Foods that may help to control diarrhea include bananas, applesauce, potatoes, and cheese.
   d) Foods that may help control odor or gas include buttermilk and fresh parsley.
   e) Foods that may contribute to diarrhea include licorice, high-sugar foods, alcohol, cabbage, and broccoli.

7. What nutritional problems may be seen in clients with ileostomy following extensive ileal resection?

_____
_____
_____
_____
_____
_____
_____
_____
_____
_____
_____
_____
_____
_____
_____

8. Determine if the following characteristics are usually present (YES) or not (NO) for each type of intestinal resection.

CHARACTERISTICS OF THE REMAINING INTESTINE AFTER INTESTINAL RESECTION		
Characteristics of the Remaining Intestine	Jejunal Resection (More than one-quarter jejunum remaining)	Extensive Distal Ileal Resection, Ileocecal Valve Preserved (>39 Inches or >100 cm of Terminal Ileum Excised)
Adequate energy absorption		
Adequate fluid absorption		
Malabsorption of bile acids		
Good adaptation of remaining bowel		
Normal intestinal transit time		
Fat malabsorption		
Possible calcium malabsorption		
Possible lactose malabsorption		
Malabsorption of vitamin B_{12}		
Possible folate malabsorption		
Overall good prognosis		

9. Which statement about the short bowel syndrome is **false**?

a) Hypersecretion of gastric acid occurs early after intestinal resection and may persist.
b) Acid in the intestinal lumen impairs digestion by denaturing pancreatic enzymes.
c) Unabsorbed fatty acids in the intestinal lumen may bind calcium and impair its absorption.
d) Bacterial overgrowth in the small intestine is usually due to the loss of the pyloric sphincter.
e) Bile salts can be deconjugated by bacteria present in the small intestine.

10. Following jejunal resection, adaptation of the remaining ileum is _____ and nutrient

absorption is _____ .

a) poor; poor   c) fair; the same as before   e) nonexistent; very poor
b) good; good   d) excellent; increased

11. Which statement is **false** about bowel resection?

a) Intestinal adaptation after resection is low in elderly patients
b) In patients with a colon, a higher percent of kilocalories (kilojoules) are absorbed from a high-fat diet than from a high-carbohydrate diet.
c) The most frequent underlying condition responsible for bowel resection is Crohn's disease.
d) Loss of the colon results in rapid gastric emptying.
e) Acid hypersecretion may cause intestinal fluid losses, diarrhea, and peptic ulcer disease.

12. Can constipation be an issue for ostomates with an end-colostomy? If so, give the dietary recommendations to help treat it.

_____

_____

_____

_____

_____

_____

13. Why is assessment and behavioral counseling by a multidisciplinary health care team required before <u>and</u> after bariatric surgery?

_____

_____

_____

_____

_____

_____

_____

_____

_____

_____

_____

_____

_____

_____

CHALLENGE YOUR LEARNING

CASE STUDY

Objectives

This case will help you reconsider the anatomy and physiology of the gastrointestinal tract and understand how surgical modifications to its anatomy will impair the normal physiology of digestion of food and absorption of nutrients. It will also help you recognize that clients who have undergone extensive gastrointestinal resection are at high risk of malnutrition, and foresee that they will require long-term nutrition support and monitoring.

Description

N.D. is a frail, 6′ tall, 53-year-old man who looks much older than his age. He had been battling Crohn's disease most of his life and was diagnosed with ileal cancer 6 months ago. He developed an enteroenteral fistula and required emergency surgery, during which 35.4 inches (90 cm) of his distal ileum was excised. His ileocecal valve was spared, but he was in septic shock for days due to contamination of his peritoneal cavity with intestinal content leaking from the fistula site. Following the surgery, he continued taking antibiotics and was given antimotility agents. In addition, he received both radiation therapy and chemotherapy. He lost 30 lb from his already lean body. N.D.'s usual body weight was only 140 lb and he has a medium bone frame.

1. What is your interpretation of N.D.'s UBW?

2. What is N.D.'s ideal body weight range?

3. What was N.D.'s usual BMI? Give your interpretation.

4. What is your interpretation of N.D.'s body weight change in the last 6 months?

5. What is your interpretation of N.D.'s percent UBW?

6. What is an enteroenteral fistula?

7. What is septic shock?

8. How would you have fed N.D. presurgery <u>and</u> postsurgery?

9. What is the long-term prognosis for N.D. after resection of about 35.4 inches (90 cm) of his distal ileum?

10. What nutritional problems is N.D. at risk of encountering following this partial distal ileal resection?

Case Follow-up

Eight months after the end of his cancer treatment, N.D.'s Crohn's disease was under control, but he developed profuse diarrhea due to acute radiation enteritis. The surgeons had to remove the rest of his ileum and anastomose his jejunum to his ascending colon. He took octreotide to help reduce his fast intestinal transit. However, he developed chronic fat malabsorption, and later on, urolithiasis and osteoporosis. Elevated concentrations of oxalate were found in his urine.

11. Define urolithiasis.

12. Explain why clients like N.D. are at risk of developing urolithiasis.

13. What complications may result from the absence of an ileocecal valve?

14. What are the long-term dietary recommendations for N.D. following his extensive intestinal resection?

15. Prepare an education handout for N.D. including a list of foods high in oxalate (more than 10 mg oxalate per serving of ½ cup or 118 mL) for him to avoid.

16. Explain why clients with a short bowel and colon may benefit from the carbohydrate salvage pathway.

Case Follow-up

Three years later, N.D. presented at the emergency department with an acute abdomen. They discovered that his colon was necrotic and had to be removed immediately. There was bacterial translocation into his peritoneal cavity. He had a subtotal colectomy and jejunosigmoid anastomosis.

17. What is intestinal bacterial translocation?

18. Should N.D. continue to follow a low-oxalate diet? Why or why not?

19. What dietary recommendations would you give N.D. now that he has lost his colon and has a short bowel?

7.12 Wasting Disorders

REVIEW THE INFORMATION

1. Define wasting.

_____

_____

2. Give some examples of wasting disorders.

_____

_____

3. Where do the following blood constituents originate?

a) Erythrocytes: _____

b) White blood cells: _____

c) Platelets: _____

d) Albumin: _____

e) Transferrin: _____

f) Prealbumin: _____

4. How long is the average life of an erythrocyte?

a) 60 days　　b) 80 days　　c) 100 days　　d) 120 days　　e) 140 days

5. Distinguish between leukocytes, granulocytes, monocytes, lymphocytes, macrophages, T cells, and immunoglobulins.

_____

_____

_____

_____

_____

_____

_____

_____

_____

_____

_____

_____

_____

_____

_____

_____

_____

_____

_____

_____

_____

_____

_____

_____

_____

_____

_____

_____

_____

6. Normal body temperature is about _____ °C or _____ °F.

    a) 34.0; 93.2   b) 35.0; 95.0   c) 36.0; 96.8   d) 37.0; 98.6   e) 38.0; 100.4

7. A person is considered to be running a fever when body temperature measured orally is over _____ °C _____ °F.

    a) 35.7; 96.3   b) 36.7; 98.1   c) 37.7; 99.9   d) 38.7; 101.7   e) 39.7; 103.5

8. Use this grid to help you find the appropriate medical terms defined below that relate to wasting disorders.

Terms Related to Wasting Disorders

a) A _____ (*word of 6 letters*) is a malignant tumor. It is an abnormal and uncontrolled proliferation of cells that has the potential to expand and invade tissues.

b) _____ (*word of 8 letters*) is the knowledge and science related to cancer and its management.

c) An _____ (*word of 10 letters*) is a physician specialized in cancer management.

d) A _____ (*word of 10 letters*) is a substance that can produce cancer.

e) A _____ (*word of 5 letters*) is an abnormal cell proliferation, which can be cancerous or noncancerous.

f) A _____ (*word of 10 letters*) is the spread of cancer cells from an initial site (primary site) to another part of the body (secondary site) by direct extension or through blood or lymph.

g) An _____ (*word of 11 letters*) is a substance that scavenges free radicals and thereby protects tissue from the damage they would cause.

h) _____ (*word of 6 letters*) means vomiting.

i) Aphthous _____ (*word of 10 letters*) is an inflammation of the mouth with painful ulcers or canker sores.

j) _____ (*word of 9 letters*) refers to the inflammation of a mucous membrane.

k) _____ (*word of 9 letters*) is the impairment or dysfunction of the sense of taste.

l) _____ (*word of 10 letters*) is a decreased perception of taste.

m) _____ (*word of 10 letters*) means dry mouth and is caused by a lack of salivary secretion.

n) _____ (*word of 6 letters*) is a state of low blood erythrocyte count or low blood hemoglobin concentration, with clinical signs of pallor, weakness, and shortness of breath.

o) _____ (*word of 9 letters*) is inflammation of the bowel, the small bowel in particular.

p) A _____ (*word of 7 letters*) is an abnormal connection or passage between two epithelial surfaces.

q) _____ (*word of 9 letters*) is a problem with chewing and/or swallowing.

r) _____ (*word of 6 letters*) refers to matter expectorated from an infected respiratory system, such as mucus and pus.

s) _____ (*word of 6 letters*) is abundant mucus expectorated from the respiratory passages.

t) _____ (*word of 7 letters*) means difficult or laborious breathing, causing shortness of breath.

u) _____ (*word of 10 letters*) care is therapy meant to help reduce the severity of the symptoms of a disease, not cure the disease.

v) _____ (*word of 9 letters*) qualifies a severe, invasive, and destructive condition, which may be fatal.

w) Cell _____ (*word of 13 letters*) is the rapid reproduction of cells.

x) Cell _____ (*word of 15 letters*) is the maturation of cells, through which cells acquire their specialized function.

y) Lymph _____ (*word of 5 letters*) are small, round, glandular structures found along lymphatic vessels, which filtrate lymph.

z) _____ (*word of 7 letters*) prevention focuses on the avoidance of disease before it develops by promoting healthy lifestyle, which reduces the risk of disease.

aa) _____ (*word of 9 letters*) prevention focuses on the screening, recognition, and early management of disease before complications from the disease appear.

bb) A _____ (*word of 9 letters*) is the likely outcome of a disease or the probable chance of a recovery.

cc) _____ (*word of 6 letters*) qualifies a mild or nonmalignant disease condition.

dd) _____ (*word of 8 letters*) is the death of some cells or tissue.

ee) _____ (*word of 6 letters*) is the feeling that one is going to vomit.

ff) _____ (*word of 8 letters*) is the condition of having frequent, liquid or semiliquid bowel movements.

gg) Chemo-_____ (*word of 7 letters*) is treatment of disease (e.g., cancer, mental disorders) using chemical agents.

hh) _____ (*word of 5 letters*) -therapy is the use of high-energy rays (e.g., x-rays) in disease management.

9. Cancer is the _____ most frequent cause of death in North America.

   a) first   b) second   c) third   d) fourth   e) fifth

10. In North America, about _____ of women and nearly _____ of men will develop some sort of cancer during their life.

   a) half; a third   b) a third; half   c) a third; a quarter   d) a quarter; a third   e) one fifth; a quarter

11. What do the abbreviations AIDS and HIV stand for?

   _____

   _____

12. More than _____ million people have already died from AIDS worldwide.

   a) 2   b) 5   c) 10   d) 15   e) 20

13. How is HIV transmitted?

   _____

   _____

   _____

   _____

UNDERSTAND THE CONCEPTS

1. Explain the meaning of these medical terms related to cancer.

   a) Neoplasm: _____

   _____

   b) Antineoplastic agent: _____

   _____

   c) Malignant tumor: _____

   _____

   d) Benign tumor: _____

   _____

   e) Oncogene: _____

   _____

f) Ageusia: _____

_____

g) Trismus: _____

_____

h) Febrile: _____

_____

i) Afebrile: _____

_____

j) Pharmacotherapy: _____

_____

k) Phytochemical: _____

_____

l) Staging: _____

_____

m) Remission: _____

_____

n) Stem cells: _____

_____

2. Select in the list below the appropriate medical term corresponding to each definition.

lymphoma	neutropenia	adenocarcinoma	leukocytosis
carcinoma	leukopenia	thrombocytosis	myeloma
leukemia	erythropoiesis	hematopoiesis	sarcoma

a) A/an _____ is a malignant tumor that originates from epithelial cells.

b) A/an _____ is a malignant tumor that originates from glandular tissue.

c) A/an _____ is a malignant tumor that originates from connective tissue (e.g., cartilage) or supportive tissue (e.g., muscle, bone).

d) A/an _____ is a malignant tumor that originates from lymphoid tissue.

e) _____ is a cancer that originates from the blood-forming organs and causes proliferation of abnormal white blood cells.

f) _____ is a malignant tumor that originates from bone marrow.

g) _____ is the generation of blood cells.

h) _____ is the production of red blood cells.

i) _____ is a condition of reduced white blood cells in blood.

j) _____ is a condition of reduced number of mature white blood cells in blood.

k) _____ is a condition of increased blood leukocyte count.

l) _____ is a condition of increased blood platelet count.

3. What do the following abbreviations related to cancer and AIDS stand for?

a) CA: _____

b) Mets: _____

c) TNM: _____

d) IFN-γ: _____

e) IL: _____

f) TNF-α: _____

g) IGF: _____

h) SOB: _____

i) COPD: _____

j) ELISA: _____

k) HAART: _____

l) CMV: _____

m) HIVAN: _____

n) MAC: _____

4. How does cancer develop?

_____

_____

_____

_____

_____

_____

_____

_____

_____

_____

5. Give examples of some common cancer-causing chemical carcinogens, including occupational carcinogens, lifestyle carcinogens, and drug carcinogens.

a) Occupational carcinogens

_____

_____

b) Lifestyle carcinogens

_____

_____

c) Drug carcinogens

_____

_____

6. Which of the following types of cancer has the highest incidence in North America?

a) Colorectal cancer   b) Liver cancer   c) Pancreatic cancer   d) Stomach cancer   e) Breast cancer

7. What are the most prevalent types of cancers in developed/affluent areas, compared to underdeveloped areas of the world?

_____

_____

_____

_____

8. Fill in each blank space with the appropriate word. A cancer is named after the body part from where it

a) _____. The type of cells of the tissue of b) _____

determines the type of cancer and the therapy. Breast cancer and lung cancer are c) _____

tumors, whereas leukemia and lymphoma are d) _____ tumors. The therapy

depends on the type of cancer and the e) _____ of the cancer.

9. In the TNM cancer classification system, what would "$T_1 N_0 Mx$" stand for?

T_1 _____

N_0 _____

Mx _____

10. What therapies are used in cancer care?

_____

_____

_____

11. Explain the role of medical nutrition therapy through the different stages of the continuum of cancer care.

a) Primary prevention

_____

_____

_____

_____

_____

b) Diagnosis and pretreatment

_____

_____

_____

_____

_____

c) Treatment

_____

_____

_____

_____

_____

   d) Posttreatment and rehabilitation

   _____

   _____

   _____

   _____

   _____

   e) Recurrence and retreatment

   _____

   _____

   _____

   _____

   _____

   f) Palliation

   _____

   _____

   _____

   _____

   _____

12. Gastrointestinal tumors, depending on their localization, can have detrimental effects on the nutritional status of clients by causing all sorts of signs and symptoms. List the signs and symptoms commonly experienced by clients with a gastrointestinal tumor.

   _____

   _____

   _____

   _____

   _____

   _____

   _____

   _____

   _____

   _____

   _____

13. Give three main nutrition goals for cancer patients who have undergone gastrointestinal tract surgery.

   a) _____

   b) _____

   c) _____

14. What five practical dietary recommendations would you give to a cancer patient who has oral and esophageal mucositis?

    a) _____

    b) _____

    c) _____

    d) _____

    e) _____

15. What five practical dietary recommendations would you give to a cancer patient suffering from xerostomia?

    a) _____

    b) _____

    c) _____

    d) _____

    e) _____

16. The first line of defense in cancer treatment is

    a) surgery   c) radiation therapy   e) hormonal therapy
    b) chemotherapy   d) blood and bone marrow transplant

17. _____ is used to destroy a solid tumor mass but can also "burn" and damage surrounding tissues.

    a) Surgery   c) Chemotherapy   e) Hormonal therapy
    b) Immunotherapy   d) Radiation therapy

18. The use of tamoxifen in the management of breast cancer is an example of

    a) surgical treatment   c) immunotherapy   e) chemotherapy
    b) hormonal therapy   d) radiation therapy

19. Possible adverse effects resulting from radiation therapy to the oral cavity include the following, <u>except</u>

    a) trismus   c) xerostomia   e) esophagitis
    b) dysphagia   d) mucositis

20. These are common side effects of chemotherapy, <u>except</u>

    a) dysgeusia   c) anemia   e) nausea
    b) diarrhea   d) trismus

21. What side effect is frequently seen when narcotics are used in cancer management?

    a) Diarrhea   c) Dysphagia   e) Nausea and vomiting
    b) Lactose intolerance d) Constipation

22. About _____% of cancer patients die from cancer-induced or treatment-related malnutrition.

    a) 15   b) 30   c) 45   d) 60   e) 75

23. Emaciation occurs when patients have lost more than _____% of their body weight. _____% of clients with widespread cancer die as a result of severe emaciation.

    a) 15; 5   b) 30; 10   c) 45; 15   d) 60; 20   e) 75; 25

24. Explain the consequences of acute radiation enteritis.

    _____

    _____

    _____

    _____

25. Approximately _____ % of cancer patients use complementary and alternative therapies, and

    _____ % do not inform their physicians about it.

    a) 30–50; 40   b) 40–60; 50   c) 50–70; 60   d) 60–80; 70   e) 70–90; 80

26. HIV can be transmitted by the following body fluids, <u>except</u>

    a) blood   b) breast milk   c) vaginal fluid   d) saliva   e) amniotic fluid

27. HIV may be transmitted during the following events, <u>except</u>

    a) giving birth   c) shaking hands   e) sharing needles
    b) transfusing blood or blood products   d) having unprotected anal or vaginal intercourse

28. Which CD antigens are found on the following T cells?

    a) Helper T cells: _____

    b) Suppressor T cells: _____

    c) Natural killer cells: _____

29. How does HIV infection affect immunity?

    _____

    _____

    _____

30. What type of virus is the human immunodeficiency virus?

    _____

    _____

    _____

31. List the four stages of HIV infection and describe how the infection develops in clients at each stage.

    1- Stage: _____

    Description: _____

    _____

    _____

    _____

    _____

    _____

    _____

    2- Stage: _____

    Description: _____

    _____

    _____

    _____

    _____

    _____

3- Stage: _____

Description: _____

_____

_____

_____

_____

_____

_____

4- Stage: _____

Description: _____

_____

_____

_____

_____

_____

_____

32. Clients infected with HIV are at risk of suffering from multiple opportunistic infections or malignancies during the course of their disease, which further impair their nutritional status and immunity.

1) Use the table below to identify some of the most common pathogens affecting clients with HIV.
2) Identify the type of pathogen as bacterium, virus, fungus, or protozoa, or otherwise as malignancy.
3) Name the disease condition(s) caused by each pathogen.
4) Give some of the clinical manifestations for each disease condition.

PATHOGENS AND DISEASES CONDITIONS ASSOCIATED WITH AIDS.			
Pathogen	Type of Pathogen	Disease Condition	Manifestations of Disease
e.g., *Coccidioidomycosis*	Fungus	Meningitis	Flu-like S&S, fever, cough, anorexia, fatigue, malaise, weight loss
1-			
2-			
3-			
4-			
5-			

(continued)

PATHOGENS AND DISEASES CONDITIONS ASSOCIATED WITH AIDS. *(continued)*			
Pathogen	Type of Pathogen	Disease Condition	Manifestations of Disease
6-			
7-			
8-			
9-			
10-			
11-			
12-			
13-			
14-			
15-			
16-			
17-			
18-			

33. What is the most common gastrointestinal symptom in patients with HIV infection?

a) Dysphagia   b) Constipation   c) Diarrhea   d) Mouth ulcers   e) Anorexia

INTEGRATE YOUR LEARNING

1. These are carcinogens, <u>except</u>

a) cigarette smoke   c) dietary saturated fatty acids   e) betel nuts
b) chewing tobacco   d) polycyclic aromatic hydrocarbons (e.g., benzene)

2. Cancer is the _____ cause of death in North America and the _____ cause of premature death.

a) leading; leading   c) second; leading   e) third; second
b) leading; second   d) second; second

3. Which of the following is an example of a systemic type of tumor?

   a) Breast cancer   c) Leukemia   e) Colon cancer with liver metastases
   b) Lung cancer   d) Esophageal cancer

4. Which statement about cancer is **false**?

   a) Tumors can be benign or cancerous.   d) Metastasis is when tumor cells change locations.
   b) Cancer is a word derived from Latin for "crab." e) None of the above
   c) Cancers are also called neoplasms.

5. In the TNM cancer classification system, what would $T_4 N_1 M_1$ stand for?

   a) Carcinoma in situ, no distant metastasis, large regional metastasis
   b) Primary tumor large in size, small number and size of regional lymph node metastasis, presence of distant metastasis
   c) Primary tumor large in size, undifferentiated stage of nodal metastasis, assessment of presence of distant metastasis not required at the present
   d) Well-differentiated primary tumor, regional lymph node metastasis not assessed, no distant metastasis
   e) Primary tumor small in size, no regional lymph node metastasis, presence of distant metastasis

6. The role of medical nutrition therapy during the _____ stage of the continuum of cancer care is to manage symptoms and to help maintain the patient's nutritional status and health.

   a) Diagnosis/pretreatment   c) Posttreatment/rehabilitation   e) End-stage of palliation
   b) Treatment   d) Early stage of palliation

7. Systemic neoplastic disease can cause the following metabolic abnormalities, <u>except</u>

   a) increased lipoprotein lipase activity   d) free fatty acid hyperlipidemia
   b) insulin resistance   e) increased protein synthesis
   c) increased lipolysis

8. Possible nutrition problems associated with the presence of neoplastic disease are unlikely to include

   a) glucose intolerance   c) bowel obstruction   e) organ hyperfunction
   b) taste changes   d) fat malabsorption

9. _____ can be given externally or internally, such as by intravenous therapy.

   a) Surgery   c) Chemotherapy   e) Hormonal therapy
   b) Immunotherapy   d) Radiation therapy

10. _____ is a progressive condition associated with weight loss, significant lean body mass depletion, early satiety, increased basal metabolic rate, weakness, and malnutrition. This syndrome is seen in some clients with chronic disorders like cancer, AIDS, congestive heart failure, and COPD.

    a) Starvation   b) Wasting   c) Cachexia   d) Anorexia   e) Emaciation

11. _____ chemotherapy is given before surgery or radiation therapy to reduce the size of the tumor.

    a) Combination   c) Palliative   e) Ablative
    b) Adjuvant   d) Neoadjuvant

12. Radiation therapy to the head and neck may cause the following, <u>except</u>

    a) reflux   c) dental caries   e) vomiting
    b) odynophagia   d) lack of smell

13. Which statement about weight loss in cancer patients is **false**?

    a) Weight loss is the best indicator of nutritional status in cancer clients.
    b) More than 80% of clients with hematologic cancer experience weight loss.
    c) Up to 40% of clients with breast cancer experience weight loss.
    d) A pretreatment weight loss, even of $<5\%$, increases the risks of morbidity and mortality.
    e) Forty-five percent of hospitalized adult cancer clients have lost 10% of their body weight pre-illness.

14. What is the most common secondary diagnosis in cancer clients?

    a) Bacterial infection   c) Protein-energy malnutrition   e) Dysphagia
    b) Depression   d) Radiation enteritis

15. Nutrition therapy is _____ when it is actually a part of the therapeutic regimen.

    a) definitive   b) adjunctive   c) supportive   d) none of the above

16. Which of the following is an <u>appropriate</u> suggestion to improve oral intake in cancer clients?

    a) Offer hot foods if the client has taste changes.
    b) Offer cold foods if the client is sensitive to smell.
    c) Offer foods with a strong aroma if the client has early satiety.
    d) Introduce nutritional supplements close to treatment time to avoid aversion.
    e) Use plastic utensils if the client is sensitive to smell.

17. What type of cancer originates in the colon and propagates to the liver and pancreas?

    _____

18. What are the most common AIDS-associated cancers?

    _____

    _____

19. Define the following terms associated with HIV infection.

    a) Viral count: _____

    _____

    b) Myalgia: _____

    _____

    c) Lymphadenopathy: _____

    _____

    d) Adenopathy: _____

    _____

    e) Seropositive: _____

    _____

    f) Thrush: _____

    _____

    g) Bacteremia: _____

    _____

    h) Hemoptysis: _____

    _____

    i) Hematemesis: _____

    _____

    j) Leukoplakia: _____

    _____

20. These factors are possible causes of dysphagia in clients infected with HIV, <u>except</u>

    a) *Clostridium difficile* infection   c) tumors in the mouth or esophagus   e) dementia
    b) Kaposi's sarcoma   d) oral or esophageal lesions

21. These factors may be the cause of diarrhea in clients infected with HIV, <u>except</u>

    a) *Candida albicans* infection   c) medication interactions   e) villous atrophy
    b) low serum albumin levels   d) bacterial overgrowth

22. What is HAART?

    _____

    _____

    _____

    _____

    _____

23. State the main goals of medical nutrition therapy for clients infected with HIV.

    _____

    _____

    _____

    _____

    _____

    _____

    _____

    _____

24. What are the diagnostic criteria for the HIV wasting syndrome?

    _____

    _____

    _____

    _____

    _____

    _____

    _____

    _____

25. Explain the HIV lipodystrophy syndrome.

    _____

    _____

    _____

    _____

    _____

    _____

    _____

    _____

26. What type of diet is generally recommended for cancer and AIDS clients?

a) Low-fat, low-cholesterol diet
b) High-energy, high-protein diet
c) Low-carbohydrate, high-fat diet
d) Low-protein, high-carbohydrate diet
e) High-fiber, high-carbohydrate diet

CHALLENGE YOUR LEARNING

CASE STUDY

Objectives

This case will help you consider the ABCD findings and other relevant data available to assess the nutritional status of an outpatient cancer client.

It will also help you perceive the limitations of the data on which your nutrition assessment is based and identify what information is required for a more comprehensive assessment.

In addition, it will help you set realistic goals of nutrition care for a client in a palliative care situation.

Description

Mr. B.K. is a 70-year-old, ex-heavy cigarette smoker, who was diagnosed with lung cancer last October 15. The cancer type is a squamous non–small cell carcinoma, which is located in the upper right lobe of his lung. The oncologist has classified his malignant lung tumor as $T_4 N_0 M_0$ and stage III, which means that his 5-year survival rate is <5%.

Mr. B.K. started to smoke cigarettes with his siblings at 16 years old. Although he is not smoking anymore, he smoked an average of 10 cigarettes a day during most of his adult life. One of his brothers, who died of lung cancer three years ago, convinced him to stop smoking.

Mr. B.K. presented with many signs and symptoms secondary to his lung cancer, including right chest pain, shortness of breath, cough with phlegm, chronic airway limitation, chronic obstructive pulmonary disease (COPD), tenderness and swelling in the right dorsal and paravertebral regions, occasional hemoptysis, numbness of the left hand, weakness, fatigue, and mild depression.

Mr. B.K. has been progressively losing weight, from a usual body weight of 165 lb (75.0 kg) prior to diagnosis. At his second visit to the regional cancer center, on November 16, his body weight was 154 lb (70.0 kg), and he weighed 145 lb (65.8 kg) at his third visit on January 4. Mr. B.K. measures 5′6″ and has a medium bone frame.

His laboratory blood work as of October 15 was the following: (Note: laboratory result values are presented in conventional units, followed by international system units in parentheses [SI units]. Normal or reference range values are shown in italic):

Complete blood count (CBC) and differential counts:
- White blood cell (WBC; leukocyte) count and differential counts:
  ○ Total leukocyte (LKC) count: $8.7 \times 10^3/\mu L$ ($8.7 \times 10^9/L$)
    ■ *Normal: $4.8–10.8 \times 10^3/\mu L$ (or $4.8–10.8 \times 10^9/L$)*

  ○ Neutrophil count: $4.5 \times 10^3/\mu L$ ($4.5 \times 10^9/L$)
    ■ *Normal: $2.0–7.5 \times 10^3/\mu L$ (or $2.0–7.5 \times 10^9/L$)*

  ○ Lymphocyte count: $2.8 \times 10^3/\mu L$ ($2.8 \times 10^9/L$)
    ■ *Normal: $1.5–4.0 \times 10^3/\mu L$ (or $1.5–4.0 \times 10^9/L$)*

  ○ Monocyte count: $0.7 \times 10^3/\mu L$ ($0.7 \times 10^9/L$)
    ■ *Normal: $0.2–0.8 \times 10^3/\mu L$ (or $0.2–0.8 \times 10^9/L$)*

○ Eosinophil count: $0.6 \times 10^3/\mu L$ ($0.6 \times 10^9/L$)
  ▪ *Normal: $0.0–0.4 \times 10^3/\mu L$ (or $0.0–0.4 \times 10^9/L$)*

○ Basophil count: $0.1 \times 10^3/\mu L$ ($0.1 \times 10^9/L$)
  ▪ *Normal: $0.0–0.1 \times 10^3/\mu L$ (or $0.0–0.1 \times 10^9/L$)*

- Red blood cell (RBC; erythrocyte) count: $4.09 \times 10^6/\mu L$ ($4.09 \times 10^{12}/L$)
  ▪ *Normal for men: $4.7–6.1 \times 10^6/\mu L$ (or $4.7–6.1 \times 10^{12}/L$)*

- Red blood cell indices:
  ○ Mean corpuscular volume (MCV): $90.7 \mu^3$ (90.7 fL)
    ▪ *Normal for men: $80–94 \mu^3$ (or 80–94 fL)*

  ○ Mean corpuscular hemoglobin (MCH): 29 pg (0.45 fmol)
    ▪ *Normal: 27–31 pg (or 0.42–0.48 fmol)*

  ○ Mean corpuscular hemoglobin concentration (MCHC): 33 g/dL (330 g/L)
    ▪ *Normal: 33–37 g/dL or % (or 330–370 g/L)*

  ○ Red blood cell distribution width (RDW): 13.9%
    ▪ *Normal: 12%–15%*

- Hemoglobin (Hb, Hgb): 12.1 g/dL (121 g/L or 1.88 mmol/L)
  ▪ *Normal for men: 14.0–18.0 g/dL (or 140–180 g/L or 2.17–2.79 mmol/L)*

- Hematocrit (Hct; packed RBC volume): 37% (0.37)
  ▪ *Normal for men: 42%–52% (or 0.42–0.52) volume fraction*

- Platelet (thrombocyte) count: $406 \times 10^3/\mu L$ ($406 \times 10^9/L$)
  ▪ *Normal: $130–400 \times 10^3/\mu L$ (or $130–400 \times 10^9/L$)*

- Mean platelet volume (MPV): $8.2 \mu^3$ (8.2 fL)
  ▪ *Normal: $7.4–10.4 \mu^3$ (or 7.4–10.4 fL)*

Blood proteins:
- Total protein: 7.6 g/dL (76 g/L)
  ▪ *Normal: 6.4–8.3 g/dL (or 64–83 g/L)*

- Albumin: 3.1 g/dL (31 g/L)
  ▪ *Normal over 60 y.o.: 3.2–4.6 g/dL (or 32–46 g/L)*

- Globulins (α-, β-, and γ-globulins, including Ig and lipoproteins): 0.26 g/dL (2.6 g/L)
  ▪ *Normal: 0.23–0.34 g/dL (or 2.3–3.4 g/L)*

Metabolic panel:
- Blood electrolyte panel:
  ○ Potassium (K): 4.6 mEq/L (4.6 mmol/L)
    ▪ *Normal in adults: 3.5–5.1 mEq/L (or 3.5–5.1 mmol/L)*

  ○ Sodium (Na): 143 mEq/L (143 mmol/L)
    ▪ *Normal: 136–145 mEq/L (or 136–145 mmol/L)*

  ○ Chloride (Cl): 102 mEq/L (102 mmol/L)
    ▪ *Normal: 98–107 mEq/L (or 98–107 mmol/L)*

  ○ Carbon dioxide (CO_2) content: 27 mEq/L (27 mmol/L)
    ▪ *Normal for adults: 23–30 mEq/L (or 23–30 mmol/L)*

- Random blood glucose: 101 mg/dL (5.6 mmol/L)
  ▪ *Normal: 61–199 mg/dL (or 3.4–11.0 mmol/L)*

- Blood calcium (Ca): 11.3 mg/dL (2.83 mmol/L)
  ▪ *Normal: 8.6–10 mg/dL (or 2.15–2.50 mmol/L)*

- Blood phosphate (PO_4, inorganic): 3.0 mg/dL (0.98 mmol/L)
  ▪ *Normal in adults: 2.7–4.5 mg/dL (or 0.87–1.45 mmol/L)*

- Blood urea nitrogen (BUN): 17.5 mg/dL (6.2 mmol/L)
    - *Normal for adults: 10–20 mg/dL (or 3.6–7.1 mmol/L)*

- Blood creatinine: 0.77 mg/dL (68 μmol/L)
    - *Normal in men: 0.7–1.3 mg/dL (or 62–115 μmol/L)*

- Total blood bilirubin: 0.38 mg/day (6.5 μmol/L)
    - *Normal: 0.3–1.0 mg/dL (or 5.1–17.0 μmol/L)*

Mr. B.K. has completed radiation therapy and is now starting chemotherapy. Surgery was not an option due to the site of his neoplasm. Mr. B.K. is receiving palliative care to maintain his quality of life.

Mr. B.K. is a white Caucasian man, who comes from a large family. He used to own the family car dealership with his three brothers. Mr. B.K. lives with his wife in town, where he grew up. His wife and daughter prepare a variety of healthy meals for him; however, his appetite has been poor since the start of his cancer treatment. Mr. B.K. is presently taking the following medications: Cisplatin, Etoposide, Tylenol No. 3, Alprazolam, Lactulose, Colace, Morphine sulfate, Codeine, Dexamethasone, and multivitamin.

You met briefly with Mr. B.K. and his wife at his third visit to the regional cancer center. Mr. B.K. had been experiencing anorexia, aphthous stomatitis, swallowing difficulties, nausea, xerostomia, and constipation. He feels tired and spends most of his day sitting or lying down. He presently has a fever of 100.4°F.

You perform a quick dietary assessment and estimate that his daily intake is presently about 1700 kcal (7106 kJ), 60 g protein, and 1⅛ quarts (41⅔ fluid oz, ~5 cups, 1250 mL) fluid. He still tries to have three meals and two snacks a day. His breakfast usually includes a fruit juice and a plain yogurt, followed by a black coffee. His lunch is often a chicken noodle soup and a cheese sandwich. His dinner tends to be meat, potatoes or rice, and a colorful vegetable. His snacks alternate between a homemade dessert and a fruit.

1. What does $T_4 N_0 M_0$ mean?

2. What is the main cause of lung cancer?

3. What is your assessment of Mr. B.K.'s usual body weight prior to diagnosis?

4. What is your assessment of Mr. B.K.'s weight change since diagnosis?

5. What is your assessment of Mr. B.K.'s biochemical data?

6. Is Mr. B.K. suffering from anemia? Explain your answer.

7. What is his body temperature in degrees Celsius?

8. What is your evaluation of Mr. B.K.'s current dietary intake?

9. List the medications Mr. B.K. is taking and indicate the type of each medication.

10. Which clinical signs and symptoms negatively impact Mr. B.K.'s dietary intake and nutritional status? Give the possible cause(s) of each sign and symptom.

11. What are limitations of the ABCD findings and other information available about Mr. B.K.? What other data do you need to assess his nutritional status in a more comprehensive way?

12. What is your overall assessment of Mr. B.K.'s nutritional status?

13. Outline the overall goal and specific objectives of nutrition care for Mr. B.K. according to your nutritional assessment of his condition.

14. What are the nutritionally relevant side effects of the chemotherapy agents Mr. B.K. is taking?

15. Give examples of appetite stimulants used for the management of cancer cachexia.

7.13 Renal Disease

REVIEW THE INFORMATION

1. What is the unit of kidney structure and function?

   _____

2. What are the main functions of the kidneys?

   _____
   _____
   _____
   _____
   _____
   _____
   _____
   _____
   _____
   _____
   _____
   _____

3. Approximately one in _____ North American adults has chronic kidney disease.

   a) three   b) six   c) nine   d) 12   e) 15

4. People in these population groups have increased risk of developing chronic renal disease due to high rates of hypertension and/or diabetes mellitus, <u>except</u>

   a) First Nations   b) Jewish   c) Pacific Islanders   d) Hispanics   e) African Americans

5. What is creatinine and how is it excreted?

   _____
   _____
   _____
   _____

6. How does the body catabolize the nitrogen group of amino acids?

   _____
   _____
   _____
   _____

7. What is the active form of vitamin D and where is it activated?

   _____
   _____

8. Sketch a nephron in the space below and identify its main parts.

9. What is the separation of molecules in solution by diffusion through a selectively permeable membrane on the basis of molecule size and concentration gradient?

   _____

10. In a healthy individual, the 24-hour urinary excretion of _____ is proportionate to the skeletal muscle mass of the individual. It can therefore be used as a tool to help estimate body protein status.

11. Underline foods rich in phosphorus and highlight foods rich in potassium from the list below.

milk	cottage cheese	banana	applesauce	grape juice
tomato	fudge ice cream	lima beans	prune juice	orange
pork	cooked mushrooms	salmon	seeds	nuts
margarine	baked potato	avocado	oil	honey
lentils	baked beans	winter squash	veal liver	molasses
chocolate	cola beverages	potato chips	cantaloupe	butter
cucumber	French fries	dried fruits	kiwifruit	peach
popcorn	whole wheat bread	sweet potato	egg	nectarine
yogurt	peanut butter	pea soup	tofu	soy milk
granola cereal	corn tortilla	sardines	pancake	beer
bran cereals	salt substitutes	vanilla cake	cranberry juice cocktail	

12. Record in the following table the quantity of sodium found in a serving of common foods, and indicate if these foods are high (**H**), moderate (**M**), or low (**L**) in sodium. Then, suggest lower sodium substitutes.

SODIUM CONTENT OF COMMON FOODS

Foods	Serving Size	Sodium Content (mg/serving) [mg/100 g or 3.6 oz]	High, Moderate, or Low in Sodium*	Lower Sodium substitutes
1- Canned tomato juice	½ cup, 4 fluid oz, or 118 mL (126 g, 4½ oz)			
2- Seasoned commercial bread crumbs	¼ cup or 59 mL (27 g, ~1 oz)			
3- Instant, cinnamon-flavored oatmeal cereal	1 packet (46 g, 1.6 oz)			
4- Beef bologna	1 slice (23 g or 0.9 oz)			
5- Minced lunchmeat ham	1 slice (21 g or 0.8 oz)			
6- Plain omelet prepared with milk and butter	1 (61 g or 2.2 oz)			
7- Pork breakfast sausage, cooked	1 link (13 g or ½ oz)			
8- American cheese spread	1 Tbsp or 15 mL (15 g or ½ oz)			
9- Cooked bacon	4 pieces (32 g or 1.2 oz)			
10- Smoked Chinook salmon	3 oz (85 g)			
11- Chicken nuggets	5 pieces (75 g or 2.7 oz)			
12- Cooked kidney beans (not canned)	½ cup or 118 mL (88 g or 3.1 oz)			
13- Seasoned peanuts	1 oz (28 g)			
14- Pickled green olives, without pits	1 (4 g or 0.1 oz)			
15- Cabbage sauerkraut	½ cup or 118 mL (118 g or 4.2 oz)			
16- Pumpernickel bread	1 piece (26 g or 0.9 oz)			
17- Canned tomato sauce	½ cup or 118 mL (122 g or 4.4 oz)			

(continued)

SODIUM CONTENT OF COMMON FOODS *(continued)*

Foods	Serving Size	Sodium Content (mg/serving) [mg/100 g or 3.6 oz]	High, Moderate, or Low in Sodium*	Lower Sodium substitutes
18- Canned green peas	½ cup or 118 mL (74 g or 2.6 oz)			
19- Soy sauce	1 Tbsp or 15 mL (18 g or 0.6 oz)			
20- Yellow prepared mustard	1 Tbsp or 15 mL (16 g or 0.6 oz)			
21- Sweet pickle relish	1 Tbsp or 15 mL (15 g or ~½ oz)			
22- Worcestershire sauce	1 Tbsp or 15 mL (14 g or ½ oz)			
23- Raisins, seedless	½ cup or 118 mL (72 g or 2.6 oz)			
24- Chocolate milk, 2% fat	1 cup, 8 fluid oz, or 237 mL (250 g or 8.9 oz)			
25- Pretzel sticks	48 pieces (28 g or 1 oz)			
26- Regular butter	1 tsp or 5 mL (5 g or 0.2 oz)			
27- Hotdog (with bun)	1 (98 g or 3½ oz)			
28- Large double cheeseburger with condiments and vegetables	1 (258 g or 9.2 oz)			
29- Vegetarian soy burger	1 (74 g or 2.6 oz)			
30- Pepperoni and cheese pizza	1 slice, ⅛ of a 12-inch pizza (125 g or 4½ oz)			
31- Canned cream of mushroom soup, prepared with milk	1 cup or 237 mL (248 g or 8.9 oz)			
32- Barbecue potato chips	1 oz (28 g)			

* High in sodium defined as >400 mg sodium per 100 g (3.6 oz) food, moderate in sodium as 200–400 mg/100 g, and low in sodium as <200 mg/100 g.

13. What is the accumulation of excess body fluids in cells, tissues, or serous cavities, often causing swelling of the extremities, such as the feet, hands, legs, and face?

    a) Dehydration   b) Euvolemia   c) Overhydration   d) Edema   e) Ascites

14. _____ is the most abundant intracellular cation.

    a) Potassium   b) Sodium   c) Chloride   d) Calcium   e) Phosphorus

15. Why is high blood potassium concentration considered to be a dangerous state?

    _____

    _____

    _____

    _____

    _____

16. How are the fluid needs of healthy adults estimated?

    _____

    _____

    _____

    _____

    _____

    _____

    _____

17. Give the DRI recommendations (RDA or AI and UL) for the following nutrients for 31- to 50-year-old men and women.

    a) Calcium: _____

    b) Sodium: _____

    c) Phosphorus: _____

    d) Potassium: _____

    e) Chloride: _____

    f) Magnesium: _____

18. Which cost-effective nutrition assessment tool, based on medical history and physical examination, is often used to assess the nutritional status of renal clients, given the confounding effect of renal disease on many biochemical laboratory measures?

    _____

19. What type of diet is recommended for the management of hypercholesterolemia?

    _____

    _____

    _____

    _____

    _____

UNDERSTAND THE CONCEPTS

1. What are the main types of renal disorders?

_____

_____

_____

2. Use this grid to help you fill in the text with appropriate terms related to kidney function and disorders.

Terms Related to Kidney Function and Disorders.

Each one of the kidneys includes approximately a *a)*_____ (*word of 7 letters*)nephrons. Each nephron has a *b)*_____ (*word of 9 letters*) containing a glomerulus that acts as a blood-filtering unit, which is covered by a Bowman's capsule. Glomerular filtration

*c)*_____ (*word of 8 letters*) is the quantity of milliliters of filtrate produced by the kidneys per minute. It is used to evaluate the renal *d)*_____ (*word of 8 letters*) of clients and the stage of their renal disease. Normal glomerular filtration rate in healthy adults is between 90 and

139 mL per *e)*_____ (*word of 6 letters*) per 1.73 m^2.

The physician calculates the glomerular filtration rate of clients based on their estimated serum

*f)*_____ (*word of 10 letters*) concentration. There is an *g)*_____ (*word of 7 letters*) relationship between serum creatinine concentration and a client's glomerular filtration rate.

Since kidneys have several important functions, renal diseases are usually *h)*_____ (*word of 7 letters*) disorders. Renal disease most often has an *i)*_____ (*word of 6 letters*) on the two kidneys.

Furthermore, testing the concentrations of serum and urine creatinine, urine protein, and serum urea

*j)*_____ (*word of 8 letters*) and measuring blood pressure allows for the presence of chronic renal disease to be detected.

Chronic renal disease is defined as renal damage with *k)*_____ (*word of 11 letters*) or glomerular filtration rate below 60 mL/min/1.73 m² for 3 months. Warning signs of chronic kidney disease include frequent urination, especially at night, painful or difficult urination, and *l)*_____ (*word of 5 letters*). Hypertension may cause *m)*_____ (*word of 7 letters*) renal disease and vice versa, creating a vicious circle. *n)*_____ (*word of 7 letters*) individuals, and those with type 2 diabetes mellitus or a family history of kidney disease, are also at risk for the development of chronic renal disease. Other causes of kidney diseases include glomerulonephritis, inherited kidney diseases (e.g., polycystic kidney disease), systemic lupus erythematous, recurrent urinary tract *o)*_____ (*word of 10 letters*) (e.g., causing pyelonephritis), congenital malformations, and kidney obstruction (e.g., by renal calculi or a tumor). Glomerulonephritis is an inflammation and damage of the glomeruli, while *p)*_____ (*word of 14 letters*) is a urinary reflux to the kidneys with infection of nephrons.

Renal damage may progress slowly and *q)*_____ (*word of 8 letters*) over many years before the person becomes aware of the problem. A considerable amount of *r)*_____ (*word of 8 letters*) may have already been damaged at diagnosis.

Complications of chronic renal disease include hypertension, poor nutritional *s)*_____ (*word of 6 letters*), proteinuria, anemia, renal *t)*_____ (*word of 4 letters*) disease, nerve damage, diabetes mellitus, cardiovascular disease, and renal failure.

End-stage renal disease is defined as advanced, irreversible kidney *u)*_____ (*word of 7 letters*). It is characterized by a glomerular filtration rate below 15 mL/min/1.73 m², which is life threatening and requires hemodialysis, *v)*_____ (*word of 10 letters*) dialysis, or kidney transplantation. Medical nutrition therapy is carefully adjusted to the needs of each client and his or her *w)*_____ (*word of 5 letters*) of chronic renal disease. Appropriate dietary modifications may help clients slow the *x)*_____ (*word of 4 letters*) of renal function.

3. The following are definitions of medical terms relevant to kidney pathophysiology. Find the correct term(s) corresponding to each definition.

a) _____ is the branch of medicine studying kidney anatomy, physiology, and pathology.

b) _____ are specialists of the kidneys, their diseases, and medical management.

c) _____ is a general term referring to an abnormal condition of the kidneys due to disease.

d) _____ is kidney inflammation, which can be acute or chronic.

e) _____ is kidney pain.

f) _____ is when the renal tissue is hardened with reduced blood flow. It is often caused by hypertension.

g) _____ is a disease condition of the kidneys, such as nephrotic syndrome, altering the function of nephrons (e.g., increasing glomerular permeability due to epithelium degeneration) but without causing inflammation.

h) _____ is an abnormal kidney condition causing clinical signs of edema, marked proteinuria, low blood albumin concentration, and hyperlipidemia due to increased glomerular permeability as a result of glomerular injury.

i) _____ is a clinical state of severe glomerulonephritis with blood in urine, high blood pressure, and kidney failure.

j) _____ qualifies a state of excess urea in blood.

k) _____ is an abnormally high amount of protein in urine.

l) _____ is the abnormal presence of albumin in the urine.

m) _____ is the abnormal presence of blood or erythrocytes in the urine.

n) _____ means high blood sodium concentration.

o) _____ means high blood potassium concentration.

p) _____ is the analysis of urine using biochemical tests, including determination of urine pH; specific gravity; presence of blood, glucose, ketones, nitrite, and leukocyte esterase in urine; and concentration of bilirubin, protein, and urobilinogen of urine.

q) The _____ is the liquid collected after dialysis that went through the selectively permeable membrane.

r) A _____ is an apparatus or piece of equipment to accomplish dialysis and that contains dialyzing membranes.

s) _____ is the radiography of kidneys.

t) _____ is the excision of both kidneys by surgery.

4. Give the meaning of the following abbreviations related to nephrology.

- CKD _____

- ESRD _____

- ARF _____

- CRF _____

- UTI _____

- ATN _____

- BUN _____

- SUN _____

- UA _____

- UUN _____

- UNA _____

- Osm _____

- UOsm _____

- mEq _____

- GFR _____

- URR _____

- RTA _____

- Cr _____

- Urine ACR _____

- EPO _____

- PTH _____

- PNA _____

- nPNA _____

- DPI _____

- HBV _____

- MDRD _____

- CAPD _____
- APD _____
- CPD _____
- MD _____
- HD _____
- MHD _____
- CAVH _____
- CAVHD _____
- CVVH _____
- CVVHD _____
- CRRT _____
- IDWG _____
- ACEI _____
- ARB _____
- CCB _____
- KDOQI guidelines _____

5. The kidneys are responsible for maintaining blood pH at

   a) 7.20–7.30　　b) 7.35–7.45　　c) 7.50–7.60　　d) 7.65–7.75　　e) 7.80–7.90

6. Which clients are susceptible to developing acute renal failure?

   _____

   _____

   _____

   _____

7. What metabolic abnormalities are seen in clients with acute renal failure?

   _____

   _____

   _____

   _____

8. There are three categories of acute renal failure, based on the etiology of the problem affecting the kidneys. What are they?

   a) _____

   b) _____

   c) _____

9. What type of diet is recommended for clients with acute renal failure?

   _____

   _____

   _____

   _____

_____

_____

_____

10. What factors should you keep in mind when making nutritional recommendations for clients with acute renal failure?

_____

_____

_____

_____

_____

_____

_____

_____

11. Explain the five stages of the development of chronic kidney disease.

1- _____

_____

2- _____

_____

3- _____

_____

4- _____

_____

5- _____

_____

12. Adult clients with a serum creatinine concentration over _____ µmol/L or _____ mg/dL are considered to have lost 50% of their kidney function.

a) 50–100; 0.6–1.1   c) 150–200; 1.7–2.3   e) 250–300; 2.8–3.4
b) 100–150; 1.1–1.7   d) 200–250; 2.3–2.8

13. What are the metabolic and clinical consequences of chronic kidney disease?

_____

_____

_____

_____

_____

_____

_____

_____

14. What are the symptoms caused by increased levels of urea in the blood or uremic symptoms?

_____

_____

_____

15. What are the two main goals of nutrition management for clients with pre–end-stage renal disease?

a) _____

_____

b) _____

_____

16. What type of diet is recommended for clients with pre-ESRD?

_____

_____

_____

_____

_____

17. What level of dietary protein restriction is usually required for clients with pre-ESRD?

_____

_____

_____

_____

_____

_____

_____

18. Describe the possible effects of too much or too little protein intake in clients with pre-ESRD.

EFFECTS OF INAPPROPRIATE PROTEIN INTAKE IN PRE–END-STAGE RENAL DISEASE	
Effects of Too <u>Much</u> Protein	Effects of Too <u>Little</u> Protein

19. What amount of energy, phosphorus, sodium, potassium, and calcium is generally recommended for clients with pre-ESRD?

a) Energy: _____

_____

_____

b) Phosphorus: _____

_____

_____

c) Sodium: _____

_____

_____

d) Potassium: _____

_____

_____

e) Calcium: _____

_____

_____

20. Categorize the following foods as high (**H**), moderate (**M**), or low (**L**) sources of protein, phosphorus, sodium, and potassium.

PROTEIN, PHOSPHORUS, SODIUM, AND POTASSIUM CONTENT OF COMMON FOODS

Foods	Protein[a]	Phosphorus[b]	Sodium[c]	Potassium[d]
1- **Cured ham** (roasted, 7% fat, 85 g or 3 oz)				
2- **Egg** (hard cooked, 50 g or 1.8 oz)				
3- **Lentils** (cooked, ½ cup or 118 mL, 99 g or 3½ oz)				
4- **Milk** (1 cup or 237 mL, 247 g or 8.8 oz, 1% fat)				
5- **Plain raw peanuts** (1 oz, 28 g)				
6- **Orange** (fresh, navel, ½ cup or 118 mL, 82 g or 2.9 oz)				
7- **Banana** (raw slices, ½ cup or 118 mL, 75 g or 2.7 oz)				
8- **Whole wheat bread** (1 piece, 28 g or 1 oz)				
9- **Cooked white rice** (½ cup or 118 mL, 93 g or 3.3 oz)				

(continued)

PROTEIN, PHOSPHORUS, SODIUM, AND POTASSIUM CONTENT OF COMMON FOODS
(continued)

Foods	Protein[a]	Phosphorus[b]	Sodium[c]	Potassium[d]
10- **Canola oil**				
11- **Baked ground beef** (3 oz, 85 g)				
12- **Raisins** (seedless, ½ cup or 118 mL, 72 g or 2.6 oz)				
13- **Jellybean candies** (10 pieces, 11 g or 0.4 oz)				
14- **Baked potato** (1, 284 g or 10.1 oz)				

[a] High in protein defined as >20.0 g protein per 100 g (3.6 oz), moderate in protein as 10.0–20.0 g/100 g, and low in protein as <10.0 g/100 g.
[b] High in phosphorus defined as >175 mg phosphorus per 100 g (3.6 oz), moderate in phosphorus as 50–175 mg/100 g, and low in phosphorus as <50 mg/100 g.
[c] High in sodium defined as >400 mg sodium per 100 g (3.6 oz), moderate in sodium as 200–400 mg/100 g, and low in sodium as <200 mg/100 g.
[d] High in potassium defined as >270 mg potassium per 100 g (3.6 oz), moderate in potassium as 70–270 mg/100 g, and low in potassium as <70 mg/100 g.

21. Which renal clients may require a fluid restriction?

_____

_____

_____

_____

22. It is important to be aware of the fluid inputs and outputs in clients requiring fluid restriction. List the many possible sources of fluid input and output in clients with kidney disease.

SOURCES OF FLUID INPUT AND OUTPUT IN CLIENTS WITH RENAL DISEASE

Sources of Fluid <u>Input</u>	Sources of Fluid <u>Output</u>

23. In clients with chronic renal insufficiency, the hormone _____ is no longer normally synthesized by the kidneys and may need to be given to clients to treat anemia and stimulate the formation of erythrocytes.

24. Fill in each blank space with the appropriate word related to renal bone disease and its management.

When the glomerular filtration rate falls below 20 mL of blood per minute, blood *a)*_____ concentration increases, which inhibits vitamin *b)* _____ activation by the kidneys. The result is a reduced absorption of dietary *c)* _____, leading to low blood calcium concentration.

The brain reacts by stimulating the secretion of *d)* _____ hormone, which increases blood calcium concentration by causing bone resorption. However, this leads to brittle bones and calcium depositions in soft tissues, including the kidneys, causing yet more loss of renal function.

Therefore, the number one action to prevent renal osteodystrophy in clients with chronic renal insufficiency is to control blood *e)* _____ concentration by *restricting* dietary phosphorus and asking clients to take their *f)* _____ binder medication with food, as prescribed by their physician. In addition, the intake of calcium should be adequate to help normalize blood calcium concentration, which will prevent secondary hyperparathyroidism and, consequently, stop soft tissue calcification. Calcium and *g)* _____ supplementation may be required.

25. Vitamin _____ supplementation is associated with toxicity in patients with chronic renal insufficiency.

   a) A   b) C   c) D   d) E   e) K

26. What are the goals of medical nutrition therapy for adult clients with nephrotic syndrome who are not on dialysis?

_____

_____

_____

_____

_____

27. What are the dietary recommendations for adult clients with nephrotic syndrome who are not on dialysis?

_____

_____

_____

_____

_____

_____

_____

_____

_____

28. What type of medication is given to clients with nephrotic syndrome to reduce their proteinuria and help normalize their blood pressure?

_____

29. The following signs and symptoms are associated with end-stage renal disease, <u>except</u>

   a) back pain   b) fatigue   c) high blood pressure   d) blood in the urine   e) dehydration

30. Explain the following types of dialysis and comment on how frequently they must be used for the treatment of advanced renal failure.

    a) Continuous ambulatory peritoneal dialysis: _____

    b) Hemodialysis: _____

    c) Continuous renal replacement therapy _____

31. What is interdialytic weight gain?

32. What are the two main goals of nutrition management for clients with end-stage renal disease on dialysis (hemodialysis or peritoneal dialysis)?

    a) _____

    b) _____

33. What type of diet is recommended for clients with ESRD who are on hemodialysis?

_____

_____

_____

_____

34. What type of diet is recommended for clients with ESRD who are on peritoneal dialysis?

_____

_____

_____

_____

_____

_____

_____

35. The nutritional status of renal clients can be assessed periodically using the scored PG-SGA, as well as the protein equivalent of total nitrogen appearance.

a) What is the protein equivalent of total nitrogen appearance?

_____

_____

_____

_____

_____

_____

b) What useful information is obtained by calculating the protein equivalent of total nitrogen appearance?

_____

_____

_____

_____

c) What is the normalized protein nitrogen appearance?

_____

_____

_____

_____

d) What is the adjusted edema-free body weight and how is it calculated?

_____

_____

_____

_____

_____

e) What biochemical data are required to calculate the PNA?

_____

_____

f) How is the PNA calculated?

_____

_____

_____

_____

g) What are normal values of nPNA for clients on maintenance dialysis?

_____

h) What is the urea nitrogen appearance?

_____

_____

_____

_____

36. Why is the ratio of serum urea nitrogen (SUN) concentration to serum creatinine concentration a valuable clinical tool to use with pre-ESRD clients?

_____

_____

_____

_____

_____

37. What is Kt/V and why is it calculated?

_____

_____

_____

_____

_____

_____

38. Practice converting the amount of sodium, potassium, and phosphorus in different units.

1- Convert the dietary recommendations of 1.5–2.3 g **sodium** per day (which are the AI and UL) into

a) mg   _____

b) mmol   _____

2- Convert the dietary restriction of 43–130 mmol **sodium** per day into

a) g   _____

b) mEq   _____

3- Convert the dietary restriction of 87–174 mEq **sodium** per day into

    a) mmol   _____

    b) mg   _____

4- Convert the serum (or plasma) reference range values of 136–145 mmol **sodium**/L into

    a) mEq/L   _____

5- Convert the urine reference range values of 40–220 mEq **sodium** per 24 hours into

    a) g/24 hours   _____

6- Convert the dietary recommendation of 4.7 g **potassium** per day (AI) into

    a) mg   _____

    b) mmol   _____

7- Convert the dietary restriction of 50–77 mmol **potassium** per day into

    a) g   _____

    b) mEq   _____

8- Convert the dietary restriction of 77–102 mEq **potassium** per day into

    a) mmol   _____

    b) g   _____

9- Convert the serum (or plasma) reference range values of 3.5–5.5 mmol **potassium**/L into

    a) mEq/L   _____

10- Convert the urine reference range values of 25–125 mEq **potassium** per 24 hours into

    a) g/24 hours   _____

11- Convert the dietary recommendations of 2.3 g **chloride** per day (AI) into

    a) mmol   _____

    b) mEq   _____

12- Convert the serum (or plasma) reference range values of 98–107 mmol **chloride**/L into

    a) mEq/L   _____

13- Convert the urine reference range values of 110–250 mEq **chloride** per 24 hours into

    a) g/24 hours   _____

14- Convert the dietary recommendation of 700 mg **phosphorus** per day (RDA) into

    a) g   _____

    b) mmol   _____

15- Convert the dietary restriction of 26–32 mmol **phosphorus** per day into

    a) g   _____

    b) mEq   _____

16- Convert the serum reference range values of 0.97–1.45 mmol **inorganic phosphate**/L into

    a) mEq/L   _____

    b) mg/dL   _____

17- Convert the urine reference range values of 0.4–1.3 g **phosphorus** per 24 hours into

   a) mmol/24 hours   _____

   b) mEq/24 hours   _____

18- Convert the dietary recommendation of 1.0 g **calcium** per day (AI) into

   a) mg   _____

   b) mmol   _____

19- Convert the dietary recommendation of 37.4 mmol **calcium** per day into

   a) g   _____

   b) mEq   _____

20- Convert the serum (or plasma) reference range values of 8.6–10.0 mg **calcium**/dL into

   a) mmol/L   _____

   b) mEq/L   _____

21- Convert the urine reference range values of 2.50–7.50 mmol **calcium** per 24 hours into

   a) mg/24 hours   _____

   b) mEq/24 hours   _____

22- Convert the dietary recommendation of 320–420 mg **magnesium** per day (RDA for adult women and men) into

   a) mmol   _____

23- Convert the serum reference range values of 1.6–2.6 mg **magnesium**/dL into

   a) mg/L   _____

   b) mmol/L   _____

   c) mEq/L   _____

24- Convert the urine reference range values of 3.0–5.0 mmol **magnesium** per 24 hours into

   a) mg/24 hours   _____

   b) mEq/24 hours   _____

INTEGRATE YOUR LEARNING

1. Kidneys are important for the activation of vitamin _____

   a) A   b) C   c) D   d) E   e) K

2. What is the main waste product of amino acid catabolism?

   _____

3. The two most common causes of chronic kidney disease are

   a) glomerulonephritis and hypertension
   b) diabetes mellitus and systemic lupus erythematous
   c) glomerulonephritis and urinary infections
   d) kidney obstruction and polycystic kidney disease
   e) hypertension and diabetes mellitus

4. Which of the following two healthy individuals has the highest plasma creatinine concentration: a young adult man or an elderly woman? Why?

_____

_____

_____

_____

5. Is the creatinine height index a useful tool to estimate muscle mass and protein-energy nutritional status in clients with pre–end-stage renal disease or end-stage renal disease? Why or why not?

_____

_____

_____

_____

6. Do high-protein diets cause chronic renal failure? Explain.

_____

_____

_____

7. One of your renal clients on a fluid restriction is suffering from thirst. Give 10 practical tips to help him control his fluid intake and reduce his thirst.

a) _____

b) _____

c) _____

d) _____

e) _____

f) _____

g) _____

h) _____

i) _____

j) _____

8. A low-protein, low-phosphorus diet is recommended for clients with pre-ESRD for the following reasons:

_____

_____

_____

_____

_____

9. These statements about the parathyroid hormone are true, <u>except</u>

a) it decreases bone resorption
b) it increases calcium reabsorption by the kidneys
c) it increases calcitriol production by the kidneys
d) it decreases kidney reabsorption of phosphorus
e) its production decreases in response to an increase in serum calcium concentration

10. These foods are high in potassium, <u>except</u>

    a) cola beverages   b) melons   c) seeds   d) bananas   e) baked potatoes

11. These foods are high in phosphorus, <u>except</u>

    a) liver   b) baked beans   c) oranges   d) chocolate   e) nuts

12. The protein and energy needs of clients with pre–end-stage renal disease are _____ g and

    _____ kcal/kg (2.2 lb) ideal/desirable body weight per day, respectively.

    a) 0.2; 25   b) 0.5; 30   c) 0.8; 35   d) 1.1; 40   e) 1.3; 45

13. In a catabolic client, cell breakdown releases _____, which increases in the blood.

    a) potassium   b) sodium   c) magnesium   d) chloride   e) phosphorus

14. High serum _____ concentration makes clients feel very itchy and causes muscle spasms.

    a) magnesium   b) chloride   c) potassium   d) calcium   e) phosphorus

15. These statements about the management of renal bone disease in clients with pre–end-stage renal disease are true, <u>except</u>

    a) these clients need to avoid legumes and whole grain products
    b) these clients may end up requiring a parathyroidectomy
    c) these clients need to avoid colas and chocolate
    d) these clients need to take phosphate binders between meals
    e) these clients need to avoid nuts and seeds

16. Low serum _____ concentration is the biggest predictor of morbidity and mortality in clients with renal disease.

    a) creatinine   b) urea   c) potassium   d) albumin   e) phosphorus

17. Which abnormal biochemical test values are typically seen in clients with nephrotic syndrome?

    _____

    _____

    _____

    _____

    _____

    _____

    _____

    _____

    _____

    _____

    _____

    _____

    _____

    _____

    _____

18. Which drug may help reduce protein loss in urine in clients with nephrotic syndrome?

    a) Furosemide   b) Clofibrate c) Amiloride   d) Captopril   e) Spironolactone

19. What is the only cure for clients with end-stage renal failure?

    _____

20. In clients using continuous ambulatory peritoneal dialysis, the _____ serves as a natural dialyzing membrane.

21. These are appropriate dietary recommendations for clients requiring **hemodialysis**, <u>except</u>

    a) fluid intake should be restricted to urine output plus two to four cups (500–1000 mL) per day
    b) potassium intake is usually limited to 50–77 mmol/day
    c) calcium intake should be 2.0–2.5 g/day
    d) sodium intake should be restricted to 43–130 mmol/day
    e) protein intake should be 1.2–1.3 g/kg (or per 2.2 lb) of edema-free body weight per day

22. These are accurate statements regarding clients on **peritoneal dialysis**, <u>except</u>

    a) clients with peritoneal dialysis tend to gain weight due to the presence of dextrose in the dialysis solution
    b) clients with peritoneal dialysis need a high protein diet of 1.2–1.3 g protein per kg (or per 2.2 lb) of edema-free body weight per day
    c) phosphorus intake should be 800–1000 mg/day
    d) sodium intake should be 87–174 mEq/day.
    e) potassium intake should be limited to 50 mEq/day

23. Summarize the general dietary recommendations for protein, phosphorus, sodium, and potassium that are usually appropriate for clients with the following renal diseases.

DIETARY RECOMMENDATIONS FOR CLIENTS WITH VARIOUS RENAL DISEASES*				
Nutrients → Renal Diseases ↓	Protein (g/kg/day)	Phosphorus (g/day)	Sodium (g/day)	Potassium (g/day)
1- **Pre-ESRD**				
2- **Nephrotic syndrome (without dialysis)**				
3- **Acute renal failure (without dialysis)**				
4- **ESRD with hemodialysis**				
5- **ESRD with peritoneal dialysis**				

* Dietary recommendations must be individualized to each client and his or her current medical status and situation.

24. Indicate if you would in general recommend (yes), ask to limit the amount to a minimum (limit), or not recommend (no) these common foods to clients with the following renal diseases. Justify your answers

GENERAL FOOD RECOMMENDATIONS FOR CLIENTS WITH VARIOUS RENAL DISEASES*

Renal Diseases → Foods ↓	Pre-ESRD	Nephrotic Syndrome (without dialysis)	Acute Renal Failure (without dialysis)	ESRD with Hemodialysis Dialysis	ESRD with Peritoneal
1- Cured ham					
2- Egg					
3- Lentils					
4- Milk					
5- Plain raw peanuts					
6- Orange					
7- Banana					
8- Whole wheat bread					
9- Cooked white rice					
10- Canola oil					
11- Baked ground beef					
12- Raisins					
13- Jellybean candies					
14- Baked potato					

* Food recommendations must be individualized to each client and his or her current medical status and situation.

CHALLENGE YOUR LEARNING

CASE STUDY

Objectives

This case will help you understand the complexity of renal disorders, which is partly due to the many important physiologic functions of the kidneys, and therefore, to realize that the care given to help clients is also complex and multifaceted and should be well coordinated by the different members of the multidisciplinary health care teams.

It will also help you understand how chronic systemic disorders can lead to other chronic disorders, such as kidney disorders and hyperlipidemias.

In addition, it will familiarize you with food habits of African Americans and some traditional foods they may consume, and help you become aware that clients with renal disease are susceptible to drug–nutrient interactions.

Description

Mr. M.B. is a 59-year-old African American man. He presented to the local community hospital with significant edema last Monday. His wife said: "His legs are like tree trunks and he cannot put on his shoes."

Mr. M.B. gained 9 lb in the past 4 weeks. His body weight at admission was 201 lb. He has a medium bone frame and is 5'10" tall.

Mr. M.B. has had mild systemic lupus erythematous for about 25 years. His mother had the disease too, although a more severe form of it, and passed away when Mr. M.B. was only a teenager. Due to this disease, Mr. M.B. has been suffering from nonerosive arthritis, which often limits his physical activities due to joint pain. He is taking corticosteroids and immunosuppressive medication to manage the disease. Last month, he had an exacerbation of the disease and had to stay home until he got better. As a result, he had to quit his contract job at the gas station and became unemployed. His wife and teenage daughter work at a large retail store in town, but the cost of medications for Mr. M.B. is increasing.

A 24-hour urine collection reveals that Mr. M.B. excretes 6 g protein per day. His other hematologic test values can be found in this table.

HEMATOLOGICAL TEST VALUES FOR MR. M.B.

Blood Tests	Results in Conventional Units	Reference Ranges in Conventional Units	Results in International Units	Reference Ranges in SI Units	Interpretation of Results (Normal, High, or Low)
Albumin	2.4 g/dL	3.2–5.2	g/L		
Creatinine	1.2 mg/dL	0.7–1.3	μmol/L		
Urea nitrogen	19 mg/dL	6–20	mmol/L		
Sodium	138 mEq/L	136–145	mmol/L		
Phosphate	4.02 mg/dL	2.7–4.5	mmol/L		
Potassium	4.4 mEq/L	3.5–5.1	mmol/L		

(continued)

Blood Tests	Results in Conventional Units	Reference Ranges in Conventional Units	Results in International Units	Reference Ranges in SI Units	Interpretation of Results (Normal, High, or Low)
HEMATOLOGICAL TEST VALUES FOR MR. M.B. *(continued)*					
Calcium	9.32 mg/dL	8.6–10.0	mmol/L		
Total chol.*	243 mg/dL	<200[ψζ]	mmol/L		
LDL chol.*	197 mg/dL	<100[ψ] <97[ζ]	mmol/L		
HDL chol.*	42.5 mg/dL	≥60[ψ] >50[ζ]	mmol/L		
Triglycerides*	157 mg/dL	<150[ψζ]	mmol/L		

* Fasting values.
[ψ] Desirable values for Mr. M.B., according to the Expert Panel on Detection, Evaluation, and Treatment of High Blood Cholesterol in Adults. Executive summary of the third report of the National Cholesterol Education Program (NCEP) expert panel on detection, evaluation, and treatment of high blood cholesterol in adults (Adult Treatment Panel III). JAMA 2001;19(285):2486–2497.
[ζ] Desirable values for Mr. M.B., according to Genest J, Frohlich J, Fodor G, et al. (The Working Group on Hypercholesterolemia and other Dyslipidemias). Recommendations for the management of dyslipidemia and the prevention of cardiovascular disease: 2003 update. Can Med Assoc J 2003;168(9):921–924.

Mr. M.B.'s diet history shows that he usually has a good appetite. He eats protein at each meal in the form of bacon, eggs, boiled peanuts, country ham, and homemade deep-fried chicken and catfish. He is lactose intolerant and prefers carbonated beverages to milk. He likes fried cornbread or corn pone, string beans, succotash, coleslaw, and homestyle fried potatoes. He tries not to add too much salt at the table, but he snacks on potato chips, benne seed candy, Crenshaw pie, and cola beverages at night.

The physician right away readjusted Mr. M.B.'s medication for his systemic lupus erythematous and prescribed torsemide, ramipril, and atorvastatin.

1. Why is Mr. M.B.'s wife saying that his legs are like "tree trunks"?

2. What was Mr. M.B.'s weight prior to the last 4 weeks?

3. Give your interpretation of Mr. M.B.'s BMI prior to the last 4 weeks.

4. What is systemic lupus erythematous?

5. Complete the table of **hematologic test values of Mr. M.B.** by converting the data from conventional units into international units and giving your interpretation of Mr. M.B.'s test results compared to the reference ranges.

6. What is your interpretation of Mr. M.B.'s renal disorder based on the biochemical and clinical data?

7. Is there a link between Mr. M.B.'s renal disorder and his systemic lupus erythematous? Explain your answer.

8. Why do clients with this kidney disorder develop hyperlipidemia?

9. What other factors could be contributing to Mr. M.B.'s hyperlipidemia?

10. Determine the glomerular filtration rate of Mr. M.B., based on his serum creatinine concentration, age, sex, and ethnicity. (*Tip: Visit the Web site of the National Kidney Foundation and use the online GFR calculator, which can be found at http://www.kidney.org/professionals/tools/.*)

11. Give your interpretation of Mr. M.B.'s glomerular filtration rate.

12. Explain the following foods commonly eaten by African Americans like Mr. M.B.

    a) Boiled peanuts:

    b) Country ham:

    c) Deep-fried catfish:

    d) Cornbread:

    e) Corn pone:

    f) String beans:

    g) Succotash:

    h) Benne seed candy:

    i) Crenshaw pie:

13. What is your interpretation of Mr. M.B.'s usual diet from his diet history?

14. What are the main possible side effects of taking corticosteroids?

15. What is torsemide and why is it prescribed to Mr. M.B.?

16. What is ramipril and why is it prescribed to Mr. M.B.?

17. What is atorvastatin and why is it prescribed to Mr. M.B.?

18. What are the effects of torsemide and ramipril on potassium metabolism?

19. What information would be useful to better assess Mr. M.B.'s nutritional status?

20. Provide four goals of medical nutrition therapy appropriate for Mr. M.B.

    1)

    2)

    3)

    4)

21. Is a high-protein diet indicated for Mr. M.B.? Why or why not?

22. What type of diet would you recommend for Mr. M.B.? Justify in detail each element of your dietary recommendation.

7.14 Neurologic and Psychiatric Disorders

REVIEW THE INFORMATION

1. The _____ system is likely the most complex and remarkable anatomic and functional component of the human body.

2. What are the two main parts of the nervous system?

    a) _____

    b) _____

3. Give the term(s) corresponding to each definition.

   a) _____ are psychiatric conditions characterized by unhealthy feeding behaviors leading to malnutrition and/or an increased risk of disease. They may include frequent fasting or overeating, binge-eating episodes, obsession with food and body shape, excessive control or lack of control over eating, and/or eating nonfood substances.

   b) _____ is an eating disorder characterized by repeated occurrence of binge-eating episodes followed by repeatedly inappropriate compensations to avoid weight gain (two or more times a week for ≥3 months), and disturbance of body image.

   c) _____ is an abnormal and obsessive ingestion of dirt or clay.

   d) _____ is an eating disorder characterized by food restriction, underweight, and refusal to maintain normal/healthy body weight or to gain weight during growth, extreme fear of gaining weight and being fat, excessive desire to be thin, disturbance of body image, and amenorrhea.

   e) _____ is an eating disorder characterized by repeated occurrence of binge-eating episodes, but not followed by repeatedly inappropriate compensations to avoid weight gain as in clients with bulimia nervosa.

   f) _____ is an abnormal compulsion to ingest substances of little or no nutritional value over a sustained period of time.

   g) _____ are characterized by disordered food intake patterns that do not correspond to the criteria of other specific eating disorders, such as anorexia nervosa and bulimia nervosa.

   h) _____ is defined as chronic excessive and/or compulsive alcohol consumption leading to frequent intoxication and dependence, and resulting in the impairment of an individual's nutritional status and health, as well as in the individual's ability to work or fulfill social obligations.

4. Two structures form the central nervous system. What are they?

   a) _____

   b) _____

5. The central nervous system is composed of specialized cells called _____. These cells are considered to be the nervous system's units of structure and function.

   a) astrocytes   b) dendrites   c) neurons   d) synapses   e) axons

6. The peripheral nervous system is made up of cranial and spinal _____ and corresponding ganglia.

7. The a) _____ part of the nervous system regulates the body's involuntary structures like the heart, glands, and smooth muscles, whereas the b) _____ part of the nervous system controls the body's voluntary activities.

8. Which part of the brain is in charge of the autonomic nervous system and is a major regulator of the body's homeostasis?

   a) The gray matter   c) The white matter   e) The occipital lobe
   b) The corpus callosum   d) The hypothalamus

9. The a) _____ component of the autonomic nervous system is in charge of the body's emergency and defense reactions, while its b) _____ component works to keep and restore the body's energy.

10. Which cranial nerve innervates a large part of the alimentary tract, including the pharynx, esophagus, stomach, liver, and pancreas, as well as the heart, larynx, trachea, and lungs?

   _____

11. What is myelin and where is it found?

   _____

   _____

12. What source of energy does the brain rely almost exclusively on?

13. Indicate in this table which nutrient deficiencies negatively impact the brain.

EFFECT OF NUTRIENT DEFICIENCIES ON THE BRAIN	
Negative Effects on the Brain	**Nutrient Deficiencies**
a) Brain lesions due to beriberi	
b) Cretinism	
c) Degeneration of brain tissue	
d) Wernicke's encephalopathy	
e) Dementia	
f) Short attention span, withdrawal, developmental delays	

14. Aging itself is associated with a gradual decrease of blood supply to the brain and a reduction of the number of neurons, which causes a progressive decrease in

    a) hearing and speech   c) balance and posture   e) all of the above
    b) memory   d) cognitive function

15. Which mental disorder is a senile type of dementia causing degeneration of the brain, memory loss, and structural changes in neuron networks?

UNDERSTAND THE CONCEPTS

1. List the functions of the nervous system.

2. Define the following terms related to the nervous system and mental functions.

    a) Neurology:

    b) Psychiatry:

    c) Psychology:

d) Cognition: _____

e) Intelligence: _____

f) Mental health: _____

g) Mental illness: _____

h) Activities of daily living: _____

i) Degenerative disorders of the nervous system: _____

j) Demyelinating diseases: _____

k) Myelopathy: _____

l) Dementia : _____

m) Psychosis: _____

n) Neurosis: _____

o) Hallucination: _____

p) Illusion: _____

q) Delusion: _____

r) Atrophy: _____

s) Paresis: _____

t) Hemiparesis: _____

u) Agnosia: _____

v) Echolalia: _____

w) Anomia: _____

_____

3. List the main psychiatric disorders.

_____

_____

_____

_____

_____

_____

_____

_____

4. What are the two main causes of irreversible dementia?

a) _____

b) _____

5. Does overdose of micronutrients have a negative impact on the brain? Justify your answer.

_____

_____

_____

_____

_____

6. Name four degenerative disorders of the nervous system.

a) _____

b) _____

c) _____

d) _____

7. What is the most frequent origin of dementia in the elderly?

_____

8. Many psychiatric disorders affect the limbic system. What is the limbic system?

_____

_____

9. What are the main demyelinating diseases?

_____

_____

10. What is the most frequent central nervous system disorder that affects young adults in North America?

_____

11. Recognize the disorders affecting the nervous system from this list.

_____ Amyotrophic lateral sclerosis (ALS)   _____ Parkinson's disease   _____ Multiple sclerosis

_____ Huntington's disease   _____ Schizophrenia   _____ Leukodystrophy

a) A group of psychotic disorders characterized by delusions, hallucinations, aberrant behavior, loss of contact with others and the environment, inappropriate expression of feelings, inability to function in daily life, isolation, and paranoia

b) A chronic, autoimmune, demyelinating disorder of the central nervous system producing inflammation and scarring of myelin sheaths and formation of hardened plaques in the brain's white matter and in the spinal cord

c) A chronic, degenerative, neurologic disorder associated with reduced levels of dopamine causing tremor, slow and rigid movements, lack of balance, shuffling gait, and weary posture

d) A progressive, fatal, degenerative disorder of the spinal cord resulting in increasing muscular atrophy, convulsive muscle irritability, and widespread muscular weakness; also called Lou Gehrig's disease

e) A group of chronic demyelinating diseases, some of which are inherited, resulting in absence or progressive degenerative disorders of myelin in the central nervous system

f) An autosomal dominant inherited degenerative disorder of the central nervous system causing chorea and dementia

12. The intake in protein and amino acids is important for the synthesis of neurotransmitters. The amino acid _____ is the precursor of serotonin, a neurotransmitter involved in appetite and mood regulation.

   a) methionine   b) lysine   c) arginine   d) tryptophan   e) phenylalanine

13. The brain is composed of _____ % structural lipids.

   a) 30   b) 40   c) 50   d) 60   e) 70

14. What is the impact of Alzheimer's disease on the nutritional status of clients? Why?

INTEGRATE YOUR LEARNING

1. Which micronutrient is the most important for the prevention of mental health disorders worldwide from a public health perspective?

   a) Zinc   b) Iodine   c) Iron   d) Selenium   e) Calcium

2. Is it normal for elderly individuals to develop Alzheimer's disease? Explain.

   _____

   _____

3. What is the effect of deficiency of the following nutrients on the brain?

   a) Iodine

   _____

   _____

   _____

   _____

   b) Iron

   _____

   _____

   _____

   _____

c) Zinc

_____

_____

_____

_____

d) Thiamin

_____

_____

_____

_____

e) Niacin

_____

_____

_____

_____

f) Cyanocobalamin

_____

_____

_____

_____

4. What other micronutrient deficiencies may alter normal brain development and function?

_____

_____

_____

_____

5. How do the following disorders affect food intake?

a) Anorexia nervosa

_____

_____

b) Marijuana addiction

_____

_____

c) Depression

_____

_____

d) Schizophrenia

_____

_____

6. What are important goals of nutrition care in clients with disorders of the nervous system due to nutritional deficiency or overdose?

_____

_____

_____

_____

_____

_____

_____

_____

_____

7. What are important goals of nutrition care for clients with chronic disorders of the nervous system?

_____

_____

_____

_____

_____

_____

_____

_____

_____

8. Your clients with dementia have the following eating behaviors, which negatively impact their food intake, nutritional status, and well-being. How can you help each of them?

Client A

Problem behavior: Very slow eater

Suggestions:

_____

_____

_____

_____

_____

_____

_____

_____

Client B

Problem behavior: Plays with food instead of eating

Suggestions:

_____

_____

_____

_____

_____

_____

_____

_____

Client C

Problem behavior: Thinks food has been poisoned by someone spying on him (paranoia)

Suggestions:

_____

_____

_____

_____

_____

_____

_____

_____

9. What types of medications are commonly used to manage psychiatric disorders? Give some examples for each type.

_____

_____

_____

_____

_____

_____

_____

_____

_____

_____

_____

_____

CHALLENGE YOUR LEARNING

CASE STUDY

Objectives

This case will raise your awareness of the fact that clients with chronic disorders of the nervous system are often at risk of malnutrition as their disease progresses.

It will also help you understand the importance of quality of life for clients with degenerative disorders of the nervous system.

Description

Mrs. V.R. is a 49-year-old woman. She has been admitted to the neurology unit of St. Andrew's Hospital 3 days ago due to an exacerbation of her multiple sclerosis.

Mrs. V.R. is Italian. She was a dance artist who immigrated at age 20 with her husband. She taught ballet and jazz at a dance studio and performed as part of a few theatrical productions. She had a busy social life until she was diagnosed with relapsing-remitting multiple sclerosis in 1990. This gradually brought her artistic career to an end.

Furthermore, her husband left her 3 years ago and she has since been living on her own in an apartment with minimal financial resources and no family support. Mrs. V.R. has been depressed and has been blaming her disease for her recent years of misery. She finds it less painful to live in the past. She frequently spends her afternoons listening to music and daydreaming. She also likes snacking and watching television.

Prior to her hospital admission, she received regular visits from community health support services to assist her with activities of daily living. A personal support worker came in the morning to help her get in her wheelchair, clean herself, take her medications, and prepare some meals for the day. Mrs. V.R. enjoyed the company and talked about her dancing years. Mrs. V.R. is wheelchair bound, as she cannot move her legs and feet. She weighs 204 lb and measures 5′4″.

At admission, Mrs. V.R. was complaining of headaches, diplopia, and hip pain. She had urinary incontinence. She looked tired and pale, and her face was puffy with edema. Her speech was slow and hard to understand. She was depressed and had poor appetite. Dysarthria, nystagmus, facial numbness, paresthesia, alopecia, and an infected pressure sore at the left hip were also noted at physical examination. Her serum albumin concentration was 2.8 g/dL (28 g/L) and serum transthyretin concentration, 10 mg/dL (100 mg/L).

The nutrition assistant who visited her at mealtime noticed that Mrs. V.R. masticated very slowly, ate very little, and coughed after drinking. She reported that Mrs. V.R.'s voice had a gurgly sound.

To make things worse, her landlord took her apartment away from her while Mrs. V.R. was at the hospital. Mrs. V.R. had mood changes and rarely remembered to pay her rent. Social workers are presently trying to sort out this situation and find Mrs. V.R. a place in a long-term care institution, where she can be transferred when she is discharged from the acute care hospital.

1. Define multiple sclerosis.

2. List the different types of multiple sclerosis, according to the rate of progression of the disease. Explain each type.

3. What are typical signs and symptoms of multiple sclerosis?

4. Do you think Mrs. V.R. has dysphagia? Justify your answer.

5. What signs and symptoms of multiple sclerosis is Mrs. V.R. experiencing?

6. What are diplopia, nystagmus, dysarthria, alopecia, and paresthesia?

7. Calculate Mrs. V.R.'s BMI and give its interpretation.

8. Give your assessment of Mrs. V.R.'s protein status based on the data provided.

9. Is Mrs. V.R. at nutritional risk? Why or why not?

10. What would you do for Mrs. V.R. if you were the dietitian at the neurology unit of St. Andrew's Hospital referred to the case by the physician in charge? Give a list of your top five priorities of action for Mrs. V.R.

   1)

   2)

   3)

   4)

   5)

7.15 Nutrition Support

REVIEW THE INFORMATION

1. Explain what "giving nutrition support" means.

2. What are oral nutritional supplements?

3. What is enteral nutrition?

4. What is parenteral nutrition?

5. What are fructooligosaccharides and why are they added to some oral and enteral nutrition formulas?

_____

_____

_____

6. What type of oral nutritional supplements can be offered to clients on a clear liquid diet?

_____

_____

7. What is the danger with pulmonary aspiration?

_____

_____

_____

_____

8. The _____ is a metabolic syndrome caused by overly aggressive nourishment of malnourished clients and resulting in potentially fatal complications. The group of symptoms, due to abnormal serum electrolyte concentrations (mainly low potassium, phosphorus, and magnesium levels), include lethargy, fatigue, lightheadedness, cardiac arrhythmia, muscle weakness, and hemolysis.

9. Provide the meaning for these abbreviations.

a) i.v. or I.V. _____

b) MCT _____

c) LCT _____

d) EFA _____

e) FOS _____

f) HN _____

g) Lytes _____

h) CBC _____

i) NPO _____

j) GI _____

k) PEG _____

l) EN _____

m) PN _____

n) TPN _____

o) Abd _____

p) CNSD _____

q) ICU _____

r) NICU _____

10. Fill in the blank space with the appropriate term corresponding to each definition.

a) A _____ is an abnormal passage or connection between one epithelium and another, such as between an organ and an adjacent structure like the skin, vessel, or another organ.

b) A _____ is a mouth or opening, possibly created through medical intervention.

c) A _____ is an artificial opening between the stomach and the skin surface created by surgery.

d) A _____ is a slight or partial paralysis of the stomach that impairs its emptying.

e) A _____ is an artificial opening between the jejunum and the skin surface created by surgery.

f) Intestinal _____ is the erosion of the structure (reduction of the length of finger-like projections) and impairment of the function (decreased number of transporters per cell) of the intestinal villi cells causing maldigestion, malabsorption of nutrients, and faster intestinal transit.

UNDERSTAND THE CONCEPTS

1. Give examples of homemade oral nutritional supplements.

_____

_____

_____

_____

_____

_____

2. What do the following abbreviations stand for?

a) TF _____

b) LFT _____

c) CPN _____

d) PPN _____

e) TNA _____

f) PEJ _____

g) PICC _____

h) NG _____

i) NGT _____

j) HEN _____

k) HPN _____

l) PEG-G or PEG/G _____

m) PEG-J or PEG/J _____

3. Define these terms related to nutrition support and its complications.

a) Ileus: _____

_____

b) Hypercapnia: _____

_____

c) Excoriation: _____

_____

d) Gastric residuals: _____

_____

e) Atresia: _____
_____

f) Epistaxis: _____
_____

g) Empyema: _____
_____

4. Describe these three main types of commercial oral and enteral nutritional supplements and give some examples of each.

a) Complete nutritional formulas: _____
_____

Examples: _____
_____

b) Noncomplete nutritional formulas: _____
_____

Examples: _____
_____

c) Nutrient supplements (or modular formulas): _____
_____

Examples: _____
_____

5. Differentiate between *polymeric* and *monomeric* oral or enteral nutritional formulas. Provide some examples.
_____
_____
_____
_____
_____
_____
_____
_____
_____

6. Compare the osmolality of elemental and polymeric formulas and explain why it is usually different.
_____
_____
_____
_____
_____
_____
_____

7. Give examples of low-residue, lactose-free polymeric oral or enteral nutritional formulas that are standard, enriched in energy, enriched in nitrogen, or enriched in energy and nitrogen.

   a) Standard formulas: _____

   _____

   _____

   b) Formulas enriched in energy: _____

   _____

   _____

   c) Formulas enriched in nitrogen: _____

   _____

   _____

   d) Formulas enriched in energy and nitrogen: _____

   _____

   _____

8. Find examples of oral or enteral nutritional formulas specifically designed for these situations:

   a) Diabetes mellitus: _____

   _____

   _____

   b) Pulmonary disease: _____

   _____

   _____

   c) Renal disease: _____

   _____

   _____

   d) Liver disease: _____

   _____

   _____

   e) Critical care: _____

   _____

   _____

   f) Trauma and metabolic stress: _____

   _____

   _____

   g) Crohn's disease: _____

   _____

   _____

h) Dysphagia: _____

_____

_____

i) Constipation: _____

_____

_____

j) Fat malabsorption: _____

_____

_____

k) Immune support: _____

_____

_____

l) Pediatric disorders: _____

_____

_____

9. Identify when it is indicated or contraindicated to give enteral or parenteral nutrition support.

INDICATIONS AND CONTRAINDICATIONS FOR ENTERAL OR PARENTERAL NUTRITION		
Possible Symptoms	Indications	Contraindications
Enteral Nutrition		
Parenteral Nutrition		

10. List the advantages and disadvantages of enteral versus parenteral nutrition support.

ADVANTAGES AND DISADVANTAGES OF ENTERAL VERSUS PARENTERAL NUTRITION		
Type of Nutrition Support	Advantages	Disadvantages
Enteral Nutrition		
Parenteral Nutrition		

11. Which factors should be taken into consideration when choosing the type of enteral nutrition formula to use?

_____

_____

_____

_____

_____

12. Identify what enteral feeding routes can be used for administration of enteral nutrition formula.

_____

_____

_____

_____

_____

_____

13. What factors influence the selection of an enteral feeding route?

_____

_____

_____

14. What are the different methods of administration for enteral nutrition formulas?

15. How should hospitalized clients receiving enteral nutrition be monitored?

16. Why are gastric residuals monitored when feeding enterally?

17. A client with a daily energy need of 2000 kcal and fluid need of 2000 mL is being fed exclusively with an enteral nutrition formula with an energy density of 1.2 kcal/mL and containing 82% free water. The client is receiving continuous feeding and IV medication containing 50 mL water per day. He is also given 250 mL water orally per day. How much extra water should this client receive in flushes every 4 hours?

18. What mechanical, gastrointestinal, and metabolic complications may arise when providing enteral nutrition support?

- Mechanical complications:

_____

_____

_____

_____

_____

_____

- Gastrointestinal complications:

_____

_____

_____

_____

- Metabolic complications:

_____

_____

_____

_____

19. What type of enteral feeding route and method of administration should be used for clients with gastroparesis or history of aspiration?

_____

_____

_____

_____

_____

20. List the different routes of PN delivery available.

_____

_____

_____

_____

_____

_____

_____

_____

21. What source of carbohydrate is used for PN and what is its energy density?

_____

_____

22. The two micronutrients <u>not</u> routinely included in TPN formulas are

a) sodium and biotin   c) cyanocobalamin and chromium   e) iodine and pantothenic acid
b) iron and vitamin K   d) selenium and manganese

23. Clients receiving parenteral nutrition support are at risk of which metabolic complications?

_____

_____

_____

_____

_____

24. Give three complications resulting from carbohydrate overfeeding in TPN patients.

a) _____

b) _____

c) _____

25. The gastrointestinal tract more easily tolerates enteral nutrition support formulas that are iso-osmotic to serum or have an osmolality of about _____ mOsm or mmol/kg.

a) 180–210   b) 280–310   c) 300–420   d) 480–700   e) 1000–1300

26. The maximum feeding rate with intestinal feeding tubes is _____ mL/hr.

a) 25   b) 75   c) 125   d) 175   e) 250

27. _____ is an immunonutrient that may provide specific benefits to the immune system when added to the enteral nutrition support formula of patients with burns or trauma, or postsurgery.

a) Arginine   b) Alanine   c) Glycine   d) Glutamine   e) Cysteine

28. Which nutrient is "bacteriostatic"?

a) Selenium   b) Zinc   c) Iron   d) Cyanocobalamin   e) Magnesium

29. In TPN patients, the most common electrolyte and mineral imbalances are related to

a) phosphorus, sodium, and potassium   d) magnesium, phosphorus, and potassium
b) potassium, calcium, and sodium   e) sodium, magnesium, and calcium
c) sodium, magnesium, and phosphorus

30. TPN may be contraindicated or needs to be carefully monitored in clients with _____ allergy, depending on the severity of the allergy.

a) peanut   b) egg   c) milk   d) fish   e) soy

31. When ICU patients are unfed, each gram of nitrogen lost means that _____ g of lean body tissue have been catabolized.

a) 20   b) 30   c) 40   d) 50   e) 60

32. ICU patients lose an average of _____ g of nitrogen daily when NPO, which represents a loss of about _____ kg or _____ lb of lean body tissue per day.

   a) 5; 0.1; 0.2   b) 10; 0.2; 0.4   c) 25; 0.3; 0.7   d) 20; 0.4; 0.9   e) 15; 0.5; 1.1

33. Under optimal nutrition conditions, nutrition support can only provide a maximum of _____ g of true nitrogen retention to ICU clients, which translates to _____ mg of lean tissue synthesis per day.

   a) 1–2; 60   b) 2–3; 100   c) 3–4; 140   d) 4–5; 180   e) 5–6; 220

34. Terminal and irreversible malnutrition occurs when _____ % of the lean body mass has been lost.

   a) 10   b) 20   c) 30   d) 40   e) 50

35. There is a significant increase in protein requirements during critical illness and ICU clients often require _____ g protein per kg (or per 2.2 lb) body weight per day.

   a) 1.0–1.5   b) 1.5–2.0   c) 2.0–2.5   d) 2.5–3.0   e) 3.0–3.5

36. The use of _____ is hardly useful as a nutrition assessment tool in the ICU, as most clients have a short stay.

   a) nitrogen balance
   b) serum transthyretin concentration
   c) serum albumin concentration
   d) creatine height index
   e) bioelectric impedance analysis

37. _____ is the nutrition assessment tool providing the most accurate method of determining protein needs in ICU clients.

   a) Nitrogen balance
   b) Serum transthyretin concentration
   c) Serum albumin concentration
   d) Creatine height index
   e) Bioelectric impedance analysis

38. _____ is the nutritional parameter most consistently associated with improved outcomes in ICU clients.

   a) Nitrogen balance
   b) Serum transthyretin concentration
   c) Serum albumin concentration
   d) Creatine height index
   e) Bioelectric impedance analysis

39. ICU clients often have an "increase of third-space fluid." What does this mean?

   _____

   _____

   _____

40. Some ICU clients need a _____ supplement to support optimal protein synthesis and wound healing. Clients will not reach a positive nitrogen balance if they are deficient in this micronutrient, which is essential for protein synthesis.

INTEGRATE YOUR LEARNING

1. Which clients may require the use of parenteral nutrition support due to their medical condition?

   _____

   _____

   _____

   _____

   _____

_____
_____
_____
_____
_____
_____
_____
_____
_____
_____

2. Explain how an enteral formula with high osmolality can adversely affect the gastrointestinal tolerance of some clients.

_____
_____
_____
_____
_____
_____

3. One of your clients exclusively fed through enteral nutrition support has diarrhea. What are some possible reasons why clients receiving enteral nutrition may have diarrhea?

_____
_____
_____
_____
_____
_____
_____
_____

4. These statements about tube feeding administrations are true, <u>except</u>

a) clients can stand, sit, or lie flat on their bed when tube feeding
b) gastric feeding tubes allow continuous, intermittent, or bolus feeding schedules
c) the bolus feeding schedule often mimics meal times
d) a feeding pump is required for continuous feeding schedule, whereas bolus feeding is usually given using the gravity method
e) the tube has to be flushed before and after medication is administered to avoid drug–nutrient interactions or clogging of the tube

5. In which situation is enteral nutrition indicated?

   a) High-output proximal gastrointestinal fistula
   b) Terminal illness
   c) Intractable diarrhea
   d) Severe gastrointestinal hemorrhage
   e) Hepatic failure

6. Enteral nutrition is given if a normally nourished client is expected to be NPO for more than _____ days

   or if a malnourished client is expected to be NPO for more than _____ days.

   a) 2–3; 1–2   b) 3–5; 2–3   c) 5–7; 3–5   d) 7–9; 5–7   e) 9–11; 7–9

7. M.V. is a cancer client receiving enteral nutrition support through continuous nasogastric tube feeding. M.V.'s total energy requirement is presently 2446 kcal (10,225 kJ)/day and the enteral formula he needs contains 1.06 kcal/mL. What volume of formula will you (progressively increase toward and) ultimately give M.V. per hour to meet his entire energy requirement?

   _____

   _____

   _____

   _____

   _____

   _____

   _____

   _____

   _____

   _____

8. Which statement about enteral feeding tube placements is **incorrect**?

   a) A gastric feeding tube placement makes use of the whole intestine.
   b) An intestinal feeding tube placement reduces the risk of aspiration.
   c) Gastric emptying rate is not an issue with an intestinal feeding tube placement.
   d) An intestinal feeding tube placement allows for bolus feeding.
   e) A gastric feeding tube placement is easier to put in place than an intestinal feeding tube placement.

9. These statements about enteral formulas are true, <u>except</u>

   a) they meet daily micronutrient requirements in 1.1–5.3 quarts (1.0–1.5 liters)
   b) elemental formulas are used for impaired digestion or absorption
   c) elemental formulas are low in residues and tend to be hyperosmolar
   d) polymeric formulas can be administered into the stomach and duodenum, but not the jejunum
   e) some polymeric formulas contain MCT oil, fiber, or fructooligosaccharides

10. Which statement about nasogastric tubes is **false**?

    a) Patients may pull them out.
    b) They do not require surgery and they are comfortable.
    c) They are used short term (<6 weeks).
    d) There is risk of aspiration.
    e) There is risk of sinusitis.

11. Hepatology formulas (like Nutrihep and Hepatic AID II) are lower in

    a) aromatic amino acids   c) energy   e) phosphorus
    b) potassium   d) branched-chain amino acids

12. Which statement about nutrition support is **false**?

   a) Enteral nutrition is safer than parenteral nutrition.
   b) Prophylactic insertion of a parenteral nutrition tube in clients with head and neck cancer is standard procedure.
   c) Enteral nutrition is more cost effective than parenteral nutrition.
   d) Parenteral nutrition is used when the risk of starvation outweighs the risk associated with the administration of parenteral nutrition in malnourished clients.
   e) Parenteral nutrition is less physiologic than enteral nutrition.

13. Define the PICC route of PN delivery and explain its three main advantages compared to other PN routes.

   _____

   1) _____

   2) _____

   3) _____

14. Which TPN patients have increased electrolyte requirements?

   a) Malnourished patients with refeeding syndrome   d) Patients with congestive heart failure
   b) Patients with renal failure   e) Patients with diabetes mellitus
   c) Patients with liver disease

15. What are criticisms to protocols usually used to initiate enteral nutrition support in ICU clients?

   _____

   _____

   _____

   _____

   _____

   _____

16. The most common cause of diarrhea in ICU patients is

   a) the high strength of the tube feed   d) the high osmolality of the tube feed
   b) the lack of use of a starter regimen for the tube feed   e) an altered GI flora due to antibiotic use
   c) the high rate of the tube feed

17. The following are potential complications of nasoenteric tube feeding, <u>except</u>

   a) otitis media   c) myocardial infarction   e) epistaxis
   b) ileal perforation   d) empyema

CHALLENGE YOUR LEARNING

CASE STUDY

Objectives

This case will help you assess the nutritional status of a client, outline nutrition care plan goals for her, and plan the detail of her enteral nutrition support regimen.

It will also help you realize that nutrition support requires well-developed practice skills and knowledge.

Description

Mrs. M.C. is a 65-year-old Chinese woman who has been residing at the Long Point Long-Term Care facility for the last 5 years. On December 24, she was taken to the emergency room of St. Paul's Hospital in the morning, after regurgitating formula and pulling out her nasogastric tube.

During the past 3 years, Mrs. M.C. has been fed exclusively by enteral nutrition because of her severe dysphagia, which resulted from her history of cerebrovascular accidents. She cannot tolerate any oral fluids or food intake. Other consequences of her cerebrovascular accidents, which she had at 60 and 62 years of age, are aphasia, limited understanding of her environment, and very reduced overall mobility. Mrs. M.C. has been gaining weight steadily since her first cerebrovascular accident, from a usual body weight of 155 lb. In addition, Mrs. M.C.'s medical history shows that she has hypercholesterolemia, hypertriglyceridemia, and hypothyroidism. In the past, she used to drink heavily and smoke a pack of cigarettes a week.

Mrs. M.C. started to experience fever, agitation, and mild distress in the days before her arrival at St. Paul's Hospital. The physician who examined her observed that she had a congested chest, difficulty breathing, partial airway obstruction with mucopurulent secretions, accumulation of fluids in the sacral area, and nasolabial irritation.

Mrs. M.C. received antibiotics, Lasix, and intravenous fluids (D_5/0.45 saline with 20 KCl at 125 mL/hr) until a PEG-J tube could be put in place. Unfortunately, because of limited staffing resources and an overload of clients at that time of the year, Mrs. M.C. received intravenous fluids for 15 days until her PEG-J was finally put in place this morning for her tube feed to be started. Mrs. M.C. weighed 185 lb at admission to the hospital, and she presently weighs 180 lb. During this period, her serum transthyretin concentration dropped from 16 to 11 mg/dL (160 to 110 mg/L).

1. What should be done when a client on enteral nutrition support is regurgitating?

2. Give possible reasons why Mrs. M.C. was regurgitating.

3. Why do you think Mrs. M.C. has a fever and congested chest?

4. Why do you think Mrs. M.C. pulled her feeding tube out?

5. Given that Mrs. M.C. is 5'1" tall, what is your interpretation of her usual body weight?

6. What was her weight change in the last 5 years? How can this be explained?

7. What is your interpretation of her body weight at hospital admission?

8. Why was Mrs. M.C. given Lasix?

9. How much energy was Mrs. M.C. receiving through her intravenous fluid infusion?

10. Why did the intravenous solution contain KCl?

11. What is your interpretation of Mrs. M.C.'s current nutritional status?

12. What is Mrs. M.C.'s adjusted body weight?

13. Calculate Mrs. M.C.'s current energy needs (TEE) using the modified Harris-Benedict method.

    Reminder: *BEE for women (kcal/day) = 655 + 9.56 W + 1.85 H − 4.7 A*
    or
    BEE for women (kJ/day) = 2743 + 40 W + 7.7 H − 19.7 A

14. Determine Mrs. M.C.'s current protein needs.

15. Determine Mrs. M.C.'s current fluid needs.

16. Why do you think a PEG-J was selected as the feeding route for Mrs. M.C. this time?

17. What type of enteral nutrition formula would you give Mrs. M.C.?

18. Select a formula and determine the amount of formula that Mrs. M.C. needs per day to meet her energy and protein needs.

19. What method of administration would you select to tube feed Mrs. M.C. right now? Why?

20. What would be your infusion rate goal to meet Mrs. M.C.'s daily nutritional needs (according to the formula you selected in question 18)?

21. How would you initiate and increase the rate of infusion of the enteral formula for Mrs. M.C.? Why?

22. What parameters will you monitor?

23. How much water will be given through regular flushes if the intravenous fluids are no longer administered, but 200 mL water per day is required to administer medications (and according to the formula you selected in question 18)?

24. What are the short-term goals of nutrition care for Mrs. M.C.?

7.16 Food/Nutrient–Drug Interactions

REVIEW THE INFORMATION

1. Define polypharmacy.

   _____

   _____

   _____

2. Who is at risk of polypharmacy?

   _____

   _____

   _____

   _____

   _____

   _____

   _____

3. Long-term intake of _____ for the management of inflammation increases the need for calcium and vitamin D, as chronic intake of these drugs is associated with a loss of bone density and osteoporosis, and increases the risk of spontaneous fractures.

   a) antacids   c) antibiotics   e) antihistamines
   b) corticosteroids   d) diuretics

4. _____ increase stomach pH and reduce the bioavailability of iron, calcium, folate, thiamin, and vitamin A.

   a) Antacids   c) Antibiotics   e) Antihistamines
   b) Corticosteroids   d) Diuretics

5. Clients taking coumarin drugs should be instructed to keep their intake of _____ consistent, so that the dosage of their anticoagulant can be adjusted to prevent nutrient–drug interactions.

6. Which of the following drugs are used to stimulate appetite in clients with cachexia?

   a) Megace   c) Marinol   e) All of the above
   b) Dexamethasone   d) Cyproheptadine

UNDERSTAND THE CONCEPTS

1. Define the following terms.

a) Pharmacy: _____

_____

_____

b) Pharmacology: _____

_____

_____

c) Pharmacodynamics: _____

_____

_____

d) Pharmacokinetics: _____

_____

_____

e) Interaction: _____

_____

_____

f) Drug–drug interaction: _____

_____

_____

g) Drug–nutrient interaction: _____

_____

_____

h) Toxicology: _____

_____

_____

i) Bioavailability: _____

_____

_____

j) Biotransformation: _____

_____

_____

k) Half-life: _____

_____

_____

l) Side effect: _____

_____

_____

m) Precipitation: _____

_____

_____

n) Chelation: _____

_____

_____

2. What is the first-pass metabolism of drugs?

_____

_____

_____

_____

3. Which individuals are at increased risk of adverse drug–nutrient interactions?

_____

_____

_____

_____

_____

_____

_____

_____

_____

_____

4. How may drugs negatively affect the metabolism of nutrients and the nutritional status of individuals?

_____

_____

_____

_____

_____

_____

_____

_____

_____

_____

_____

5. How may food or nutrients have a negative impact on the pharmacokinetics and pharmacodynamics of medications?

_____

_____

_____

_____

_____

_____

_____

_____

_____

_____

_____

6. What is the effect of alcohol intake on the metabolism of medications?

_____

_____

_____

_____

7. Which medications used for the management of psychiatric disorders are often associated with significant weight gain?

a) Clorazepine, olanzapine, and quetiapine   c) Divalproex sodium   e) All of the above

b) Amitriptyline   d) Lithium carbonate

INTEGRATE YOUR LEARNING

1. Explain briefly what adverse drug–nutrient interactions are commonly seen with the following drugs and what preventative action should be taken.

a) Angiotensin-converting enzyme inhibitors

_____

_____

_____

_____

_____

_____

_____

b) Systemic corticosteroids

_____
_____
_____
_____
_____
_____
_____

c) Antacids

_____
_____
_____
_____
_____
_____
_____
_____

d) Thiazide diuretics

_____
_____
_____
_____
_____
_____
_____

2. Explain briefly what adverse food/nutrient–drug interactions are commonly seen with the following food components and what preventative action should be taken.

a) Grapefruit juice

_____
_____
_____
_____
_____
_____
_____

b) Vitamin K

c) Dietary potassium

d) Tyramine and phenylethylamine

3. Which foods contain tyramine and are limited or avoided as part of the tyramine-controlled diet?

_____

_____

_____

_____

_____

_____

_____

_____

_____

_____

CHALLENGE YOUR LEARNING

CASE STUDY

Objectives

This case will help you recognize which individuals are at risk of adverse food/nutrient–drug interactions.

It will also ask you to investigate and identify the presence of adverse food/nutrient–drug interactions in individuals at risk, and to help prevent food/nutrient–drug interactions or manage them when they occur.

Description

Mr. J.T. is a 71-year-old man of Indonesian and Caucasian American descent. He was admitted to the intensive care unit with pneumonia and acute respiratory failure last night. He was immediately put on a ventilator. Enteral nutrition support was initiated this morning.

Mr. J.T.'s medical history includes Parkinson's disease for the last 12 years, chronic depression and anxiety, lifelong asthma, epilepsy, longstanding hypercholesterolemia, chronic constipation, and pedal edema.

He is presently receiving the following drugs: Claforan, Cleocin, Motilium, Ventolin, Calciparine, MS Contin, Sinemet, Tylenol, Zantac, Colace, Lipitor, Dilantin, and Lasix.

Prior to his hospital admission, his wife, daughter, and son-in-law were taking care of him at home. He had bradykinesia and facial rigidity. According to his wife, he had difficulty eating minced foods and had a reduced appetite. His favorite foods are toast, curried rice, and citrus fruits. He refuses to eat pureed foods.

1. What is Parkinson's disease?

2. Define bradykinesia.

3. What may have caused Mr. J.T.'s pneumonia?

4. List the reasons why Mr. J.T. is at high risk of adverse drug–nutrient interactions.

5. For each drug Mr. J.T. is taking, provide the generic name, the class of drug, why it was prescribed to Mr. J.T. (indication), and the main nutrition-related side effects (adverse food/nutrient–drug interactions).

a) **Claforan**

- Generic name:

- Class:

- Indication:

- Adverse food/nutrient–drug interactions

b) **Cleocin**

- Generic name:

- Class:

- Indication:

- Adverse food/nutrient–drug interactions

c) **Motilium**

- Generic name:

- Class:

- Indication:

- Adverse food/nutrient–drug interactions

d) **Ventolin**

- Generic name:

- Class:

- Indication:

- Adverse food/nutrient–drug interactions

e) **Calciparine**

- Generic name:

- Class:

- Indication:

- Adverse food/nutrient–drug interactions

f) **MS Contin**

- Generic name:

- Class:

- Indication:

- Adverse food/nutrient–drug interactions

g) **Sinemet**

- Generic name:

- Class:

- Indication:

- Adverse food/nutrient–drug interactions

h) **Tylenol**

- Generic name:

- Class:

- Indication:

- Adverse food/nutrient–drug interactions

i) **Zantac**

- Generic name:

- Class:

- Indication:

- Adverse food/nutrient–drug interactions

j) **Colace**

- Generic name:

- Class:

- Indication:

- Adverse food/nutrient–drug interactions

k) **Lipitor**

- Generic name:

- Class:

- Indication:

- Adverse food/nutrient–drug interactions

l) **Dilantin**

- Generic name:

- Class:

- Indication:

- Adverse food/nutrient–drug interactions

m) **Lasix**

- Generic name:

- Class:

- Indication:

- Adverse food/nutrient–drug interactions

UNITS CONVERSION FACTORS

Energy Units

1 kilocalorie (kcal)	= 4.18 kilojoules (kJ)
1 kJ	= 0.239 kcal
1 g (gram) protein	= about 4 kcal or 17 kJ
1 g carbohydrate	= about 4 kcal or 17 kJ
1 g fat	= about 9 kcal or 37 kJ
1 g alcohol	= about 7 kcal or 29 kJ

Length / Height Units

1 cm (centimeter)	= 0.394 in (inch) = 0.01 m (meter)
1 m	= 39.37 in = 100 cm = 1000 mm (millimeters)
1 in	= 2.54 cm
1 ft (foot)	= 12 inches = 30.48 cm

Volume Measures

1 fl. oz. (fluid ounce)	= 2 Tbsp (tablespoons) = ⅛ c (cup) = 29.6 mL (milliliters) or about 30 mL
¼ cup	= 2 fl. oz. = 4 Tbsp = 59.1 mL
⅓ cup	= 5 Tbsp + 1 tsp. (teaspoon) = 78.9 mL
½ cup	= 4 fl. oz. = 8 Tbsp = 118.3 mL
1 cup	= 8 fl. oz. = 16 Tbsp = 237 mL
1 tsp.	= 5 mL
3 tsp.	= ½ fl. oz. = 1 Tbsp = 15 mL
1 Tbsp	= ½ fl. oz. = 3 tsp. = 15 mL
1 mL	= 1 cc (cubic centimeter) = 0.001 L (liter) = 0.01 dL (deciliter)
	= 0.1 cL (centiliter) = 1000 μL (microliter) = 0.034 fl. oz.
1000 mL	= 1 L = 10 dL = 100 cL = 34 fl. oz.
1 L	= 1000 mL = 100 cL = 10 dL = 1.06 qt (quart) = 0.85 imperial gal (gallon)
1 qt	= 4 cups = 2 pints = 32 fl. oz. = 0.95 L
1 gal	= 4 qt = 3.79 L

Weight Units

1 g	= 1000 mg = 1,000,000 mcg (micrograms) = 0.035 oz. = 0.001 kg (kilogram)
454 g	= 1 lb (pound) = 16 oz. = 0.454 kg
1 mg	= 1000 mcg = 0.001 g
1 mcg (μg)	= 0.001 mg
1 oz.	= 28.35 g or about 28 g
16 oz.	= 1 lb = 454 g = 0.454 kg
1 kg	= 1000 g = 2.2 lb
1 lb	= 454 g = 0.454 kg

Adapted from Hands, E.S. 2000. "Conversion Factors for Measures" in: *Nutrients in Food.* Lippincott, Williams & Wilkins, Baltimore, MD, p. 17.

Dietary Reference Intakes (DRIs): Recommended Intakes for Individuals, Vitamins
Food and Nutrition Board, Institute of Medicine, National Academies

Life Stage Group	Vit A (µg/d)[a]	Vit C (mg/d)	Vit D (µg/d)[b,c]	Vit E (mg/d)[d]	Vit K (µg/d)	Thiamin (mg/d)	Riboflavin (mg/d)	Niacin (mg/d)[e]	Vit B6 (mg/d)	Folate (µg/d)[f]	Vit B12 (µg/d)	Pantothenic Acid (mg/d)	Biotin (µg/d)	Choline[g] (mg/d)
Infants														
0–6 mo	400*	40*	5*	4*	2.0*	0.2*	0.3*	2*	0.1*	65*	0.4*	1.7*	5*	125*
7–12 mo	500*	50*	5*	5*	2.5*	0.3*	0.4*	4*	0.3*	80*	0.5*	1.8*	6*	150*
Children														
1–3 y	300	15	5*	6	30*	0.5	0.5	6	0.5	150	0.9	2*	8*	200*
4–8 y	400	25	5*	7	55*	0.6	0.6	8	0.6	200	1.2	3*	12*	250*
Males														
9–13 y	600	45	5*	11	60*	0.9	0.9	12	1.0	300	1.8	4*	20*	375*
14–18 y	900	75	5*	15	75*	1.2	1.3	16	1.3	400	2.4	5*	25*	550*
19–30 y	900	90	5*	15	120*	1.2	1.3	16	1.3	400	2.4	5*	30*	550*
31–50 y	900	90	5*	15	120*	1.2	1.3	16	1.3	400	2.4	5*	30*	550*
51–70 y	900	90	10*	15	120*	1.2	1.3	16	1.7	400	2.4[i]	5*	30*	550*
>70 y	900	90	15*	15	120*	1.2	1.3	16	1.7	400	2.4[i]	5*	30*	550*
Females														
9–13 y	600	45	5*	11	60*	0.9	0.9	12	1.0	300	1.8	4*	20*	375*
14–18 y	700	65	5*	15	75*	1.0	1.0	14	1.2	400[i]	2.4	5*	25*	400*
19–30 y	700	75	5*	15	90*	1.1	1.1	14	1.3	400[i]	2.4	5*	30*	425*
31–50 y	700	75	5*	15	90*	1.1	1.1	14	1.3	400[i]	2.4	5*	30*	425*
51–70 y	700	75	10*	15	90*	1.1	1.1	14	1.5	400	2.4[h]	5*	30*	425*
>70 y	700	75	15*	15	90*	1.1	1.1	14	1.5	400	2.4[h]	5*	30*	425*

Pregnancy													
14–18 y	**750**	**80**	5*	**15**	75*	**1.4**	**1.4**	**18**	**1.9**	**600**[j]	**2.6**	6*	450*
												30*	
19–30 y	**770**	**85**	5*	**15**	90*	**1.4**	**1.4**	**18**	**1.9**	**600**[j]	**2.6**	6*	450*
												30*	
31–50 y	**770**	**85**	5*	**15**	90*	**1.4**	**1.4**	**18**	**1.9**	**600**[j]	**2.6**	6*	450*
												30*	
Lactation													
14–18 y	**1,200**	**115**	5*	**19**	75*	**1.4**	**1.6**	**17**	**2.0**	**500**	**2.8**	7*	550*
												35*	
19–30 y	**1,300**	**120**	5*	**19**	90*	**1.4**	**1.6**	**17**	**2.0**	**500**	**2.8**	7*	550*
												35*	
31–50 y	**1,300**	**120**	5*	**19**	90*	**1.4**	**1.6**	**17**	**2.0**	**500**	**2.8**	7*	550*
												35*	

NOTE: This table (taken from the DRI reports, see www.nap.edu) presents Recommended Dietary Allowances (RDAs) in **bold type** and Adequate Intakes (AIs) in ordinary type followed by an asterisk (*). RDAs and AIs may both be used as goals for individual intake. RDAs are set to meet the needs of almost all (97 to 98 percent) individuals in a group. For healthy breastfed infants, the AI is the mean intake. The AI for other life stage and gender groups is believed to cover needs of all individuals in the group, but lack of data or uncertainty in the data prevent being able to specify with confidence the percentage of individuals covered by this intake.

[a] As retinol activity equivalents (RAEs). 1 RAE = 1 μg retinol, 12 μg β-carotene, 24 μg α-carotene, or 24 μg β-cryptoxanthin. The RAE for dietary provitamin A carotenoids is twofold greater than retinol equivalents (RE), whereas the RAE for preformed vitamin A is the same as RE.

[b] As cholecalciferol. 1 μg cholecalciferol = 40 IU vitamin D.

[c] In the absence of adequate exposure to sunlight.

[d] As α-tocopherol. α-Tocopherol includes *RRR*-α-tocopherol, the only form of α-tocopherol that occurs naturally in foods, and the *2R*-stereoisomeric forms of α-tocopherol (*RRR*-, *RSR*-, *RRS*-, and *RSS*-α-tocopherol) that occur in fortified foods and supplements. It does not include the *2S*-stereoisomeric forms of α-tocopherol (*SRR*-, *SSR*-, *SRS*-, and *SSS*-α-tocopherol), also found in fortified foods and supplements.

[e] As niacin equivalents (NE). 1 mg of niacin = 60 mg of tryptophan; 0–6 months = preformed niacin (not NE).

[f] As dietary folate equivalents (DFE). 1 DFE = 1 μg food folate = 0.6 μg of folic acid from fortified food or as a supplement consumed with food = 0.5 μg of a supplement taken on an empty stomach.

[g] Although AIs have been set for choline, there are few data to assess whether a dietary supply of choline is needed at all stages of the life cycle, and it may be that the choline requirement can be met by endogenous synthesis at some of these stages.

[h] Because 10 to 30 percent of older people may malabsorb food-bound B_{12}, it is advisable for those older than 50 years to meet their RDA mainly by consuming foods fortified with B_{12} or a supplement containing B_{12}.

[i] In view of evidence linking folate intake with neural tube defects in the fetus, it is recommended that all women capable of becoming pregnant consume 400 μg from supplements or fortified foods in addition to intake of food folate from a varied diet.

[j] It is assumed that women will continue consuming 400 μg from supplements or fortified food until their pregnancy is confirmed and they enter prenatal care, which ordinarily occurs after the end of the periconceptional period—the critical time for formation of the neural tube.

Dietary Reference Intakes (DRIs): Recommended Intakes for Individuals, Elements
Food and Nutrition Board, Institute of Medicine, National Academies

Life Stage Group	Calcium (mg/d)	Chromium (µg/d)	Copper (µg/d)	Fluoride (mg/d)	Iodine (µg/d)	Iron (mg/d)	Magnesium (mg/d)	Manganese (mg/d)	Molybdenum (µg/d)	Phosphorus (mg/d)	Selenium (µg/d)	Zinc (mg/d)	Potassium (g/d)	Sodium (g/d)	Chloride (g/d)
Infants															
0–6 mo	210*	0.2*	200*	0.01*	110*	0.27*	30*	0.003*	2*	100*	15*	2*	0.4*	0.12*	0.18*
7–12 mo	270*	5.5*	220*	0.5*	130*	11	75*	0.6*	3*	275*	20*	3	0.7*	0.37*	0.57*
Children															
1–3 y	500*	11*	340	0.7*	90	7	80	1.2*	17	460	20	3	3.0*	1.0*	1.5*
4–8 y	800*	15*	440	1*	90	10	130	1.5*	22	500	30	5	3.8*	1.2*	1.9*
Males															
9–13 y	1,300*	25*	700	2*	120	8	240	1.9*	34	1,250	40	8	4.5*	1.5*	2.3*
14–18 y	1,300*	35*	890	3*	150	11	410	2.2*	43	1,250	55	11	4.7*	1.5*	2.3*
19–30 y	1,000*	35*	900	4*	150	8	400	2.3*	45	700	55	11	4.7*	1.5*	2.3*
31–50 y	1,000*	35*	900	4*	150	8	420	2.3*	45	700	55	11	4.7*	1.5*	2.3*
51–70 y	1,200*	30*	900	4*	150	8	420	2.3*	45	700	55	11	4.7*	1.3*	2.0*
> 70 y	1,200*	30*	900	4*	150	8	420	2.3*	45	700	55	11	4.7*	1.2*	1.8*
Females															
9–13 y	1,300*	21*	700	2*	120	8	240	1.6*	34	1,250	40	8	4.5*	1.5*	2.3*
14–18 y	1,300*	24*	890	3*	150	15	360	1.6*	43	1,250	55	9	4.7*	1.5*	2.3*
19–30 y	1,000*	25*	900	3*	150	18	310	1.8*	45	700	55	8	4.7*	1.5*	2.3*
31–50 y	1,000*	25*	900	3*	150	18	320	1.8*	45	700	55	8	4.7*	1.5*	2.3*
51–70 y	1,200*	20*	900	3*	150	8	320	1.8*	45	700	55	8	4.7*	1.3*	2.0*
> 70 y	1,200*	20*	900	3*	150	8	320	1.8*	45	700	55	8	4.7*	1.2*	1.8*
Pregnancy															
14–18 y	1,300*	29*	1,000	3*	220	27	400	2.0*	50	1,250	60	12	4.7*	1.5*	2.3*
19–30 y	1,000*	30*	1,000	3*	220	27	350	2.0*	50	700	60	11	4.7*	1.5*	2.3*
31–50 y	1,000*	30*	1,000	3*	220	27	360	2.0*	50	700	60	11	4.7*	1.5*	2.3*
Lactation															
14–18 y	1,300*	44*	1,300	3*	290	10	360	2.6*	50	1,250	70	13	5.1*	1.5*	2.3*
19–30 y	1,000*	45*	1,300	3*	290	9	310	2.6*	50	700	70	12	5.1*	1.5*	2.3*
31–50 y	1,000*	45*	1,300	3*	290	9	320	2.6*	50	700	70	12	5.1*	1.5*	2.3*

NOTE: This table presents Recommended Dietary Allowances (RDAs) in **bold type** and Adequate Intakes (AIs) in ordinary type followed by an asterisk (*). RDAs and AIs may both be used as goals for individual intake. RDAs are set to meet the needs of almost all (97 to 98 percent) individuals in a group. For healthy breastfed infants, the AI is the mean intake. The AI for other life stage and gender groups is believed to cover needs of all individuals in the group, but lack of data or uncertainty in the data prevent being able to specify with confidence the percentage of individuals covered by this intake.

SOURCES: *Dietary Reference Intakes for Calcium, Phosphorous, Magnesium, Vitamin D, and Fluoride* (1997); *Dietary Reference Intakes for Thiamin, Riboflavin, Niacin, Vitamin B6, Folate, Vitamin B12, Pantothenic Acid, Biotin, and Choline* (1998); *Dietary Reference Intakes for Vitamin C, Vitamin E, Selenium, and Carotenoids* (2000); *Dietary Reference Intakes for Vitamin A, Vitamin K, Arsenic, Boron, Chromium, Copper, Iodine, Iron, Manganese, Molybdenum, Nickel, Silicon, Vanadium, and Zinc* (2001); and *Dietary Reference Intakes for Water, Potassium, Sodium, Chloride, and Sulfate* (2004). These reports may be accessed via http://www.nap.edu.

Dietary Reference Intakes (DRIs): Tolerable Upper Intake Levels (UL[a]), Vitamins
Food and Nutrition Board, Institute of Medicine, National Academies

Life Stage Group	Vitamin A (µg/d)[b]	Vitamin C (mg/d)	Vitamin D (µg/d)	Vitamin E (mg/d)[c,d]	Vitamin K	Thiamin	Ribo-flavin	Niacin (mg/d)[d]	Vitamin B6 (mg/d)	Folate (µg/d)[d]	Vitamin B12	Pantothenic Acid	Biotin	Choline (g/d)	Carote-noids[e]
Infants															
0–6 mo	600	ND[f]	25	ND	ND	ND	ND	ND	ND	ND	ND	ND	ND	ND	ND
7–12 mo	600	ND	25	ND	ND	ND	ND	ND	ND	ND	ND	ND	ND	ND	ND
Children															
1–3 y	600	400	50	200	ND	ND	ND	10	30	300	ND	ND	ND	1.0	ND
4–8 y	900	650	50	300	ND	ND	ND	15	40	400	ND	ND	ND	1.0	ND
Males, Females															
9–13 y	1,700	1,200	50	600	ND	ND	ND	20	60	600	ND	ND	ND	2.0	ND
14–18 y	2,800	1,800	50	800	ND	ND	ND	30	80	800	ND	ND	ND	3.0	ND
19–70 y	3,000	2,000	50	1,000	ND	ND	ND	35	100	1,000	ND	ND	ND	3.5	ND
> 70 y	3,000	2,000	50	1,000	ND	ND	ND	35	100	1,000	ND	ND	ND	3.5	ND
Pregnancy															
14–18 y	2,800	1,800	50	800	ND	ND	ND	30	80	800	ND	ND	ND	3.0	ND
19–50 y	3,000	2,000	50	1,000	ND	ND	ND	35	100	1,000	ND	ND	ND	3.5	ND
Lactation															
14–18 y	2,800	1,800	50	800	ND	ND	ND	30	80	800	ND	ND	ND	3.0	ND
19–50 y	3,000	2,000	50	1,000	ND	ND	ND	35	100	1,000	ND	ND	ND	3.5	ND

[a]UL = The maximum level of daily nutrient intake that is likely to pose no risk of adverse effects. Unless otherwise specified, the UL represents total intake from food, water, and supplements. Due to lack of suitable data, ULs could not be established for vitamin K, thiamin, riboflavin, vitamin B12, pantothenic acid, biotin, carotenoids. In the absence of ULs, extra caution may be warranted in consuming levels above recommended intakes.

[b]As preformed vitamin A only.

[c]As α-tocopherol; applies to any form of supplemental α-tocopherol.

[d]The ULs for vitamin E, niacin, and folate apply to synthetic forms obtained from supplements, fortified foods, or a combination of the two.

[e]β-Carotene supplements are advised only to serve as a provitamin A source for individuals at risk of vitamin A deficiency.

[f]ND = Not determinable due to lack of data of adverse effects in this age group and concern with regard to lack of ability to handle excess amounts. Source of intake should be from food only to prevent high levels of intake.

SOURCES: *Dietary Reference Intakes for Calcium, Phosphorous, Magnesium, Vitamin D, and Fluoride* (1997); *Dietary Reference Intakes for Thiamin, Riboflavin, Niacin, Vitamin B6, Folate, Vitamin B12, Pantothenic Acid, Biotin, and Choline* (1998); *Dietary Reference Intakes for Vitamin C, Vitamin E, Selenium, and Carotenoids* (2000); and *Dietary Reference Intakes for Vitamin A, Vitamin K, Arsenic, Boron, Chromium, Copper, Iodine, Iron, Manganese, Molybdenum, Nickel, Silicon, Vanadium, and Zinc* (2001). These reports may be accessed via http://www.nap.edu.

Dietary Reference Intakes (DRIs): Tolerable Upper Intake Levels (UL[a]), Elements
Food and Nutrition Board, Institute of Medicine, National Academies

Life Stage Group	Arsenic[b]	Boron (mg/d)	Calcium (g/d)	Chromium	Copper (μg/d)	Fluoride (mg/d)	Iodine (μg/d)	Iron (mg/d)	Magnesium (mg/d)[c]	Manganese (mg/d)	Molybdenum (μg/d)	Nickel (mg/d)	Phosphorus (g/d)	Potassium	Selenium (μg/d)	Silicon[d]	Sulfate	Vanadium (mg/d)[e]	Zinc (mg/d)	Sodium (g/d)	Chloride (g/d)
Infants																					
0–6 mo	ND[f]	ND	ND	ND	ND	0.7	ND	40	ND	ND	ND	ND	ND	ND	45	ND	ND	ND	4	ND	ND
7–12 mo	ND	ND	ND	ND	ND	0.9	ND	40	ND	ND	ND	ND	ND	ND	60	ND	ND	ND	5	ND	ND
Children																					
1–3 y	ND	3	2.5	ND	1,000	1.3	200	40	65	2	300	0.2	3	ND	90	ND	ND	ND	7	1.5	2.3
4–8 y	ND	6	2.5	ND	3,000	2.2	300	40	110	3	600	0.3	3	ND	150	ND	ND	ND	12	1.9	2.9
Males,																					
Females																					
9–13 y	ND	11	2.5	ND	5,000	10	600	40	350	6	1,100	0.6	4	ND	280	ND	ND	ND	23	2.2	3.4
14–18 y	ND	17	2.5	ND	8,000	10	900	45	350	9	1,700	1.0	4	ND	400	ND	ND	ND	34	2.3	3.6
19–70 y	ND	20	2.5	ND	10,000	10	1,100	45	350	11	2,000	1.0	4	ND	400	ND	ND	1.8	40	2.3	3.6
>70 y	ND	20	2.5	ND	10,000	10	1,100	45	350	11	2,000	1.0	3	ND	400	ND	ND	1.8	40	2.3	3.6
Pregnancy																					
14–18 y	ND	17	2.5	ND	8,000	10	900	45	350	9	1,700	1.0	3.5	ND	400	ND	ND	ND	34	2.3	3.6
19–50 y	ND	20	2.5	ND	10,000	10	1,100	45	350	11	2,000	1.0	3.5	ND	400	ND	ND	ND	40	2.3	3.6
Lactation																					
14–18 y	ND	17	2.5	ND	8,000	10	900	45	350	9	1,700	1.0	4	ND	400	ND	ND	ND	34	2.3	3.6
19–50 y	ND	20	2.5	ND	10,000	10	1,100	45	350	11	2,000	1.0	4	ND	400	ND	ND	ND	40	2.3	3.6

[a]UL = The maximum level of daily nutrient intake that is likely to pose no risk of adverse effects. Unless otherwise specified, the UL represents total intake from food, water, and supplements. Due to lack of suitable data, ULs could not be established for arsenic, chromium, silicon, potassium, and sulfate. In the absence of ULs, extra caution may be warranted in consuming levels above recommended intakes.

[b]Although the UL was not determined for arsenic, there is no justification for adding arsenic to food or supplements.

[c]The ULs for magnesium represent intake from a pharmacological agent only and do not include intake from food and water.

[d]Although silicon has not been shown to cause adverse effects in humans, there is no justification for adding silicon to supplements.

[e]Although vanadium in food has not been shown to cause adverse effects in humans, there is no justification for adding vanadium to food and vanadium supplements should be used with caution. The UL is based on adverse effects in laboratory animals and this data could be used to set a UL for adults but not children and adolescents.

[f]ND = Not determinable due to lack of data of adverse effects in this age group and concern with regard to lack of ability to handle excess amounts. Source of intake should be from food only to prevent high levels of intake.

SOURCES: *Dietary Reference Intakes for Calcium, Phosphorous, Magnesium, Vitamin D, and Fluoride* (1997); *Dietary Reference Intakes for Thiamin, Riboflavin, Niacin, Vitamin B[6], Folate, Vitamin B[12], Pantothenic Acid, Biotin, and Choline* (1998); *Dietary Reference Intakes for Vitamin C, Vitamin E, Selenium, and Carotenoids* (2000); *Dietary Reference Intakes for Vitamin A, Vitamin K, Arsenic, Boron, Chromium, Copper, Iodine, Iron, Manganese, Molybdenum, Nickel, Silicon, Vanadium, and Zinc* (2001); and *Dietary Reference Intakes for Water, Potassium, Sodium, Chloride, and Sulfate* (2004). These reports may be accessed via http://www.nap.edu.

A-6

Dietary Reference Intakes (DRIs): Estimated Energy Requirements (EER) for Men and Women 30 Years of Age[a]
Food and Nutrition Board, Institute of Medicine, National Academies

Height (m [in])	PAL[b]	Weight for BMI[c] of 18.5 kg/m² (kg [lb])	Weight for BMI of 24.99 kg/m² (kg [lb])	EER, Men[d] (kcal/day)		EER, Women[d] (kcal/day)	
				BMI of 18.5 kg/m²	BMI of 24.99 kg/m²	BMI of 18.5 kg/m²	BMI of 24.99kg/m²
1.50 (59)	Sedentary	41.6 (92)	56.2 (124)	1,848	2,080	1,625	1,762
	Low active			2,009	2,267	1,803	1,956
	Active			2,215	2,506	2,025	2,198
	Very active			2,554	2,898	2,291	2,489
1.65 (65)	Sedentary	50.4 (111)	68.0 (150)	2,068	2,349	1,816	1,982
	Low active			2,254	2,566	2,016	2,202
	Active			2,490	2,842	2,267	2,477
	Very active			2,880	3,296	2,567	2,807
1.80 (71)	Sedentary	59.9 (132)	81.0 (178)	2,301	2,635	2,015	2,211
	Low active			2,513	2,884	2,239	2,459
	Active			2,782	3,200	2,519	2,769
	Very active			3,225	3,720	2,855	3,141

[a]For each year below 30, add 7 kcal/day for women and 10 kcal /day for men. For each year above 30, subtract 7 kcal/day for women and 10 kcal/day for men.
[b]PAL = physical activity level.
[c]BMI = body mass index.
[d]Derived from the following regression equations based on doubly labeled water data:
  Adult man: EER = $662 - 9.53 \times$ age (y) + PA $\times$ ($15.91 \times$ wt [kg] + $539.6 \times$ ht [m])
  Adult woman: EER = $354 - 6.91 \times$ age (y) + PA $\times$ ($9.36 \times$ wt [kg] + $726 \times$ ht [m])
Where PA refers to coefficient for PAL
PAL = total energy expenditure ÷ basal energy expenditure
  PA = 1.0 if PAL $\geq$ 1.0 < 1.4 (sedentary)
  PA = 1.12 if PAL $\geq$ 1.4 < 1.6 (low active)
  PA = 1.27 if PAL $\geq$ 1.6 < 1.9 (active)
  PA = 1.45 if PAL $\geq$ 1.9 < 2.5 (very active)

Dietary Reference Intakes (DRIs): Acceptable Macronutrient Distribution Ranges
Food and Nutrition Board, Institute of Medicine, National Academies

Macronutrient	Range (percent of energy)		
	Children, 1–3 y	Children, 4–18 y	Adults
Fat	30–40	25–35	20–35
n-6 polyunsaturated fatty acids[a] (linoleic acid)	5–10	5–10	5–10
n-3 polyunsaturated fatty acids[a] (α-linolenic acid)	0.6–1.2	0.6–1.2	0.6–1.2
Carbohydrate	45–65	45–65	45–65
Protein	5–20	10–30	10–35

[a]Approximately 10% of the total can come from longer-chain n-3 or n-6 fatty acids.

SOURCE: *Dietary Reference Intakes for Energy, Carbohydrate, Fiber, Fat, Fatty Acids, Cholesterol, Protein, and Amino Acids* (2002).

Dietary Reference Intakes (DRIs): Recommended Intakes for Individuals, Macronutrients
Food and Nutrition Board, Institute of Medicine, National Academies

Life Stage Group	Total Water[a] (L/d)	Carbohydrate (g/d)	Total Fiber (g/d)	Fat (g/d)	Linoleic Acid (g/d)	α-Linolenic Acid (g/d)	Protein[b] (g/d)
Infants							
0–6 mo	0.7*	60*	ND	31*	4.4*	0.5*	9.1*
7–12 mo	0.8*	95*	ND	30*	4.6*	0.5*	**11.0**[c]
Children							
1–3 y	1.3*	**130**	19*	ND	7*	0.7*	**13**
4–8 y	1.7*	**130**	25*	ND	10*	0.9*	**19**
Males							
9–13 y	2.4*	**130**	31*	ND	12*	1.2*	**34**
14–18 y	3.3*	**130**	38*	ND	16*	1.6*	**52**
19–30 y	3.7*	**130**	38*	ND	17*	1.6*	**56**
31–50 y	3.7*	**130**	38*	ND	17*	1.6*	**56**
51–70 y	3.7*	**130**	30*	ND	14*	1.6*	**56**
> 70 y	3.7*	**130**	30*	ND	14*	1.6*	**56**
Females							
9–13 y	2.1*	**130**	26*	ND	10*	1.0*	**34**
14–18 y	2.3*	**130**	26*	ND	11*	1.1*	**46**
19–30 y	2.7*	**130**	25*	ND	12*	1.1*	**46**
31–50 y	2.7*	**130**	25*	ND	12*	1.1*	**46**
51–70 y	2.7*	**130**	21*	ND	11*	1.1*	**46**
> 70 y	2.7*	**130**	21*	ND	11*	1.1*	**46**
Pregnancy							
14–18 y	3.0*	**175**	28*	ND	13*	1.4*	**71**
19–30 y	3.0*	**175**	28*	ND	13*	1.4*	**71**
31–50 y	3.0*	**175**	28*	ND	13*	1.4*	**71**
Lactation							
14–18 y	3.8*	**210**	29*	ND	13*	1.3*	**71**
19–30 y	3.8*	**210**	29*	ND	13*	1.3*	**71**
31–50 y	3.8*	**210**	29*	ND	13*	1.3*	**71**

NOTE: This table presents Recommended Dietary Allowances (RDAs) in **bold** type and Adequate Intakes (AIs) in ordinary type followed by an asterisk (*). RDAs and AIs may both be used as goals for individual intake. RDAs are set to meet the needs of almost all (97 to 98 percent) individuals in a group. For healthy infants fed human milk, the AI is the mean intake. The AI for other life stage and gender groups is believed to cover the needs of all individuals in the group, but lack of data or uncertainty in the data prevent being able to specify with confidence the percentage of individuals covered by this intake.

[a]*Total* water includes all water contained in food, beverages, and drinking water.
[b]Based on 0.8 g/kg body weight for the reference body weight.
[c]Change from 13.5 in prepublication copy due to calculation error.

Dietary Reference Intakes (DRIs): Additional Macronutrient Recommendations
Food and Nutrition Board, Institute of Medicine, National Academies

Macronutrient	Recommendation
Dietary cholesterol	As low as possible while consuming a nutritionally adequate diet
Trans fatty acids	As low as possible while consuming a nutritionally adequate diet
Saturated fatty acids	As low as possible while consuming a nutritionally adequate diet
Added sugars	Limit to no more than 25% of total energy

SOURCE: *Dietary Reference Intakes for Energy, Carbohydrate, Fiber, Fat, Fatty Acids, Cholesterol, Protein, and Amino Acids* (2002)

Dietary Reference Intakes (DRIs): Estimated Average Requirements for Groups
Food and Nutrition Board, Institute of Medicine, National Academies

Life Stage Group	CHO (g/d)	Protein (g/d)a	Vit A (µg/d)b	Vit C (mg/d)	Vit E (mg/d)c	Thiamin (mg/d)	Riboflavin (mg/d)	Niacin (mg/d)d	Vit B6 (mg/d)	Folate (µg/d)b	Vit B12 (µg/d)	Copper (µg/d)	Iodine (µg/d)	Iron (mg/d)	Magnesium (mg/d)	Molybdenum (µg/d)	Phosphorus (mg/d)	Selenium (µg/d)	Zinc (mg/d)
Infants																			
7–12 mo		9*												6.9					2.5
Children																			
1–3 y	100	11	210	13	5	0.4	0.4	5	0.4	120	0.7	260	65	3.0	65	13	380	17	2.5
4–8 y	100	15	275	22	6	0.5	0.5	6	0.5	160	1.0	340	65	4.1	110	17	405	23	4.0
Males																			
9–13 y	100	27	445	39	9	0.7	0.8	9	0.8	250	1.5	540	73	5.9	200	26	1,055	35	7.0
14–18 y	100	44	630	63	12	1.0	1.1	12	1.1	330	2.0	685	95	7.7	340	33	1,055	45	8.5
19–30 y	100	46	625	75	12	1.0	1.1	12	1.1	320	2.0	700	95	6	330	34	580	45	9.4
31–50 y	100	46	625	75	12	1.0	1.1	12	1.1	320	2.0	700	95	6	350	34	580	45	9.4
51–70 y	100	46	625	75	12	1.0	1.1	12	1.4	320	2.0	700	95	6	350	34	580	45	9.4
> 70 y	100	46	625	75	12	1.0	1.1	12	1.4	320	2.0	700	95	6	350	34	580	45	9.4
Females																			
9–13 y	100	28	420	39	9	0.7	0.8	9	0.8	250	1.5	540	73	5.7	200	26	1,055	35	7.0
14–18 y	100	38	485	56	12	0.9	0.9	11	1.0	330	2.0	685	95	7.9	300	33	1,055	45	7.3
19–30 y	100	38	500	60	12	0.9	0.9	11	1.1	320	2.0	700	95	8.1	255	34	580	45	6.8
31–50 y	100	38	500	60	12	0.9	0.9	11	1.1	320	2.0	700	95	8.1	265	34	580	45	6.8
51–70 y	100	38	500	60	12	0.9	0.9	11	1.3	320	2.0	700	95	5	265	34	580	45	6.8
> 70 y	100	38	500	60	12	0.9	0.9	11	1.3	320	2.0	700	95	5	265	34	580	45	6.8

Pregnancy																	
14–18 y	135	50	530	66	12	1.2	14	1.6	520	2.2	785	160	23	335	40	1,055	49	10.5
19–30 y	135	50	550	70	12	1.2	14	1.6	520	2.2	800	160	22	290	40	580	49	9.5
31–50 y	135	50	550	70	12	1.2	14	1.6	520	2.2	800	160	22	300	40	580	49	9.5
Lactation																	
14–18 y	160	60	885	96	16	1.3	13	1.7	450	2.4	985	209	7	300	35	1,055	59	10.9
19–30 y	160	60	900	100	16	1.3	13	1.7	450	2.4	1,000	209	6.5	255	36	580	59	10.4
31–50 y	160	60	900	100	16	1.3	13	1.7	450	2.4	1,000	209	6.5	265	36	580	59	10.4

NOTE: This table presents Estimated Average Requirements (EARs), which serve two purposes: for assessing adequacy of population intakes, and as the basis for calculating Recommended Dietary Allowances (RDAs) for individuals for those nutrients. EARs have not been established for vitamin D, vitamin K, pantothenic acid, biotin, choline, calcium, chromium, fluoride, manganese, or other nutrients not yet evaluated via the DRI process.

[a]For individual at reference weight (Table 1-1). *indicates change from prepublication copy due to calculation error.

[b]As retinol activity equivalents (RAEs). 1 RAE = 1 μg retinol, 12 μg β-carotene, 24 μg α-carotene, or 24 μg β-cryptoxanthin. The RAE for dietary provitamin A carotenoids is two-fold greater than retinol equivalents (RE), whereas the RAE for preformed vitamin A is the same as RE.

[c]As α-tocopherol. α-Tocopherol includes *RRR*-α-tocopherol, the only form of α-tocopherol that occurs naturally in foods, and the *2R*-stereoisomeric forms of α-tocopherol (*RRR*-, *RSR*-, *RRS*-, and *RSS*-α-tocopherol) that occur in fortified foods and supplements. It does not include the *2S*-stereoisomeric forms of α-tocopherol (*SRR*-, *SSR*-, *SRS*-, and *SSS*-α-tocopherol), also found in fortified foods and supplements.

[d]As niacin equivalents (NE). 1 mg of niacin = 60 mg of tryptophan.

[e]As dietary folate equivalents (DFE). 1 DFE = 1μg food folate = 0.6 μg of folic acid from fortified food or as a supplement consumed with food = 0.5 μg of a supplement taken on an empty stomach.

SOURCES: *Dietary Reference Intakes for Calcium, Phosphorous, Magnesium, Vitamin D, and Fluoride* (1997); *Dietary Reference Intakes for Thiamin, Riboflavin, Niacin, Vitamin B⁶, Folate, Vitamin B¹², Pantothenic Acid, Biotin, and Choline* (1998); *Dietary Reference Intakes for Vitamin C, Vitamin E, Selenium, and Carotenoids* (2000); *Dietary Reference Intakes for Vitamin A, Vitamin K, Arsenic, Boron, Chromium, Copper, Iodine, Iron, Manganese, Molybdenum, Nickel, Silicon, Vanadium, and Zinc* (2001), and *Dietary Reference Intakes for Energy, Carbohydrate, Fiber, Fat, Fatty Acids, Cholesterol, Protein, and Amino Acids* (2002). These reports may be accessed via www.nap.edu.

Diet/Calorie Count Form

Food	Portion	Number of Portions	CHO (g)	Protein (g)	Fat (g)
Starch/bread	½ cup, 118 mL or 1 slice (1 oz, 28 g)		15	3	
Fruit	½ cup, 118 mL or 1 small		15		
Vegetable	½ cup or 118 mL		7	2	
Milk:	½ cup, 4 fluid oz or 118 mL				
- **Nonfat**			6	4	0
- **1% fat**			6	4	1
- **2% fat**			6	4	2
- **Whole**			6	4	4
Meat:	1 oz or 28 g				
- **Very lean**				7	0–1
- **Lean**				7	3
- **Medium fat**				7	5
- **High fat**				7	8
Fat	1 tsp or 5 mL				5
Sugar	1 tsp or 5 mL			5	
Others:					
Total (g)					
			× 4 kcal/g or 17 kJ/g	× 4 kcal/g or 17 kJ/g	× 9 kcal/g or 37 kJ/g
Total					
TOTAL ENERGY	= _____				
% of Energy					

Birth to 36 months: Boys
Length-for-age and Weight-for-age percentiles

NAME _____

RECORD # _____

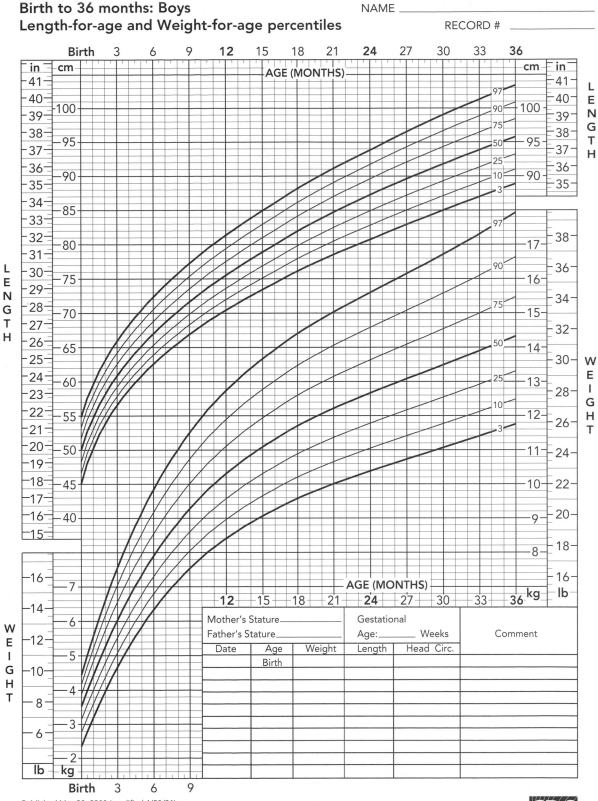

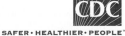

Published May 30, 2000 (modified 4/20/01).
SOURCE: Developed by the National Center for Health Statistics in collaboration with
the National Center for Chronic Disease Prevention and Health Promotion(2000).
http://www.cdc.gov/growthcharts

Birth to 36 months: Boys length-for-age and weight-for-age percentiles. (Developed by the National Center for Health Statistics in collaboration with the National Center for Chronic Disease Prevention and Health Promotion [2000]. http://www.cdc.gov/growthcharts.)

Birth to 36 months: Boys
Head circumference-for-age and
Weight-for-length percentiles

NAME _____

RECORD # _____

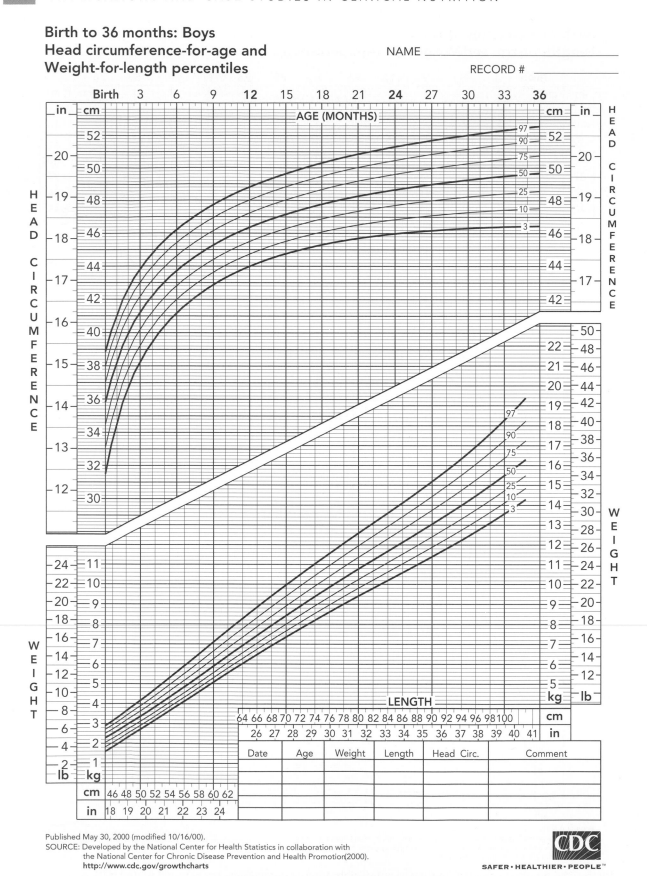

Published May 30, 2000 (modified 10/16/00).
SOURCE: Developed by the National Center for Health Statistics in collaboration with
the National Center for Chronic Disease Prevention and Health Promotion (2000).
http://www.cdc.gov/growthcharts

CDC
SAFER • HEALTHIER • PEOPLE™

Birth to 36 months: Boys head circumference-for-age and weight-for-length percentiles. (Developed by the National Center for Health Statistics in collaboration with the National Center for Chronic Disease Prevention and Health Promotion [2000]. http://www.cdc.gov/growthcharts.)

Birth to 36 months: Girls
Length-for-age and Weight-for-age percentiles

NAME _____

RECORD # _____

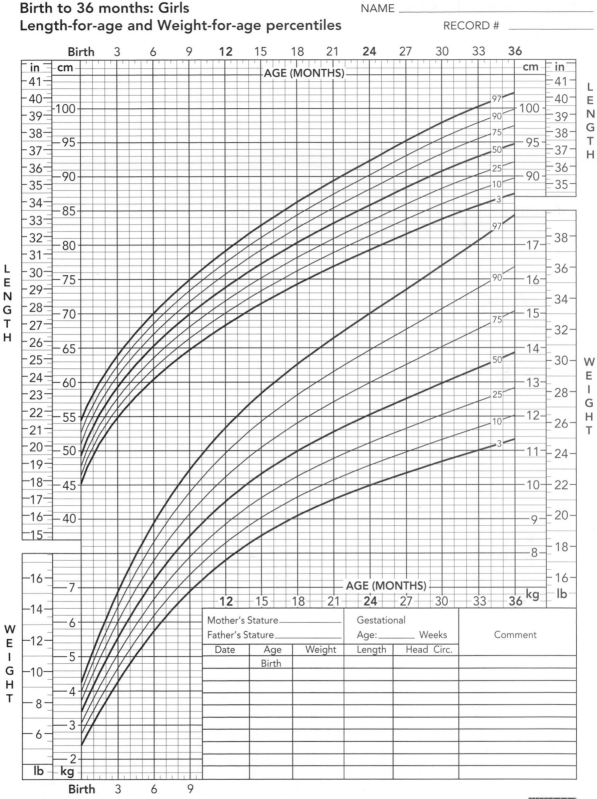

Published May 30, 2000 (modified 4/20/01).
SOURCE: Developed by the National Center for Health Statistics in collaboration with
the National Center for Chronic Disease Prevention and Health Promotion(2000).
http://www.cdc.gov/growthcharts

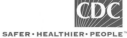

SAFER · HEALTHIER · PEOPLE™

Birth to 36 months: Girls length-for-age and weight-for-age percentiles. (Developed by the National Center for Health Statistics in collaboration with the National Center for Chronic Disease Prevention and Health Promotion [2000]. http://www.cdc.gov/growthcharts.)

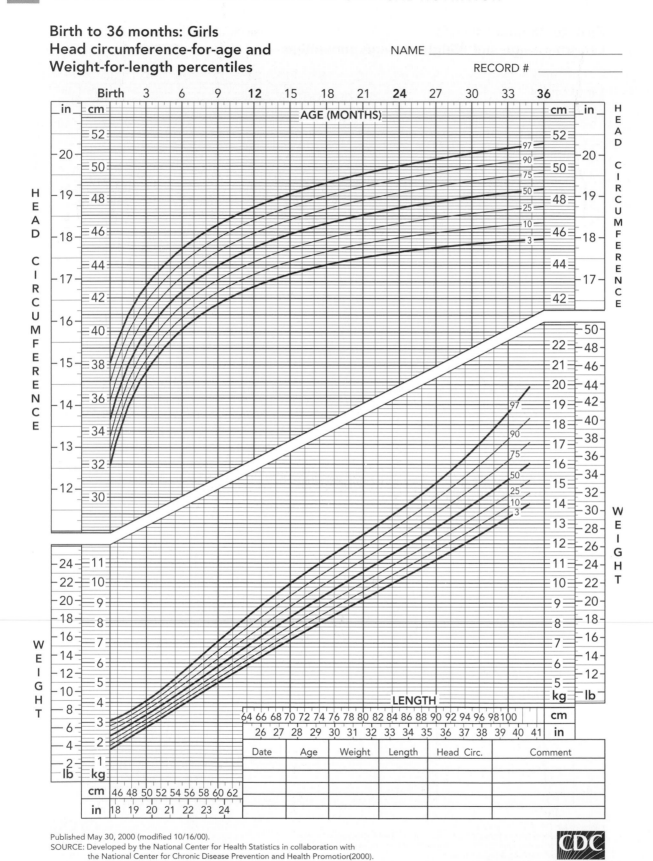

Birth to 36 months: Girls head circumference-for-age and weight-for-length percentiles. (Developed by the National Center for Health Statistics in collaboration with the National Center for Chronic Disease Prevention and Health Promotion [2000]. http://www.cdc.gov/growthcharts.)

2 to 20 years: Boys
Stature-for-age and Weight-for-age percentiles

NAME _____

RECORD # _____

Mother's Stature _____ Father's Stature _____

Date	Age	Weight	Stature	BMI*

*To Calculate BMI: Weight (kg) ÷ Stature (cm) ÷ Stature (cm) x 10,000
or Weight (lb) ÷ Stature (in) ÷ Stature (in) x 703

AGE (YEARS)

STATURE

WEIGHT

Published May 30, 2000 (modified 11/21/00).
SOURCE: Developed by the National Center for Health Statistics in collaboration with
the National Center for Chronic Disease Prevention and Health Promotion(2000).
http://www.cdc.gov/growthcharts

CDC
SAFER · HEALTHIER · PEOPLE™

2 to 20 years: Boys stature-for-age and weight-for-age percentiles. (Developed by the National Center for Health Statistics in collaboration with the National Center for Chronic Disease Prevention and Health Promotion [2000]. http://www.cdc.gov/growthcharts.)

2 to 20 years: Boys
Body mass index-for-age percentiles

NAME _____

RECORD # _____

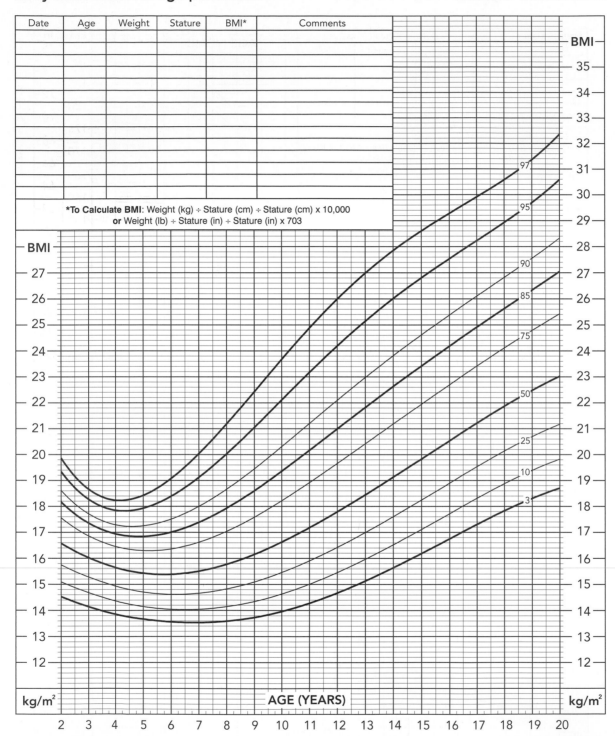

Date | **Age** | **Weight** | **Stature** | **BMI*** | **Comments**

***To Calculate BMI**: Weight (kg) ÷ Stature (cm) ÷ Stature (cm) x 10,000
or Weight (lb) ÷ Stature (in) ÷ Stature (in) x 703

AGE (YEARS)

kg/m²

BMI

Published May 30, 2000 (modified 10/16/00).
SOURCE: Developed by the National Center for Health Statistics in collaboration with
the National Center for Chronic Disease Prevention and Health Promotion (2000).
http://www.cdc.gov/growthcharts

SAFER • HEALTHIER • PEOPLE™

2 to 20 years: Boys body mass index-for-age percentiles. (Developed by the National Center for Health Statistics in collaboration with the National Center for Chronic Disease Prevention and Health Promotion [2000]. http://www.cdc.gov/growthcharts.)

2 to 20 years: Girls
Stature-for-age and Weight-for-age percentiles

NAME _____

RECORD # _____

Mother's Stature _____ Father's Stature _____

Date	Age	Weight	Stature	BMI*

*To Calculate BMI: Weight (kg) ÷ Stature (cm) ÷ Stature (cm) x 10,000
or Weight (lb) ÷ Stature (in) ÷ Stature (in) x 703

AGE (YEARS)

STATURE

WEIGHT

Published May 30, 2000 (modified 11/21/00).
SOURCE: Developed by the National Center for Health Statistics in collaboration with
the National Center for Chronic Disease Prevention and Health Promotion(2000).
http://www.cdc.gov/growthcharts

CDC
SAFER · HEALTHIER · PEOPLE™

2 to 20 years: Girls stature-for-age and weight-for-age percentiles. (Developed by the National Center for Health Statistics in collaboration with the National Center for Chronic Disease Prevention and Health Promotion [2000]. http://www.cdc.gov/growthcharts.)

2 to 20 years: Girls
Body mass index-for-age percentiles

NAME _____

RECORD # _____

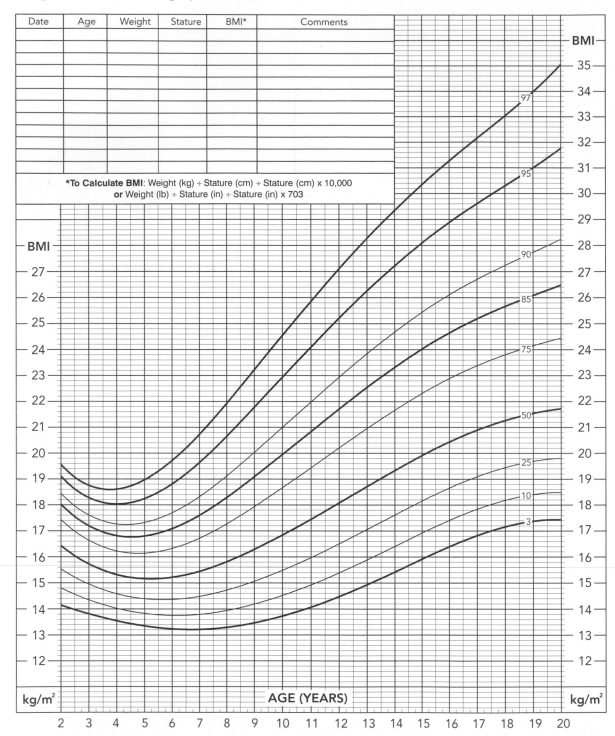

*To Calculate BMI: Weight (kg) ÷ Stature (cm) ÷ Stature (cm) x 10,000
or Weight (lb) ÷ Stature (in) ÷ Stature (in) x 703

AGE (YEARS)

Published May 30, 2000 (modified 10/16/00).
SOURCE: Developed by the National Center for Health Statistics in collaboration with
the National Center for Chronic Disease Prevention and Health Promotion(2000).
http://www.cdc.gov/growthcharts

SAFER · HEALTHIER · PEOPLE™

2 to 20 years: Girls body mass index-for-age percentiles. (Developed by the National Center for Health Statistics in collaboration with the National Center for Chronic Disease Prevention and Health Promotion [2000]. http://www.cdc.gov/growthcharts.)

NAME _____

Weight-for-stature percentiles: Boys

RECORD # _____

Date	Age	Weight	Stature	Comments

Published May 30, 2000 (modified 10/16/00).
SOURCE: Developed by the National Center for Health Statistics in collaboration with
the National Center for Chronic Disease Prevention and Health Promotion (2000).
http://www.cdc.gov/growthcharts

Boys weight-for-stature percentiles. (Developed by the National Center for Health Statistics in collaboration with the National Center for Chronic Disease Prevention and Health Promotion [2000]. http://www.cdc.gov/growthcharts.)

Weight-for-stature percentiles: Girls

NAME _____

RECORD # _____

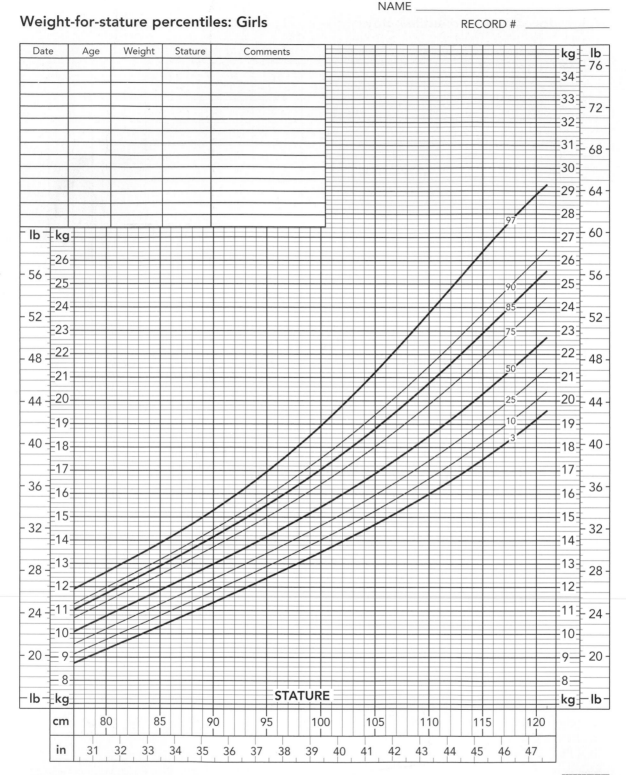

Date	Age	Weight	Stature	Comments

STATURE

Published May 30, 2000 (modified 10/16/00).
SOURCE: Developed by the National Center for Health Statistics in collaboration with
the National Center for Chronic Disease Prevention and Health Promotion(2000).
http://www.cdc.gov/growthcharts

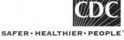

SAFER · HEALTHIER · PEOPLE™

Girls weight-for-stature percentiles. (Developed by the National Center for Health Statistics in collaboration with the National Center for Chronic Disease Prevention and Health Promotion [2000]. http://www.cdc.gov/growthcharts.)

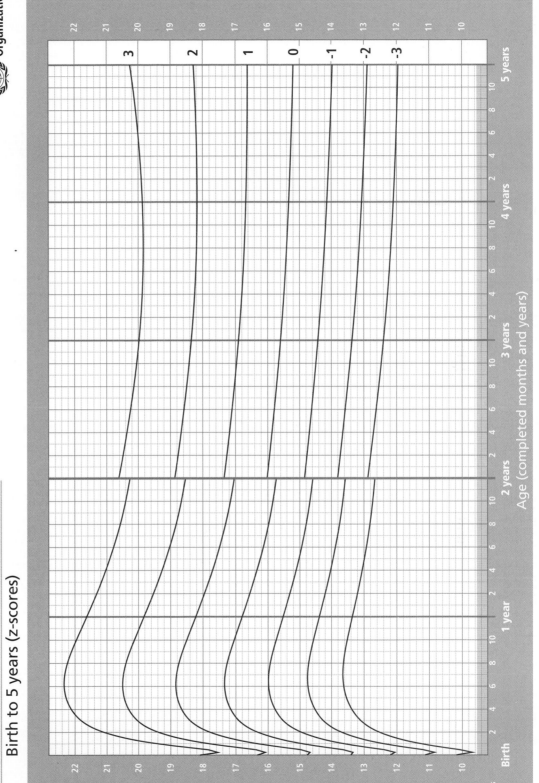

Boys BMI-for-age: Birth to 5 years (z-scores). (Reprinted with permission of the World Health Organization. http://www.who.int/nutrition/media_page/en/.)

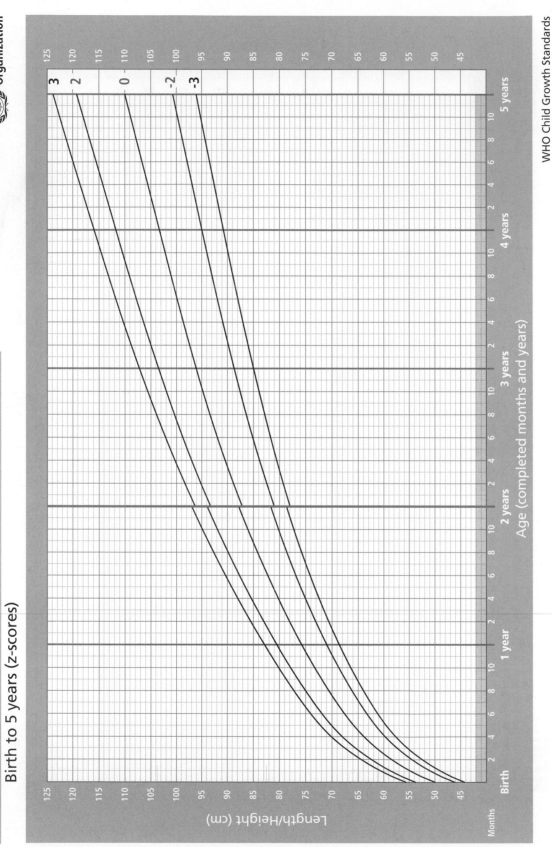

Boys length/height-for-age: Birth to 5 years (z-scores). (Reprinted with permission of the World Health Organization. http://www.who.int/nutrition/media_page/en/.)

Weight-for-age BOYS

Birth to 5 years (z-scores)

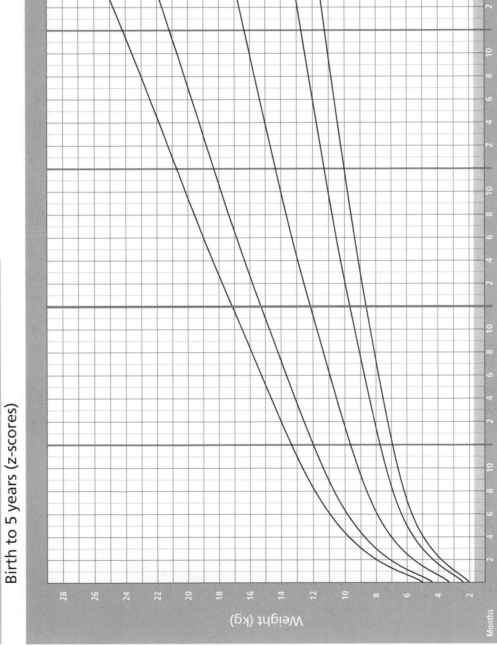

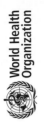
World Health
Organization

WHO Child Growth Standards

Boys weight-for-age: Birth to 5 years (z-scores). (Reprinted with permission of the World Health Organization. http://www.who.int/nutrition/media_page/en/.)

BMI-for-age GIRLS

Birth to 5 years (z-scores)

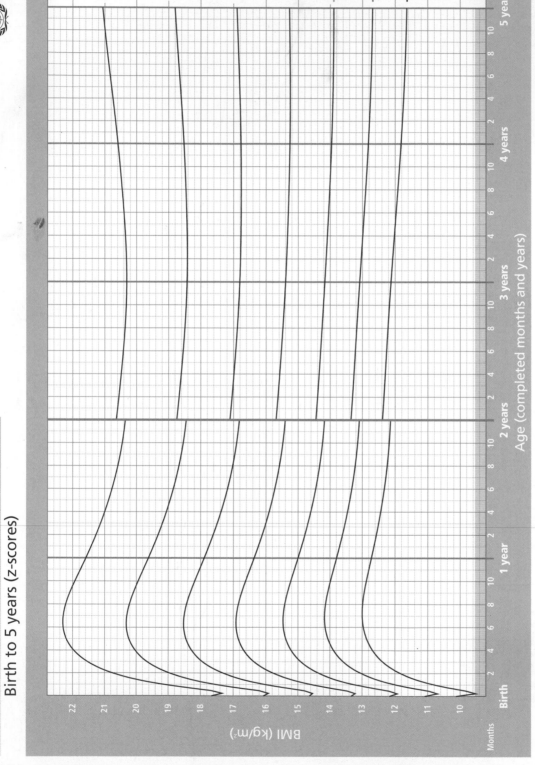

Girls BMI-for-age: Birth to 5 years (z-scores). (Reprinted with permission of the World Health Organization. http://www.who.int/nutrition/media_page/en/.)

Length/height-for-age GIRLS

Birth to 5 years (z-scores)

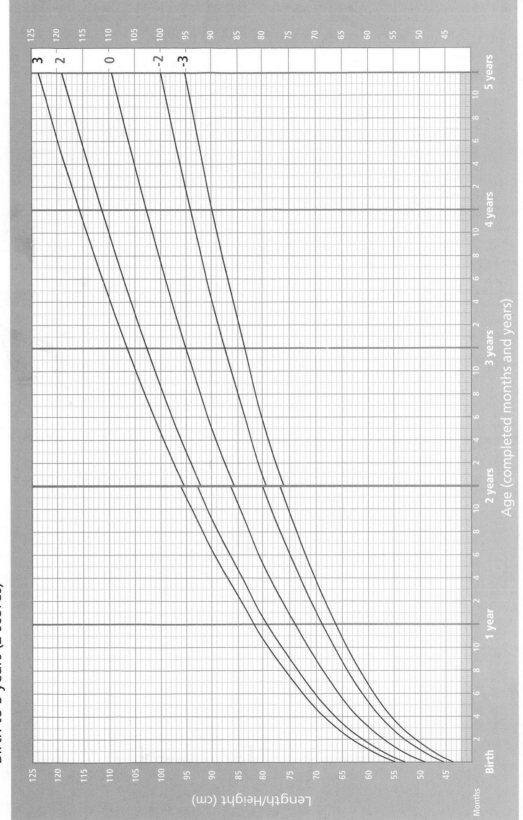

Girls length/height-for-age: Birth to 5 years (z-scores). (Reprinted with permission of the World Health Organization. http://www.who.int/nutrition/media_page/en/.)

Weight-for-age GIRLS

Birth to 5 years (z-scores)

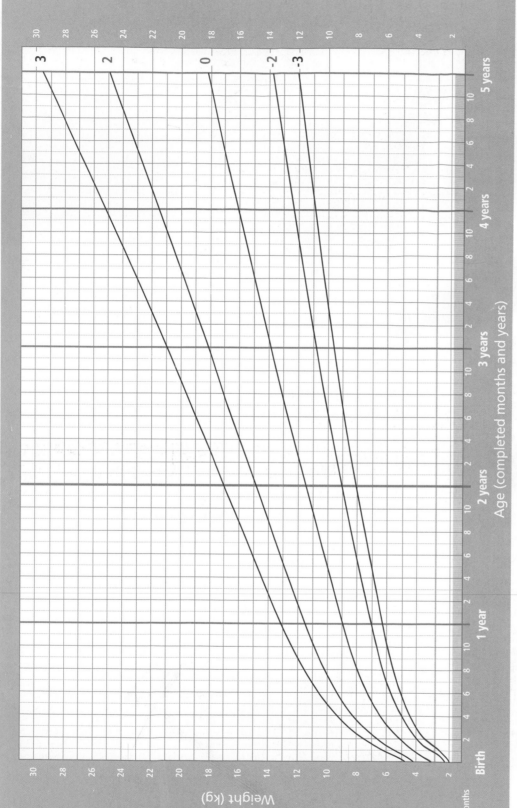

Girls weight-for-age: Birth to 5 years (z-scores). (Reprinted with permission of the World Health Organization. http://www.who.int/nutrition/media_page/en/.)